Encyclopedia of Natural Remedies

by

Louise Tenney

Encyclopedia of Natural Remedies

Published by
Woodland Publishing Inc.
P.O. Box 160
Pleasant Grove, Utah 84062

Printed in the United States of America
ISBN 0-913923-98-2

The *Encyclopedia of Natural Healing* is not intended to prescribe or diagnose in any way. The information in this book is not meant as a substitute for professional help. Diagnosing or attempting to treat an illness should come under the direction of a physician. The purpose of this book is to offer historical uses and research on herbs and nutritional supplements.

Neither the author nor the publisher directly or indirectly dispense medical advice or prescribe the use of herbs as a form of treatment. The author and the publisher assume no responsibility if an individual prescribes for themselves without a physician's approval.

CONTENTS

INTRODUCTION

Throughout history, man has been plagued by illness, deformities, and discomfort. From the beginning of time, man has sought relief from these problems. Over time and through experience, many different techniques and methods have been used. Human beings utilized whatever was available. Trial and error were employed to test effectiveness. Different methods of treatment included plants, manipulation, spiritual healing, massage, and mystical chanting.

Modern medicine has veered from the traditional methods of the past. It has opted for synthetic drug intervention and immediate surgery to cure the ills we face. According to the World Health Organization, however, approximately 80% of the four billion people on the earth rely on herbal medicines. Many doctors in Europe use herbal preparations as their primary medicines. The Asian countries use herbs regularly for treating disease. In Tawain alone, a small country one sixth the size of California, there are over 8000 herb stores.

Fortunately, times are changing. More and more of the population is looking for alternative methods of treatment for their ailments. The medical community is certainly aware of this change. Many medical doctors are incorporating the use of these natural therapies in their practices, and the population seems to appreciate their efforts. The natural approach seems to be coming back into vogue. People appreciate an alternative to synthetic drug therapies that often have debilitating side effects, while concentrating on only the symptoms associated with an illness. Modern health practices have, to some extent, taken a step backwards toward "folk remedies." In reality, natural medicine is merely the return to the center of the pendulum of medicine, which had swung too far towards technology and is now returning to the natural.

Natural health practitioners believe that prevention is the most practical approach to healthy living. If you feel fine, your doctor can do nothing for you. Come back when you are sick. Modern medicine takes the position that one must react to disease, find the cause of a problem and treat it. This narrow approach allows the physician the opportunity to track cures, and pronounce certain treatments as effective and others, ineffective.

Natural medicine looks at the individual as a whole and treats the body as a whole. The holistic approach involves keeping the body healthy by avoiding a problem before it occurs. It offers natural methods derived from natural sources as opposed to the synthesized medicines. Herbs are specialized foods that help generate vital body energy. They help the body heal itself.

Natural medicine is not intended to replace modern medicine. However, it should not be dismissed or ignored because it does not depend on modern technology or because its benefits are not readily discernable in a controlled environment. Natural medicine should be appreciated for its ability to help individuals enjoy a higher quality of life.

Research is heading out of the lab and into the wilderness. Cancer researchers have recently disclosed their efforts to look for cures in the rain forests. Scientists are looking at local folklore throughout the world to search for clues to cures. Many drugs are based on plant research and in use even now. More work is being encouraged using natural methods. The history of botanical medicine is full of drug therapies. Quinine from chichona bark, digitalis from foxglove, reserpine from periwinkle, and belladonna from the nightshade family are now used for treating malaria, heart failure, high blood pressure, psychosis, cancer and the action of the heart. Nearly 80 percent of the synthetic drugs today are chemically modified or purified versions of substances found originally in plants.

The plant kingdom has provided man with food and medicine since the beginning of time. References to the use of herbs are found throughout the Bible. Evidence of the herbal treatments by all ancient cultures has been well documented. In fact, herbs were thought to be magical and full of healing benefits. Even today, herbs are used throughout the world to provide a method of treatment in many developing countries and throughout western Europe. Folklore also offers some insight into herbal remedies and treatments. These stories were passed down to each generation as a means to heal and maintain health. Families shared their knowledge with each other and with neighbors. They took care of each other. They relied on the earth to treat ailments.

Herbs are considered to be a natural means of providing the body with essential nutrients which can aid in the healing process. Herbs feed the body as food does, and they work with the body to help strengthen and build up the body as it heals itself. Herbalists believe that the body can heal itself using natural herbal therapy to activate the body's own self-healing powers.

Herbs are plants and contain many nutritious elements. They are most effective when used in their natural balanced state. Herbalists believe that the body is readily able to receive and assimilate these nutrients. It seems to be able to utilize these herbs where and when they are needed. This strengthens and enhances the entire body.

Herbs are considered unique from drugs in that they contain elements in the amounts that nature intended. Drugs sometimes contain a single active substance, which has been extrapolated form a plant and synthesized. Herbs, on the other hand, provide a broad array of catalysts which work together harmoniously. Consequently, they work with the body to provide the complete healing network. Instead of focusing on an isolated segment of the human system, herbs can ennervate and cleanse the entire blood supply or whatever area is affected. Herbalists believe that the natural approach of using herbs can add health and vigor to the body.

Generally, the actions of the herbs require a period of time to be effective. Their action is subtle. This process is usually a gradual one while curing is taking place. In fact, major health problems are thought to be slow in healing allowing time for the body to heal throughout. Herbalists agree that this slow natural approach is ultimately more effective in offering a permanent cure to an ailment. In addition, individuals who have chosen to abuse their bodies for many years may take even longer to see changes from herbal remedies. Using herbal treatments requires us to stop what we are doing and slow down. We must focus on the immediate needs of the body.

Drugs made synthetically or extracted from plants are not used in this natural form. People are finding that drugs can often cause more problems because of side effects than they alleviate. Drugs are considered chemicals because the elements are taken from a natural state and synthesized and made stronger, to an unnatural state. Herbs generally contain natural buffers and synergistic substances which help balance and make the herb more useful. This new synthetic drug is in a form that is foreign to the body and may disrupt it's internal harmony. Herbalists feel that this is the reason for side effects associated with many prescribed and over-the-counter drugs. Indeed, every drug contains warning labels describing possible side effects. Drugs are part of the fast paced world in which we live demanding an immediate cure to a problem. We want the doctor to prescribe a pill to rid us of the symptoms that afflict our bodies. The medical community often treats the problem while neglecting the cause of the condition. The natural approach is to look at the cause while working on healing the whole body, rather than only the symptoms of an illness. In a life threatening situation, it is important to remember that any method capable of saving a life should be used. Emergencies require immediate results. There is certainly a place for the medical community in this world in which we live. Additionally, most believe that natural methods can co-exist with the modern medical therapies.

In contrast to drugs, herbs are natural and safe. They do not build up in the body producing side effects. Herbs, as with other foods, need to be used with wisdom and knowledge. Different herbs are used to help different problems. Herbs can be of value for every system of the body. Found in nature are herbs which benefit the nervous system, digestive system, circulatory system, glandular system, immune system, respiratory system, intestinal system, urinary system and the skeletal and muscular systems. The properties of each plant target specific areas of the body. Modern research has added much knowledge to the effectiveness of these herbal remedies. Herbs are believed to contain properties which can heal and build the body. Herbs are known to be rich in vitamins and minerals, which work with the body to heal specific areas.

Each herb contains many different bio-chemical constituents. They contain vitamins, minerals, auxins, hormones, enzymes, chlorophyll, essential fatty acids, fiber and many other important elements. Herbs provide the body with nutrients that it needs to strengthen the immune system and aid in healing itself.

The following are some of the properties commonly found in herbs.

2

NATURE'S PROVEN FORMULAS

Herbs have been used since the dawn of history for human illness. In early times, people didn't realize that all the chemical elements of which our bodies are composed are contained in the roots, barks, leaves, flowers and fruits of herbs. With time, their knowledge and wisdom grew by using nature's natural medicines.

Modern science has substantiated the use of these herbal medicines and has proven why they have been used successfully for thousands of years.

Herbal combinations are formulated to compliment one another. A single herb doesn't always contain the proper healing qualities that are needed to cover the symptoms being treated. By combining several herbs together, the formulas are able to treat many symptoms that one herb alone cannot always do. There are exceptions in the case of some single herbs.

BLOOD CLEANSERS

Blood cleansers can be used for all diseases. They are especially useful for chronic diseases, which are diseases that have taken years to develop. These herbs are beneficial for cleaning the blood and cells.

USED FOR

Arteriosclerosis—Asthma—Blood Poisoning—Cancer—Candida—Catarrh—Colon Diseases—Chemical Poisoning Circulatory Problems—Cysts-Polyps, and Tumors—Diabetes—Epilepsy—Endometriosis—Environmental Poisoning—Epstein-Barr Virus—Gout—Hepatitis—Herpes—Hodgkin's Disease—Hives—Immune System Disorders—Lupus — Malabsorption Syndrome — Meningitis—Multiple Sclerosis—Muscular Dystrophy—Shingles—Stroke—

1. _____
Burdock, Turkey Rhubarb, Sorrel, Holy Thistle (Milk Thistle), Slippery Elm, Cress.

This formula acts as a blood purifier. It increases the enzyme function of the body. It strengthens the immune system and hormone function so the body can heal itself. Burdock prevents inorganic minerals from accumulating in the joints. Rhubarb cleans the liver and stomach.

Slippery elm has cleansing and healing properties. Sorrel has the ability to destroy growths in the body. Milk Thistle was found to protect the liver from damage as well as repair liver disorders. The cress acts as a blood purifier and tonic and helps regulate metabolism.

2. _____
Red Clover Blossoms, Sheep Sorrel, Peach Bark, Barberry Root, Echinacea, Licorice, Oregon Grape Root, Stillingia Root, Cascara Sagrada, Sarsaparilla, Prickly Ash, Burdock, Kelp, Rosemary.

3. _____
Red Clover Blossoms, Licorice, Stillingia, Sarsaparilla, Prickly Ash, Red Beet Root, Kelp.

These formulas are excellent blood cleansers. They are beneficial for all diseases when used with a lower bowel formula. They serve to neutralize acids in the blood, and stimulates circulation, clean the liver and glands. These herbs help in the assimilation of nutrients. These combinations are beneficial to use when on cleansing diets.

4. _____
Garlic, Comfrey Root, Wormwood, Lobelia, Marshmallow, White Oak Bark, Black Walnut Hulls, Mullein, Scullcap, Uva Ursi in a base of Apple Cider Vinegar, Glycerine and Honey.

5. _____

Garlic, Marshmallow, White Oak Bark, Black Walnut Hulls, Mullein, Uva Ursi in a base of Apple Cider Vinegar, Glycerin and Honey.

These two formulas are liquid extracts and beneficial for preventing colds, flu, fevers and plagues. They are excellent for killing germs and viruses. These formulas clean the body of toxins, and poisons. A clean, healthy body will prevent disease germs from invading the system.

6. _____

Red Clover Blossoms, Sheep Sorrel, Prickly Ash Bark, Sarsaparilla Root, Buckthorn Bark, Burdock Root, Licorice Root, Peach Bark, Barberry Root, Echinacea, Cascara Sagrada, Rosemary.

This extract formula is a blood purifier. It eliminates toxins from the blood and cells. The prickly ash increases circulation and dissolves mineral deposits in the joints. It is an excellent formula for acute and chronic diseases. It neutralizes acids and toxins and strengthens the immune system.

USED FOR

Auto-intoxication — Immune System Disorders—All Chronic Diseases—AIDS— Alcoholism—Allergies—Arthritis— Bronchitis—Cancer—Childhood Diseases— Chemical Poisoning—Cold and Flu—Ear Infections—Epstein-Barr—Fasting Cleanses— Food Poisoning—Glands—Immune System Disorders—Lupus—Lymphatic System Congestion—Meningitis—Mucus—Skin Diseases—Parasites and Worms—Venereal Diseases—

GENERAL CLEANSER

7. _____

Gentian Root, Catnip, Bayberry, Golden Seal Root, Myrrh Gum, Irish Moss, Fenugreek, Chickweed, Comfrey Root, Yellow Dock, Prickly Ash, St. Johnswort, Blue Vervain, Mandrake, Evening Primrose, Cyani Flowers.

This formula is a general cleanser to use on all acute and chronic diseases. It cleans morbid matter from the stomach. The stomach is considered the seat of all diseases and needs to be clean. The digestive tract harbors toxins, parasites, worms and in order to digest and assimilate essential nutrients, these need to be eliminated. This formula also cleans the liver and spleen. The spleen filters the blood of broken and dead red blood cells and bacteria. This formula can be used with blood cleansers and colon cleansers for excellent results.

USED FOR

Acute Diseases (Allergies, Bronchitis, Colds, Flu, Hayfever, and Fevers)—Congestion of the Kidneys and Liver—Autoimmune Diseases, (AIDS, Epstein-Barr Virus, Candida, Gastritis, Herpes, Legionnaires' Disease, Lupus, Tuberculosis, Leprosy)—Chronic Diseases (Arthritis, Alzheimers Disease, Cancer, Cardiovascular Disorders, Cysts and Tumors, Diabetes, Endometriosis, Epilepsy, Indigestion, Malabsorption Syndrome, Mental Illness, Multiple Sclerosis, Radiation Poisoning, Senility, Stroke, Ulcers.)

CIRCULATORY SYSTEM FORMULAS

1. _____

Vitamin A (fish liver oil and beta carotene), Vitamin D (fish liver oil), Vitamin E (D-alphtocopherol succinate), Vitamin C, Vitamin B1, B2, B6, B12, Niacin (niacin and niacinamide), Pantothenic Acid, Glandular:

Adrenal substances, Spleen extract, Thymus substance, Essential fatty acids; Marine Fish Lipids, Chelated minerals: Iron, Copper, Zinc, Iodine, Manganese, Calcium, Magnesium, Potassium, Chromium, Selenium, Butcher's Broom, Capsicum, Hawthorn Berries, Peppermint, Ginger Root, Rutin, Citrus Bioflavonoids, Amino Acids: L-Cysteine HCI, L-Methionine.

This formula is designed to help the body eliminate toxins from the circulatory system and the veins. This formula has been designed to produce a positive influence on the circulatory, cardiovascular and glandular systems. It has a chelating effect on the circulatory system which includes the brain. People who have used these formulas report a warming effect, which demonstrates its favorable effect on circulation. The many natural nutrients found in this formula help to keep the entire body healthy and invigorated. The chelating elements work together in a bonding reaction by surrounding plaque and drawing it from the veins, much like a magnet attracts metal.

USED FOR

Arteriosclerosis—Arthritis—Autoimmune Diseases—Cholesterol—Circulatory Problems—Heart Diseases—Heavy Metal Poisoning—Immune System Disorders—Stroke—Contains all the antioxidants to protect against free radical damage that attacks DNA molecules cell nuclei disturbing the genetic blueprints that control cell division causing cancer. Free radicals also attack blood vessels causing blood platelets to clump together resulting in arteriosclerosis and coronary heart disease. These radicals can attack brain cells, causing senility and memory loss. They can damage the skin which can cause brown age spots. They attack the immune cells and depress the immune system causing autoimmune diseases such as rheumatoid arthritis and multiple sclerosis. They can also cause hardening of the arteries and cataracts.

2. _____
Vitamin A (beta-carotene), Vitamin C, E, B12, Folic Acid, Niacin, Magnesium, Zinc, Selenium, Potassium, White Willow Bark, Deodorized Garlic, Hawthorn Berry Concentrate, Ginkgo, Co-enzyme Q10, and L-Carnitine.

This formula contains all the natural ingredients to support the body's circulatory system. These nutrients are all beneficial to feed, clean and strengthen the heart, veins and brain. The formula is designed to insure efficient absorption and assimilation. This formula also contains all the antioxidants needed to protect against free radical damage.

3. _____
Capsicum, Golden Seal Root, Parsley, Ginger, Garlic, Siberian Ginseng.

This formula helps regulate blood pressure whether high or low. These natural herbs help stimulate the circulatory system and clean and dissolve plaque on the veins.

4. _____
Capsicum and Garlic.

This formula is useful for regulating blood pressure, whether high or low. It will increase circulation and help feed and nourish the heart. It will clean the veins and protect against germs and viruses. Garlic is well know for lowering blood pressure.

5. _____
Siberian Ginseng, Sage, Bee Pollen, Capsicum, Ginkgo.

This formula is excellent to strengthen brain function and increase stamina. The Capsicum helps carry all the nutrients to the brain and other parts of the body where they are needed. Capsicum is the strongest stimulant in the herbal kingdom. Bee Pollen and Ginkgo act as adaptogens, which normalize problems and regulate imbalances in the

5

body. Ginkgo is a vasoregulator, which acts to treat senility to improve mental clarity. It has also helped in tinnitus, which helps tone down the ringing in the ears. This combination will improve many conditions associated with aging.

6. _____

Fumitory (Fumaria officinalis), Jerusalem Artichoke, Persian Garlic, Onion, Strawberry Leaves, RaspberryLeaves, Garlic, Citruce (lime and orange peel), Chicory, Linn, Pear, Calcome, Fox Geranium, Grape Leaf, Licorice Root.

This formula is beneficial to reduce high blood pressure. In addition, it helps eliminate excess cholesterol. Strawberry and Raspberry leaves are rich in iron to nourish the blood. Citruce is high in bioflavonoids for healthy veins. Licorice feeds the adrenal glands.

USED FOR

Cholesterol—Diabetes—Heart Problems—High Blood Pressure—

7. _____

Purified Water, Natural Caramel Color, Glycerin, Potassium Citrate, Calcium Glycerophosphate, Potassium Glycerophosphate, Magnesium Glycerophosphate, Ferric Glycerophosphate, Iodine (potassium), Chamomile Flowers, Sarsaparilla Root, Celery Seed, Alfalfa, Dandelion Root, Horehound Root, Licorice Root, Senega Root, Passion Flower, Thyme, Gentian Root, Saw Palmetto Berry, Angelica Root, Siberian Ginseng, Gotu Kola, Cascara Sagrada, Methylparaben, Potassium Hydroxide, Propyl-paraben, Natural Mint and Anise Flavors.

This extract formula is designed for easy digestion and assimilation. It is rich in minerals essential for every body function. It strengthens the heart, muscles, and nerves. It aids in cleaning the blood and balancing the glandular system. It increases energy and stamina by providing essential nutrients to the body.

People who have taken this extract report many positive results, including a feeling of increased vitality, endurance and energy and added resistance to illness.

USED FOR

Auto-Immune Diseases—Arthritis—Cardiovascular Diseases—Mineral Imbalance—Nervous System Diseases—

COLDS, FLU, FEVERS AND ALLERGIES

ACUTE DISEASES

Colds, flu and fevers are acute diseases. They are nature's way of cleansing and healing the body. When we treat acute diseases with natural methods, using herbs in teas, extracts and capsules, we not only eliminate toxins, but prevent chronic diseases later on. Fasting is the first law of nature with acute diseases.

The body is trying to eliminate or squeezing toxins from the cells and pushing them into the stomach to be eliminated through the colon. When we eat during an acute disease, this stops the cleansing process. This hardens the toxins and they can accumulate in other parts of the body, creating the potential for chronic disease later.

1. _____

Bayberry, Ginger, White Willow, White Pine, Cloves, Capsicum.

2. _____

Horehound, Ginger, Garlic, White Willow, Licorice, Chickweed, Mullein, Echinacea, Capsicum, Wild Cherry, Rose Hips.

These formulas are excellent for all acute diseases, for aiding the body in eliminating toxins and mucus from the system. They help the body heal itself by eliminating and relieving congestion. They purify the blood and help fight infections. They are soothing to the stomach, strengthen the lungs and increase immune function.

3. _____
Comfrey Root, Fenugreek, Yerba Santa, Hyssop, Wild Cherry.

This formula is beneficial for eliminating built-up mucus any where in the body. Mucus accumulates from eating the wrong foods, eating when acute disease invade the body, and from a lack of proper elimination.

Comfrey contains allantoin to induce production of new tissue growth. Fenugreek helps dissolve hard mucus as well as heal the delicate mucous membranes. Yerba Santa is a natural decongestant. An excellent remedy for acute and chronic diseases, such as asthma and chronic bronchitis. Hyssop is good for fevers and helps produce sweating. It is good for all catarrh ailments. Wild Cherry is an effective expectorant.

4. _____
Fenugreek Seed and Thyme.

This formula is beneficial for accumulated mucus in the lungs, throat, sinuses, head, stomach and colon. It is beneficial to use with other herbal formulas for the lungs, colon and stomach. It loosens the toxic mucus and eliminates it from the body. It is especially beneficial for sinusitis.

5. _____
Mullein and Lobelia.

This formula is designed to help in acute diseases and especially in cleaning the lymphatic system. Mullein loosens mucus and eliminates it from the system, and lobelia removes obstructions in the body. Lobelia is the "thinking herb" and knows where the obstructions are located in the body. It is excellent for childhood diseases, asthma, bleeding in the bowel or lungs, bronchitis, coughs, croup, lymphatic obstructions, mumps, nervousness, pain, and pleurisy.

6. _____
Comfrey Root, Mullein, Chickweed, Marsh-mallow, Slippery Elm, Lobelia.

This formula is excellent for the respiratory system. It acts to heal, cleanse and nourish the lungs. It is beneficial by protecting and eliminating particles that lodge in the lungs from airborne pollutants. It is used for allergies, asthma, bronchitis, coughs, croup, emphysema, hay fever, lung congestion, mucus congestion, pneumonia, and sinus congestion.

7. _____
Ephedra, White Willow Bark, Valerian, Pan Pien Lien, Golden Seal, Bee Pollen, Capsicum, Peppermint.

8. _____
White Willow Bark, Ginger, Bee Pollen, Echinacea, Capsicum.

These formulas are natural decongestants. They help reduce swelling and drain nasal and sinus passages due to colds, allergies, hayfever and sinusitis. They are relaxants for the respiratory system. They contain antiseptic properties and stimulate healing.

9. _____
Ephedra, Horehound, White Willow, Licorice Root, Pan Pien Lien, Chickweed, Mullein, Echinacea, Golden Seal.

10. _____
Horehound, Ginger, Garlic, White Willow, Licorice Root, Echinacea, Chickweed, Mullein, Capsicum, Wild Cherry, Rose Hips.

These formulas are excellent to use for acute diseases such as colds, flu and fevers. They will help nature heal and remove toxins that are causing infections. They will ease lung and throat congestion. They are relaxing, cleansing and healing.

USED FOR

All Acute Diseases—Allergies—Asthma—Colds—Bronchitis-Childhood Diseases—Congestion—Ear Infections—Emphysema—Fevers—Flu—Hay Fever—Infections—Lung Congestion—Mucus Build-Up— Pneumonia—Sinusitis—Tonsillitis—

COLON CLEANSERS

1. _____
Cascara Sagrada, Barberry, Raspberry Leaves, Lobelia, Ginger, Rhubarb, Golden Seal Root, Fennel, Capsicum.

This formula is designed to restore tone to a relaxed and underactive bowel. It stimulates bile function, helps in constipation and is calming to the gastrointestinal tract. It cleans the liver and urinary tract, acts as a natural diuretic, and eliminates mucus from the bowels. This formula is good for almost all diseases. The bowels are the cause of autointoxication that enters the blood stream from congested bowels.

2. _____
Cascara Sagrada, Aloe Vera.

This formula is excellent for acute constipation and helps promote regularity. Aloe vera cleans, soothes and heals. Cascara sagrada promotes peristaltic action in the intestinal canal. It is also good for chronic constipation and is non habit forming like over the counter laxatives.

3. _____
Cascara Sagrada, Barberry, Raspberry Leaves, Fennel, Senna, Lobelia, Ginger, Golden Seal Root, Cayenne.

This colon formula is a liquid extract which is excellent to use for children and the elderly. It cleans, tones, and nourishes the lower bowels. It is used for constipation and stimulates bile function, and cleans mucus from the bowels and urinary tract. This is useful for all diseases. A congested colon is the cause of most diseases.

4. _____
Psyllium Husk, Fructose, Maltodextrin, Fructooligo Saccharide, Citrus Pectin, Natural Orange Flavor, Hibiscus, Natural Banana Flavor, Guar Gum, Caa Inhem Extract, Peppermint, Cinnamon, Papaya, Garlic, Rhubarb, Alfalfa, Fenugreek, Slippery Elm Bark Powder, Ginger, Cape Aloe, Burdock, Pumpkin Seed, Yucca, Althea, Uva Ursi, Buchu, Capsicum, Clove, Chickweed, Cornsilk, Dandelion, Echinacea, False Unicorn.

This is a high fiber formula with supportive herbs to clean and nourish the colon, urinary tract, liver, spleen, and digestive tract. Fiber is the missing link in the American diet. Lack of fiber has been linked to cancer of the bowels, obesity, diabetes, gallstones, cardiovascular diseases, and many other ailments.

5. _____
Senna, Buckthorn, Peppermint, Caa Inhem, Uva Ursi, Orange Peel, Rose Hips, Althea, Honeysuckle, Chamomile.

This formula is a natural diuretic and laxative. It assists the digestive process and helps the body get rid of unwanted fat, including cellulite. It cleans the whole system; it even eliminates mucus from the sinuses. It is in a natural tea drink form for quick assimilation. Children can take it in small quantities for irregularity.

USED FOR

All Acute Diseases—Colds—Flu—Fevers—Acute and Chronic Constipation—Bad Breath—Colitis—Colon Cleanse—Croup—Diarrhea—

Intestinal Mucus—Parasites—Worms—Cancer and All Chronic Diseases—

DIGESTIVE SYSTEM FORMULAS

1. _____

Gentian Root, Catnip, Bayberry, Golden Seal Root, Myrrh Gum, Irish Moss, Fenugreek, Chickweed, Comfrey Root, Yellow Dock, Prickly Ash, St. Johnswort, Blue Vervain, Mandrake, Evening Primrose, Cyani Flowers.

This formula is excellent to clean, nourish and eliminate toxins from the digestive system and the blood. It is good to use with any cleansing program especially on chronic diseases to promote cleansing and healing. Gentian is one of the best stomach tonics in the herbal kingdom. Gentian helps to strengthen the pancreas and the spleen. Catnip is considered nature's "Alka-Seltzer." Golden Seal helps in catarrhal conditions of the stomach. Myrrh is an antiseptic and is valuable in cleansing and healing the stomach and colon. Prickly Ash is beneficial for a weak stomach.

USED FOR

Arthritis—Cancer—Colon Cleanse—Digestive Problems—Skin Problems—Toxic Waste—Tumors—

2. _____

Peppermint, Fennel, Ginger, Wild Yam, Catnip, Cramp Bark, Spearmint, Papaya.

This formula is important to stimulate the digestive system. When used over a period of time, it soothes, heals and calms the digestive process. It is useful for healing and restoring the stomach lining. The stomach is the seat of most diseases, and this formula will help for all related ailments.

USED FOR

Appetite—Gas—Heartburn—Nervous Stomach—Poor Digestion—Helpful in all diseases to assure proper digestion and assimilation—

3. _____

Papaya, Peppermint.

This formula helps improve digestive disorders. Poor digestion is the beginning of all ailments. This formula helps to calm a nervous stomach. It is beneficial to use after vomiting to settle the stomach.

USED FOR

Acute and Chronic Ailments—Allergies—Gas—Colds—Flu—Hay Fever—Heartburn—Hiatal Hernia—Weight Problems—

4. _____

Bromelain, Chamomile Extract, Peppermint Leaves, Papain, Prolase (protease), Diastase, Amaylase, Anise Seed, Slippery Elm Bark, Golden Seal Root, Fennel Seed, Papaya Melon Extract, Papaya Leaves.

This formula is useful to promote proper digestion and assimilation of food. It stimulates the enzyme process, which is vital for complete digestion. It is soothing and healing to the digestive system. It contains enzymes for complete digestion

USED FOR

Bloating—Digestion—Gas—Stomach Upset—

5. _____

Pancreatin, N.F., Pepsin, Papain, Bromelain, Ox Bile, Betaine Hydrochloride in a base of Peppermint Leaves, Comfrey and Slippery Elm.

Incomplete protein digestion and enzyme deficiency are the main causes of degenerative diseases. Cooked food destroys enzymes and forces the pancreas and other enzyme secreting glands to work harder to supply the essential enzymes required to break down the proteins, carbohydrates and fats. This forced digestive process from the glands will result in a deficiency of enzymes needed in biochemical functions. This formula will supply the necessary enzymes and hydrochloride to protect the body and prevent illness.

USED FOR

Proper Digestion of Carbohydrates, Proteins and Fats—Allergies—Asthma—Bronchitis— Cancer—Circulatory Diseases—Diabetes— Digestion—Endocrine System—Good for breaking down protein congestion in the body and preventing diseases.

6. _____
Ginger Root, Peppermint Leaves Extract. Anise Seed, Catnip.

This is a beneficial formula to help with nausea and a weak stomach. It is good to use to prevent stomach upset. It settles, soothes and relaxes the stomach.

USED FOR

Indigestion—Motion Sickness—Nausea— Nervous Stomach—Soothing to use for the Flu—Vomiting—

ULCER FORMULA

7. _____
Echinacea, Golden Seal Root, Burdock, Dandelion Root, Capsicum.

This formula acts to cleanse and heal the entire gastrointestinal tract. It speeds the healing of ulcers, canker sores and pyorrhea. It prevents and stops internal bleeding. It cleans and nourishes the stomach and colon.

USED FOR

Bad Breath—Canker Sores—Colitis—Crohn's Disease—Diverticulosis—Dysentery— Heartburn—Hiatal Hernia—Indigestion— Mouth Sores—Pyorrhea—Thrush—Ulcers—

ENERGY AND STAMINA FORMULAS

1. _____
Chinese Herbal Tea Extract (Huang Chi, Ma Huang, We Wei Tzu, Gei Zee, Mai Tung and Wu You), Siberian Ginseng, Gotu Kila, Calcium Carbonate, Ascorbic Acid, Potassium Phosphate, Magnesium Oxide, Kelp, Zinc Gluconate, Manganese Gluconate, d-alphatocopherol succinate, Niacinamide, Copper Pantothenate, Vitamin D-3, Rose Hips, Pyridoxine HCL, Riboflavin, Thiamine Mononitrate, Folic Acid, Octacosanol, Biotin, Cyanocobalamin.

This formula provides nutrients to protect the body from stress and illness. The body's nutrients are reduced when under stress and illness, and this formula meets physiological needs necessary to strengthen and fortify the immune system. It nourishes the nervous system and the brain enabling it to cope with everyday stress. It is rich in vitamins and minerals required to meet the body's needs.

USED FOR

Depression—Nervous Disorders—Nutritional Deficienceis—Exhaustion—Mental Fatigue— Stress—Caffeine Withdrawal—

2. _____
Siberian Ginseng, Gota Kola, Bee Pollen, Capsicum.

This formula is used to increase energy and strengthen the body as well as the brain. It increases circulation to help eliminate toxins and supply essential nutrients to the brain. Gota Kola is food for the brain. Bee Pollen provides nourishment for the entire body.

USED FOR

Addictions—Diets—Drug Withdrawal—Endurance—Energy—Exhaustion—Fasting—Fatigue—Glands—Hyperactivity—(ADD)—Longevity—Memory—Senility—

3. _____

Valerian Root, Scullcap, Hops, Thiamine Mononitrate, Riboflavin, Nicotinamide, Calcium Pantothenate, Pyridoxine HCI, Ascorbic Acid, Choline Bitarate, Inositol, Paraaminobenzoic Acid, Schizandra Chinenis, Piper Methsticum, Folic Acid, Cyanocobalamin, Biotin.

This formula has essential nutrients to nourish the brain and the nervous system. When the nerves are strong, the body can handle stress and illness better. It contains nutrients necessary for clear thinking and reasoning. Stress leaches out vitamins and minerals, especially the B-complex vitamins. Lack of B-vitamins causes listlessness, irritability, edginess, feelings of persecution, depression, and lack of interest in school, work and life. This formula, along with #2, helps in treating depression.

USED FOR

Depression—Illness—Nervous Disorders—Exhaustion—Nutritional Deficiencies—Stress—Strengthens the Immune and Nervous Systems—

4. _____

Elk Antler, Canadian Ginseng, Bee Pollen, Echinacea, Ginger, Cinnamon, Capsicum.

This formula is designed to increase stamina and energy. The benefits of Elk Antler, are to promote longevity and strengthen the immune system. It increases circulation and supplies nutrients to the veins and capillaries. It is beneficial for impotency and loss of interest in sex.

USED FOR

Arthritis—Stress—Stamina—Sexual Function—Senility—Structural System—

5. _____

L-Carnitine, Zinc amino acid chelate.

This formula is designed to eliminate fat build-up, increase muscle tissue and energy. It eliminates cholesterol build-up in the veins and strengthens the heart. It protects the heart during athletic stress and is good for high cholesterol.

USED FOR

Athletes—Cholesterol—Heart Problems—Increase Stamina—Provides nutrients essential for Weight Loss—

6. _____

Gymnema Sylvestre, Papaya, Chromium Di-Nicitanate.

This formula is useful to aid in eliminating excess body fat by speeding up metabolic rate. It builds muscles similar to anabolic steroids with no side effects. It speeds up healing of wounds, improves glucose tolerance and eliminates fat and cholesterol deposits in the arteries. This is beneficial for regulating blood sugar in diabetes. Chromium has been found to be vital to good health. It is lacking in the typical American diet. It is depleted when sugar is used in excess.

USED FOR

Aging—Cholesterol—Diabetes—Eliminates Fat—Heart Disease—Hypoglycemia—Immune System—Weight Loss—

7. _____

Natural Fiber, L-Carnitine, Potassium Gluconate, Calcium glycerophosphate, T64X (special natural herbs in lactose phosphate), Vitamin C, Vitamin B1, B2, B6, B12, Siberian Ginseng, Gotu Kola, Bee Pollen.

This formula is in a powder form to be added to water to help in losing weight. It contains fiber, which is the missing link in the American diet. It creates bulk and creates a feeling of fullness. The minerals in this formula help control fluid balance. This formula helps prevent muscle cramps during exercise, and helps increase endurance and stamina in combination with vital vitamins, minerals and glucose polymers.

USED FOR

Athletes—Aging—Diets—Cholesterol— Depression — Electrolyte Depletion — Endurance—Energy—Firms Muscles—Heart Muscle—

8. _____

Complex Carbohydrates, Chelated Minerals, Vitamins, Lipotropics, Amino Acids.

This is in a liquid formula form to replace glycogen and electrolyte for easy assimilation. Glycogen is essential in sports activity. When it is depleted in the body, fatigue occurs. When natural sources of glycogen are used up in the muscle tissues, the body begins to burn muscle protein, which causes pain. This is a good formula for building muscles and stamina.

Carbohydrates and amino acids are needed when recovering from illness. They help strengthen and nourish the body to prevent illness.

USED FOR

Athletes—Builds Strength—Energy and Stamina—Supplies Electrolytes—Replenishes Nutrients when Recovering from Illness— Tissue Repair—Weight Loss—

9. _____

Glycogen, Chelated Minerals, Electrolytes, Amino Acids, Vitamins.

This formula supplies all natural supplements to build rapid muscle growth. It is rich in glycogen, other complex carbohydrates, chelated minerals, vitamins, lipotropics and amino acids. This is considered an excellent training supplement. It contains no cholesterol, fat or white sugar. This is excellent for weight lifting or fitness training programs.

USED FOR

Athletes—Fatigue—Exercise—Gymnastics— Running Programs—This provides Rapid Muscle Building Properties—

10. _____

Glycogen, Electrolyte Minerals, Potassium, Magnesium, Copper, Manganese, Iron, Zinc, and Chromium. Chinese Ephedra, Capsicum and Licorice Root, Vitamins C, D, E, B1, B6, B12, Niacinamide, D-Calcium, Pantothenate, Folic Acid and Biotin.

This formula contains glycogen from a plant source which is a complex carbohydrate. It provides a natural energy source, which gives extra energy to athletes and sustains energy through the very common afternoon burnout that effects many people. Athletes need this energy to sustain them for better performance.

USED FOR

Energy—Endurance—Stamina—Mental Alertness—

GLANDULAR SYSTEM FORMULAS

1. _____

Gymnema Sylvestre, Papaya, Chromium Di-Nicitanate.

This formula is beneficial for regulating blood sugar in diabetes. Chromium has been found to be a vital element to health. It is lacking in the typical American diet. It is depleted when sugar is eaten.

USED FOR

Aging—Diabetes—Heart Disease—Hypoglycemia—Immune System Disorders—Weight Loss—

2. _____

Cedar Berries, Licorice Root, Uva Ursi, Golden Seal Root, Mullein, Capsicum.

This formula helps to rebuild the pancreas so it can produce its own insulin. Since the pancreas doesn't work alone, it needs the help of all other glands. This is a good formula for the pituitary, pineal and adrenal glands. These herbs are also food for the glandular system. Mullein cleans and rebuilds the glands. Uva Ursi is good for diabetes and controls mucus and toxins in the bladder and kidneys. Golden Seal regulates blood sugar levels and Cedar Berries help to heal the pancreas.

USED FOR

Diabetes—Glandular Dysfunction—Balances Glandular Function—

3. _____

Licorice Root, Juniper Berries, Wild Yam, Dandelion Root, Horseradish.

This is an excellent formula for glandular health. It is very good for eliminating toxins from the liver and promoting adrenal function. It is a cleanser, builder and healer for the glands.

It is beneficial for adrenal function, energy, glands, liver, pancreas, and for a weakened body.

USED FOR

Adrenal Function—Energy—Glands—Liver—Pancreas—Weakened Body—This will help to build all the glands when one is not functioning properly—

4. _____

Alfalfa, Dandelion Root, Kelp.

This formula is beneficial to supply vitamins and minerals lacking in the diet. This formula is good for all ailments as well as a means of preventing disease.

USED FOR

Anemia—Bones—Hair Health—Mineral Imbalance—Nails—Menopause—Pregnancy—Pre-Menstrual Syndrome—Skin—

5. _____

Siberian Ginseng, Sarsaparilla, Black Cohosh, Licorice Root, Golden Seal Root, Periwinkle, Damiana, Alfalfa, Kelp.

This formula contains herbs that will feed and balance the glandular system for better function. It stimulates hormone functions. It is very rich in nutrients to nourish the adrenals, pituitary, thyroid, and the female and male glands.

USED FOR

Depression—Energy— Female Problems—Glandular Imbalance—Impotence—

6. _____

Golden Seal Root, Parsley, Marshmallow, Ginger, Capsicum, Queen of the Meadow, Juniper Berries, Uva Ursi, Lobelia.

7. _____

Parsley, Marshmallow, Ginger, Capsicum, Queen of the Meadow, Juniper Berries, Uva Ursi.

These two formulas relieve inflammation and reduce the pain of swollen glands. They contain antibiotic and antiseptic properties. They eliminate toxins from the bladder, and stimulate secretion of the liver, kidneys, and lymph glands.

USED FOR

Bladder Infections—Hormone Imbalance—Kidneys (heals and nourishes)—Liver—Spleen—Urinary Tract—

8. _____

Golden Seal Root, Myrrh Gum, Capsicum.

This formula strengthens the entire gastrointestinal system. It speeds the healing of ulcers, canker sores and pyorrhea. It prevents and stops internal bleeding and cleans and nourishes the stomach and colon. This is an excellent ulcer formula.

USED FOR

Bad Breath—Canker Sores—Colitis—Crohn's Disease—Diverticulosis—Dysentery—Heartburn—Hiatal Hernia—Indigestion—Mouth Sores— Pyorrhea—Thrush—Ulcers—

9. _____

Adrenals 4CH, Epiphyse 7CH, Hypophyse 7CH, Hypothalamus 7CH, Placenta 4CH, Thyroid 7CH, Silicea 8X, Spigelia CX, Corallium Rubrum 10X, Eleutherococcus 30X, Biotin 6X, and Graphites 4CH.

This homeopathic formula is an aid in balancing the glandular system and increasing energy throughout the body. It provides a rich hair care treatment and nourishes the body internally and externally.

IMMUNE BUILDER FORMULAS

1. _____

Vitamin C, Odorless Garlic, Zinc Gluconate, Bee Propolis, Echinacea, Pau d'Arco, Rutin, Golden Seal Root, Selenium, Peppermint, Cloves.

This formula is unique and beneficial in its ability to build and sustain the health of the immune system. The immune system is under attack from air pollution, toxins in the food and water, drugs, sugar, and heavy metals, etc.

USED FOR

Asthma—Allergies—Cancer—Lupus—Multiple Sclerosis — Immune System Disorders—

2. _____

Ginseng, Echinacea, Psyllium and vital nutrients to enhance the immune system.

Ginseng helps reduce cholesterol, relaxes the blood vessels and strengthens the body to withstand stress. Ginseng improves immune response and eliminates toxins from the liver. Echinacea is nature's protection against viral infections. Psyllium helps the body eliminate toxins.

USED FOR

Allergies — Ankylosing Spondylitis — Bacteremia—Cancer—Candida—Chylamydial Disease—Epstein-Barr Virus—Gastritis—Legionnaires' Disease— Erythematosus Lupus—Reye's Syndrome—Toxic Shock Syndrome—And many other auto-immune diseases—

3. _____

Cruciferous Vegetables and Concentrated Dietary Indoles.

This is an excellent dietary supplement containing antioxidant nutrients. These nutrients will protect as well as strengthen the immune system. This formula helps balance estrogen levels in women which helps them eliminate PMS problems.

USED FOR

Allergies—Auto-Immune Diseases—Acute Diseases such as Colds—Flu—Hay Fever—Childhood Diseases—Chronic Diseases such as Asthma—Arthritis—Cancer—Circulatory Problems—

4. _____

Caprylic Acid, Pau d'Arco, Echinacea, Vitamin E, Pure Odorless Garlic, Black Walnut, Selenium, with natural herbal essential oils as flavorings.

This formula is an excellent infection fighter. It is very effective for candida in preventing as well as healing the body. It is effective for building up the immune system. It protects against viruses and helps the liver detoxify poisons. The garlic acts as an antibiotic and the black walnut helps to kill parasites and worms. It is very useful to use if you have been on antibiotics, birth control pills or a high sugar diet.

USED FOR

Addictions—AIDS—Allergies—Anorexia Nervosa—Asthma—Bacteremia—Blood Poisoning—Cancer—Candida—Chemical Imbalance—Chemical Toxicity—Environmental Poisoning—Epstein-Barr—Fatigue—Gastritis—Hay Fever—Hepatitis—Immune System Disorders—Lupus—Mental Illness—Multiple Sclerosis—Muscular Dystrophy—Parkinson's Disease — Premenstrual Problems—Stress—

5. _____

A powdered beverage formula containing natural vitamins, minerals and fiber designed especially for children.

This is a natural drink which supplies the essential nutrients that children need to protect against germs and viruses. It is a great drink for everyone to replace cool aid drinks, soda pop, and caffeine drinks.

USED FOR

Children—To supply nutrients missing from the typical American diet—Colds—Flu—Fevers—Childhood Diseases—

6. _____

Natural extract containing Garlic, Gravel Root, Comfrey Root, Wormwood, Lobelia, Marshmallow, White Oak Bark, Black Walnut Hulls, Mullein, Scullcap, Uva Ursi in a base of Apple Cider Vinegar, Glycerine and Honey.

7. _____

Garlic, Marshmallow, White Oak Bark, Black Walnut Hulls, Mullein, Uva Ursi in a base of Apple Cider Vinegar, Glycerine and Honey.

These formulas are designed to protect the immune system and nervous system. They are a natural way to help prevent flu epidemics, viruses of unknown origins and germs. Garlic acts as a natural antibiotic. Gravel root protects the kidneys. Lobelia is relaxing and helps the body heal itself.

USED FOR

Addictions—AIDS—Alcoholism—Allergies—Bronchitis—Cancer—Childhood Diseases—Chemical Poisoning—Colds, Flu—Ear Infections—Epstein-Barr Virus— Fasting Cleanses—Food Poisoning—Glands—Immune System Builder — Lymphatic System Cleanser—Meningitis—Mucus—Parasites and Worms—Venereal Diseases—

ANTIOXIDANT SUPPLEMENT

This formula is an excellent combination of antioxidants to protect and sustain the immune system. It helps prevent toxins and poisons from invading the body and restores health diminished by the many autoimmune diseases that are plaguing us today.

8. _____
Bioflavonoids, Grapefruit Pectin, Milk Thistle Extract, Acerola Fruit, Cruciferous Vegetables.

Bioflavonoids are part of the vitamin C family. They work together synergistically for enhancing absorption. They need to be replaced daily because the body cannot reproduce or store these nutrients. This formula has anti-inflammatory, anti-allergy and anti-viral properties. It also helps the body produce its own interferon to fight off cancer and other diseases.

Grapefruit pectin is derived from the pulp and rind of the grapefruit. This pectin ingredient is one of the fibers which helps eliminate toxins from the body.

Milk thistle extract is a potent antioxidant which prevents free radical damage. It is very effective to protect the liver from the damage of cirrhosis or hepatitis. It will also help regenerate liver cells and restore normal liver function.

Acerola fruit is derived from the acerola cherry, a tropical fruit which is very high in natural vitamin C. It enhances the activity of the bioflavonoids.

Cruciferous vegetables contain a powerful indole concentrate which provides the very active indol-3-carbinol as well as ascorbigen and other indoles. Indoles are a class of phytonutrients which have been scientifically shown to balance hormone levels, detoxify the intestines and liver and reinforce the body's immune system. In addition, they combat free-radical damage.

USED FOR

Aging—Allergies—Asthma—Bacteremia—Cancer—Candida—Chylamydial Disease—Epstein-Barr Virus — Gastritis — Heart Disease—Legionnaires' Disease—Erythematosus Lupus—Reye's Syndrome—Toxic Shock Syndrome—And many other Auto-Immune Diseases—

INFECTION FIGHTING FORMULAS

1. _____
Echinacea, Myrrh Gum, Capsicum.

This formula contains antiseptic properties to eliminate infections. Echinacea improves lymphatic filtration and drainage and helps remove toxins from the blood. Myrrh ia a powerful antiseptic. Capsicum is a strong stimulant and healer.

USED FOR

Breast Infections—Blood Infections—Colds—Contagious Diseases—Earache—Fevers—Flu—Gangrene—Lymphatic Swellings—Infections—Lung Congestion—Measles—Mumps—Scarlet Fever—Sinus Infections—Throat Infections—Tonsillitis—

2. _____
Echinacea, Golden Seal Root, Burdock, Dandelion Root, Capsicum.

3. _____
Echinacea, Burdock, Dandelion, Capsicum.

These formulas are great blood cleansers to eliminate infections in the body. The herbs contain antiseptic properties. Dandelion nourishes and heals the liver for better elimination. Burdock is a great blood purifier and eliminates calcification deposits. These herbs contain antifungal and antibacterial properties.

Acne—Arthritis—Asthma—Boils—Bronchitis—Candida—Canker Sores—Cancer—Eczema—Fevers—Gout—Kidney Infections—Leprosy—Liver Purifier—Urinary Deposits—Venereal Diseases—

NERVOUS SYSTEM AND BRAIN FORMULAS

The nervous system and brain formulas are beneficial for all diseases listed under the nervous system disorders.

1. _____

Valerian, Hops, Wood Betony, Scullcap, Black Cohosh, Mistletoe, Lobelia, Capsicum, Lady's Slipper.

This formula is considered food for the nerves. It is used for relieving nervous tension and insomnia by feeding and building the nerves. The nervine herbs are excellent for all ailments. Healing takes place when the body is relaxed, and these herbs relax the nerves and strengthen the immune system. They act as a tonic for exhaustion and stress. The nerves are connected to the immune system so this formula is beneficial for all diseases.

USED FOR

Anxiety—Convulsions—Cramps—Headaches—Hyperactivity—Hysteria—Insomnia—Nervous Breakdown—Nervous Disorders—Nervous Stomach—Nightmares—Muscular Pain—Relaxant—Shock—Stress—

2. _____

Valerian Root, Hops, Chamomile Flowers, Scullcap, Passion Flower, Kava Kava, Catnip.

This formula helps to increase relaxation and induce natural sleep. These herbs help to build and nourish the nerves to increase the body's ability to relax in a natural way. This will help promote natural sleep. Nervine herbs help the body relax so that every day stresses and problems are easier to cope with.

USED FOR

Anxiety—Convulsions—Headaches—Hyperactivity—Hysteria—Insomnia—Nervous Breakdown—Stress—

3. _____

Passion Flower, Scullcap and Valerian Root.

This is an excellent formula for the nervous system. It is a natural muscle relaxant. It is very good to use before visiting a chiropractor or massage therapist to help the body relax. It helps to restore nerves and improve the immune system.

USED FOR

Anxiety—Headaches—Hysteria—Insomnia—Nervous Disorders—Relaxing for the Body—Helpful in all Muscular, and Nervous System Disorders such as Alzheimer's Disease—Anorexia—Autism—Bulimia—Depression—Down's Syndrome—Dyskinesia—Dyslexia—Epilepsy—Fatigue—Headaches—Hyperactivity—Insomnia—Manic-Depressive Disorder and all other diseases listed under The Nervous System—

NERVINE HERBAL EXTRACTS

4. _____

Scullcap, Myrrh Gum, Valerian Root, Lobelia, Black Cohosh, Capsicum, Distilled Water and Ethyl Alcohol.

This formula is easy to digest and assimilate for speedy action. It contains herbs which help the body to relax. Healing takes place faster when the body is calm and relaxed.

These herbs help build and restore the nervous system and control nervous irritations and exhaustion. They are good for insomnia caused by an overactive mind.

USED FOR

Anxiety—Convulsions—Headaches—Hyperactivity—Hysteria—Insomnia—Nervous Breakdown—Relaxant—Stress—Useful for all diseases listed under the Nervous System Disorders—

5. _____
Black Cohosh, Blue Cohosh, Blue Vervain, Scullcap, Lobelia with Distilled Water and Vegetable Glycerine.

This formula is excellent to rebuild the motor nerves. The scullcap is beneficial for renewing and feeding the spinal cord. The blue cohosh and black cohosh are very beneficial to strengthen the entire nervous system.

USED FOR

Brain Food—Depression—Epilepsy—Hearing Loss (put in ears)—Hyperactivity—Insomnia—Manic Depression—Memory—Meniere's Syndrome—Meningitis—Multiple Sclerosis — Parkinson's Disease — Poor Equilibrium—Schizophrenia—Senility—Shingles—Vertigo—

6. _____
Extract of Scullcap, Passiflora, Wild Yam Root and Valerain Root in a Sorbitol base.

This formula calms the nerves and relaxes the muscles. It contains natural sedative properties. It can be used for insomnia, restlessness, hysteria, nervous headaches and as a general relaxant for better healing.

USED FOR

Depression—Antispasmodic—Tonic—Hysteria—Insomnia—Nervous Headaches—Muscle Pain — Menstrual Cramps — Hyperactivity—Calming for Children with Colds, Flu and Fevers — Epilepsy — Schizophrenia—Senility—Shingles—

7. _____
Extract of White Willow Bark.

This herbal extract is a natural approach to pain relief. It acts as a nerve sedative without side effects. It also has antiseptic properties for infections.

USED FOR

Arthritis—Chills—Fevers—Headaches—Nerves—Pain from Backache—Premenstrual Syndrome—Arthritis—Aches and Pains any where in the body—

BRAIN FORMULAS

1. _____
Siberian Ginseng, Sage, Bee Pollen, Capsicum, Ginkgo.

This formula is excellent to strengthen brain function and increase stamina. Sage improves memory and the ability to concentrate. These herbs stimulate circulation in the veins and especially in the brain area. They act as free radical scavengers.

USED FOR

Addictions—Aging—Endurance—Exhaustion—Longevity—Memory—Stamina—It is helpful for a problem in the head area such as Eye Problems—Ear Problems—

2. _____

Siberian Ginseng, Gota Kola, Bee Pollen, Capsicum.

This formula is used to increase energy and strengthen the body and the brain. It will increase circulation to eliminate toxins and build immunity. Gota Kola is food for the brain and Bee Pollen is food for the entire body.

USED FOR

Attention Deficit Disorder—(Hyperactivity)—Diets—Addictions—Drug Withdrawal—Endurance—Energy—Exhaustion—Fasting—Fatigue—Glandular Health—Longevity—Memory—Senility—

3. _____

Valerian Root, Scullcap, Hops, Thiamine, Mononitrate, Riboflavin, Nicotinamide, Calcium Pantothenate, Pyridoxine HCL, Ascorbic Acid, Choline, Bitartrate, Inositol, Para-aminobenzoic acid, Schizandra Chinesis, Piper Methysticum, Folic Acid, Cyanocobalamin, Biotin.

USED FOR

Stress—Anxiety—Fatigue—Insomnia—Nervousness—Strengthens the Nervous System—Calming and Relaxing—

4. _____

Calcarea iodata 12X, Calcarea fluorica 12X, Magnesiacarbonica 8X, Naphtalinum 6X, Vitamin A 12X, Euphrasia 6X, Julgans regia 6X, Cornea 7CH, Pancreas 4CH, Ophtalmic Arteria 4CH, Optic Nerve 7CH, and Liver 4CH.

This is a homeopathic formula designed to improve eye conditions. It can help in vision problems and those with cataracts. It is beneficial for conditions in the head area. It is used under the tongue to supply nutrients for the eyes.

STRUCTURAL SYSTEM FORMULAS

These formulas are excellent for bones, flesh and cartilage.

1. _____

Yucca, White Willow, Hydrangea, Alfalfa, Burdock, Black Cohosh, Sarsaparilla, Parsley, Slippery Elm. Redmond Clay, Capsicum, Lobelia.

2. _____

Yucca, White Willow, Alfalfa, Burdock, Black Cohosh, Sarsaparilla, Parsley, Slippery Elm, Redmond Clay, Capsicum.

These formulas clean deep in the joints to rid the body of calcium deposits that cause arthritis, bursitis, calcification, gout, neuritis, rheumatism and tennis elbows. These formulas clean the blood, ease pain, and relax the body for proper healing. The herbs contain properties that act like cortisone to ease pain.

3. _____

White Oak Bark, Comfrey Root, Wormwood, Lobelia, Scullcap, Black Walnut, Queen of the Meadow, Marshmallow, Mullein.

4. _____

White Oak Bark, Black Walnut, Queen of the Meadow, Marshmallow, Mullein.

These formulas heal, clean and nourish the bones, flesh and cartilage. They provide protein to build muscles, heal glands to nourish the body, dissolve inorganic minerals, feeds the spinal cord, and dissolve plaque and toxins.

Acne—Arthritis—Broken Bones—Bruises—Chipped and Damaged Bones—Cell Building—Hernia—Muscles—Muscular Dystrophy—Multiple Sclerosis—Nerves—

Polio—Post Poliomyelitis—Scoliosis—Spinal Cord Damage—Stroke—

5. _____
Oatstraw, Horsetail, Comfrey Leaves, Lobelia.

This formula is a natural calcium and mineral supplement. It is useful for almost any ailment. It is rich in vitamin A, B-complex, C and E. It is also rich in calcium, and silicon which are essential for calcium assimilation. It contains an abundant supply of selenium, potassium, phosphorus and iron.

This formula is used for all structural disorders.

Allergies—Arthritis—Bursitis—Cartilage— Female Problems—Fractures—Growing Pains—High Blood Pressure—Infections— Insomnia—Nerves—Rheumatism—Teeth—

URINARY SYSTEM FORMULAS

1. _____
Juniper Berries, Golden Seal Root, Parsley, Marshmallow, Watermelon Seeds, Uva Ursi, Lobelia, Ginger.

2. _____
Juniper Berries, Echinacea, Parsley, Marshmallow, Watermelon Seeds, Uva Ursi, Ginger.

These formulas are excellent for cleaning and nourishing the bladder and kidneys. They keep the urinary tract clear from toxic mucus build-up to keep it working smoothly and prevent blockage. These herbs help dissolve mucus, clear infections and strengthen the urinary tract.

USED FOR

Bed Wetting—Bladder Infections—Bloody Urine— Diuretic—Kidney Infections—Kidney Stones—Urinary Infections—

3, _____
Uva Ursi, Juniper Berries, Shavegrass (Horsetail), Cornsilk, Parsley, Queen of the Meadow, Goldenrod, Cubeb Berries, Powdered Whole Cranberries, Watermelon Seeds.

USED FOR

Bladder Problems—Bloody Urine—Diuretic— Kidney Problems—Menstrual Problems— Prostate—Urinary Tract Problems—

4. _____
Senna, Buckthorn, Althea, Peppermint, Uva Ursi, Rose Hips, Caa' Inhem, Orange Peel, Chaparral, Honeysuckle, Chrysanthemum.

This formula helps to clear obstructions from the digestive and urinary tracts. These herbs help the body digest and assimilate nutrients from food, herbs, vitamins and minerals. This formula also helps clean and dissolve toxins from the colon. It is also designed to clear the body of excess water accumulation in the cells.

This is an excellent formula to use when going on a cleansing diet or when trying to lose weight. This formula helps nature in the healing of acute diseases. It helps in chronic diseases to clear obstructions.

USED FOR

Allergies—Acute Diseases such as Colds— Flu—Childhood Diseases—Chronic Diseases— Cleansing Programs—Constipation—Diets—

FEMALE HERBAL FORMULAS

1. _____

Oatstraw, Horsetail, Comfrey Leaves, Lobelia.

This formula is a natural calcium and mineral supplement. It is useful for female problems. It helps prevent osteoporosis, and premenstrual problems. It is excellent to use to prevent mineral deficiencies. It is rich in Vitamin A, B-complex, C and E. It is also rich in calcium, and silicon (necessary for calcium assimilation). In addition, it contains an excellent supply of selenium, potassium, phosphorus and iron.

USED FOR

Allergies—Arthritis—Bursitis—Cartilage— Female Problems—Fractures—Growing Pains (teenage girls need extra calcium)— High Blood Pressure—Infections—Insomnia— Nervous Disorders — Osteoporosis — Rheumatism—Essential for health of Bones— Teeth—Nails—

2. _____

Licorice Root, Juniper Berries, Wild Yam, Dandelion Root, Horseradish.

This formula helps in maintaining glandular health. All glands work together. When one gland is deficient as with the ovaries, the other glands take over when they are nourished properly. This formula helps nourish and clean the glands.

USED FOR

Adrenal Function—Energy—Feeds Glands— Liver—Pancreas—Weakened Body—

3. _____

False Unicorn, Black Cohosh, Blue Cohosh, Cramp Bark, Pennyroyal, Bayberry, Ginger, Squaw Vine, Uva Ursi, Raspberry Leaves, Valerian, Blessed Thistle.

4. _____

False Unicorn, Black Cohosh, Cramp Bark, Bayberry, Ginger, Squaw Vine, Uva Ursi, Raspberry Leaves, Blessed Thistle.

These formulas supply nutrients for the body to balance hormones, stimulate glandular function, strengthen the uterus and supply energy to a weakened body.

USED FOR

Child Birth (last five weeks)—Hormone Imbalance—Hot Flashes—Glandular Mal-function—Menstrual Problems—Morning Sickness — Sexual Impotence — Uterine Problems—

5. _____

Alfalfa, Dandelion Root, Kelp.

This formula is beneficial to supply vitamins and minerals to help build glandular health. The alfalfa feeds the adrenal glands and kelp feeds the thyroid gland. It is good to use for all ailments as well as a means of preventing disease.

USED FOR

Anemia—Bones—Hair Health—Mineral Imbalance—Nails—Menopause—Pregnancy— Premenstrual Syndrome—Skin—

6. _____

Turnera Aphrodisiaca, Brazilian Ginseng, Wild Yam, Passion Flower, Licorice Root, Serenoa Repens Fruit Extract, Dietary Indoles.

This formula supplies nutrients for female health. It contains nutrients to prevent excess estrogen from accumulating in the liver and causing breast or uterine problems. It is calming for the nerves and helps balance hormones.

USED FOR

Breast Diseases—Female Problems—Frigidity— Premenstrual Problems—Menopause—

7. _____

Blessed Thistle, Golden Seal Root, Red Raspberry Leaves, Squaw Vine, Ginger, Cramp Bark, Capsicum, Uva Ursi, Marshmallow, Lobelia, False Unicorn.

This formula helps regulate hormonal function. It helps the liver detoxify the excess estrogen that causes mental imbalance. It is good for all female problems. Cramp bark helps regulate heavy menstrual flow. False Unicorn helps with cramps and lower back pain.

USED FOR

Breast Tenderness — Cramps — Endometriosis—Hormone Imbalance—Morning Sickness — Sterility — Hot Flashes — Hysterectomy—Menopause—Menstrual Problems—Tumors—Uterine Infections—Vaginal Problems—

8. _____

Squaw Vine, Chickweed, Slippery Elm, Comfrey Root, Yellow Dock, Mullein, Marshmallow.

This formula will help in treating female related ailments. It aids in soothing, cleaning, and healing problems related to the uterus and vagina such as endometriosis and yeast infections.

USED FOR

Cysts—Endometriosis—Polyps—Toxemia—Tumors — Uterine Problems — Vaginal Infections—

9. _____

Dong Quai, White Willow Bark, Uva Ursi, Valerian, Juniper Berries, Licorice Root, DL Phenylalanine, Black Cohosh, Cramp Bark, Ginger.

10. _____

Dong Quai, White Willow Bark, Uva Ursi, Juniper Berries, Licorice, Black Cohosh, Cramp Bark, Ginger.

These formulas help to aid in premenstrual syndrome. There are many symptoms related to PMS and menopause, and these herbs help ease the discomfort.

USED FOR

Bloating—Cramps—Hormone Imbalance—Menstrual Discomforts—Morning Sickness—Sterility—Hot Flashes—Menopause—Uterine Problems—Water Retention—

MALE HERBAL FORMULAS

1. _____

Serenoa repens Fruit Extract, Brazilian Ginseng, Turnera Aphrodisiaca, Korean Ginseng, Wild Yam, Pumpkin Seed, Dietary Endoles.

This formula is designed to stimulate and nourish the reproductive organs in the male. It will help prevent prostate problems and balance hormones.

USED FOR

Aging — Energy — Hormone Balance — Impotence—Longevity—Prostate Problems—Senility—Sterility—

2. _____

Elk Antler, Canadian Ginseng, Bee Pollen, Echinacea, Ginger, Cinnamon, Capsicum.

This formula is useful to increase stamina in the male. It promotes longevity and strengthens the immune system. It benefits in impotency. It increases circulation in the veins and capillaries.

USED FOR

Immune Function—Stamina—Senility—Sexual Function — Stress — Weight Reduction—

3. _____

Licorice Root, Juniper Berries, Wild Yam, Dandelion Root, Horseradish.

This formula strengthens and feeds the glands. It helps to eliminate toxins from the liver and promotes adrenal function to prevent stress. It is a cleanser, builder and healer for the glandular system.

USED FOR

Adrenal Function—Energy—Glands—Liver—Pancreas—Stress—Weakened System—

4. _____

Suma, Siberian Ginseng, Damiana, Sarsaparilla, Gotu Kola, Licorice Root, Fo-Ti Herb, Saw Palmetto, Ginger Root, Ho-Shou-Wu, and Nettle.

This formula strengthens the male and female glands. It acts as a dissolvant for catarrh and uric acid and contains anti-cancer properties. It relieves stress, cleans the veins and acts as a tonic for the whole body.

USED FOR
(Male or Female)

Aphrodisiac—Energy—Hormone Imbalance—Impotence—Prostate Problems—Cancer—

5. _____

Alfalfa, Dandelion Root, Kelp.

This formula is beneficial to supply vitamins and minerals lacking in the diet. It is good to use for all ailments as well as in preventing disease. It helps balance the glandular system, and contains nutrients to build the immune system.

USED FOR

Anemia—Bones—Hair Health—Hormone Balance—Mineral Imbalance—Nails—Skin Health—Stress—

6. _____

Essence of Adrenals, Epiphyse, Hypophyse, Hypothalamus, Placenta, Thyroid, Silica, Corallium, Rubrum, Eleutheroeoccus, Biotin, Graphite.

This is a homeopathic formula to nourish the glandular system. It helps the nervous system and helps in hair loss.

USED FOR

Supplies nutrients to the Glandular System—Energy—Balding—Glandular Balance—Stimulate Hair Growth—

HERBAL GLOSSARY

ADAPTATION/ADAPTOGEN

These are immune system enhancers which help the body adjust and regulate to restore natural immune resistance. Herbs which are used for this purpose include: Chlorophyll, Ginseng, Pau D'Arco, Suma, Ginkgo, Garlic, Echinacea, Goldenseal, and Taheebo.

ALTERATIVE

Alteratives are considered useful in altering the body chemistry. They are blood purifiers which correct impurities in the blood and stimulate gradual changes in metabolism and tissue function in acute and chronic conditions. Alterative herbs include: Alfalfa, Aloe Vera, Barberry Root, Black Cohosh Root, Blue Cohosh, Blue Green Algae, Buckthorn, Burdock Root, Cascara Sagrada, Dandelion, Devil's Claw, Dong Quai, Echinacea, Elder Flowers, Elecampane, Garlic, Ginkgo, Ginseng, Gotu Kola, Golden Seal Root, Ho Shou Wu, Hops, Licorice, Marshmallow, Milk Thistle, Oregon Grape Root, Pau D'Arco, Prickley Ash Bark, Red Clover, Red Raspberry, Sarsaparilla Root, Sassafras Bark, Uva Ursi, Virginia Poke Root, Yarrow, Yellow Dock Root.

ANALGESIC

These herbs are used to relieve pain. Some of the herbs commonly used as analgesics include: Lobelia, Mullein, Pau D'Arco, Scullcap, Wood Betony, and White Willow Bark.

ANTACID

An antacid is used to neutralize acids in the stomach and intestinal tract. Herbs used for this purpose include: Dandelion, Fennel, Ginger, Kelp, Irish Moss, and Slippery Elm.

ANTHELMINTICS/VERMIFUGES

These herbs are used to expel intestinal parasites and worms. Herbs used include Blue Cohosh, Black Walnut, Gentian, Golden Seal Root, Mandrake Root, Prickly Ash, Pumpkin Seed, and Senna.

ANTI-ASTHMATIC

Anti-asthmatics are used to help relieve and ease the symptoms associated with asthma. Some of the anti-asthmatic herbs are: Cherry Bark, Elecampane, Ephedra, Gotu Kola, Lobelia, Prickly Ash, and Yerba Santa.

ANTIBIOTIC

Herbs that work as natural antibiotics help the body's immune system to destroy both viral and bacterial infections. Some herbs commonly used as natural antibiotics include: Buchu, Chaparral, Echinacea, Garlic, Golden Seal, Myrrh, Red Clover, and Yellow Dock.

ANTICATARRHAL

These are herbs which help dissolve and eliminate as well prevent the formation of mucus. Herbs that are considered to be anticatarrhal include: Ephedra, Lobelia, Comfrey, Mullein, Fenugreek, Marshmallow, Elecampane, Wild Cherry and Licorice.

ANTILITHIC

These work to prevent the formation of gravel and stones in the gall bladder and kidneys. They also help to relieve those already formed. Some herbs used for this purpose are: Buchu Leaves, Hydrangea, and Uva Ursi Leaves.

ANTIRHEUMATIC

Antirheumatic herbs help to ease and prevent arthritis and rheumatism. Some include: Alfalfa, Buchu, Buckthorn, Bugleweed, Burdock, Devil's Claw, Gravel Root, Hydrangea, Mandrake, and Yucca.

ANTISEPTIC

These help to prevent and counteract infection and the formation of pus. Herbs used are: Black Walnut, Chaparral, Echinacea, Elecampane, Garlic, Gentian, Ginkgo, Golden Seal, Myrrh, Rose Hips, Tea Tree Oil, Uva Ursi, Valerian, White Oak Bark, and Yarrow.

ANTISPASMODIC

These herbs are used to prevent or counteract spasms. Some are: Black Cohosh, Blue Cohosh, Cascara Sagrada, Catnip, Cramp Bark, Dong Quai, Gotu Kola, Hawthorn, Juniper Berries, Kava Kava, Linden Flowers, Lobelia, Mistletoe, and Scullcap.

APHRODISIAC

An aphrodisiac is used to help improve and restore normal sexual potency and function. Some herbs used as aphrodisiacs include: Astragalus, Damiana, False Unicorn, Fenugreek, Ginseng, Kava Kava, and Saw Palmetto.

ASTRINGENT

An astringent acts to contract and tighten. This constricting action can help eliminate secretions and hemorrhaging. Some herbs with astringent actions are: Amaranth, Blackberry Root, Black Walnut, Capsicum, Elecampane, Ephedra, Fenugreek, Horsetail, Hydrangea, Mullein, Oak Bark, Queen of the Meadow, Red Raspberry, Rose Hips, Schizandra, Shepherd's Purse, Slippery Elm, St. Johns Wort, Witchhazel, Yarrow, and Yellow Dock.

CARMINATIVE

Herbs which can help eliminate and expel gas from the stomach and intestines are considered carminatives. Some of the herbs commonly used are: Angelica Root, Capsicum, Caraway Seeds, Cardamon Seeds, Catnip, Chamomile Flowers, Echinacea, Fennel, Ginger, Hops, Lemon Balm, Parsley Root, Peppermint, Saffron, and Valerian.

CATHARTIC

A cathartic herb is used for purging and stimulating the action of evacuating the bowels. This action may be mild or strong depending on the need. Herbs considered to be cathartic include: Aloe Vera, Barberry Bark, Buckthorn Bark, Cascara Sagrada, Mandrake, Rhubarb Root, and Senna Leaves.

CHOLAGOGUE

This is the action of increasing the flow of bile to aid in digestion and act as a mild laxative. Herbs which are used for this purpose are: Aloe Vera, Barberry, Culver's Root, Dandelion, Goldenseal, Hops, Licorice, Oregon Grape Root, and Wild Yam.

DEMULCENT

These herbs help soothe and and protect the mucous membranes in the body. Some herbs with this property are: Aloe Vera, Burdock, Chia Seeds, Chickweed, Comfrey, Echinacea, Fenugreek, Flax Seeds, Irish Moss, Kelp, Licorice, Marshmallow, Mullein, Oatstraw, and Psyllium.

DIAPHORETIC

Diaphoretic herbs help the body produce perspiration to help the skin eliminate toxins. Herbs with diaphoretic properties include: Angelica, Blue Vervain, Boneset, Borage, Butcher's Broom, Catnip, Cayenne, Chamomile, Elder Flowers, Elecampane, Ephedra, Garlic, Hyssop, Lemon Balm Leaves, Linden Flowers, and Yarrow.

DIRUETIC

A diuretic is used to increase the flow of urine to relieve water retention. Some herbs used for this purpose are: Alfalfa, Blue Cohosh, Buchu Leaves, Burdock, Butcher's Broom, Corn Silk, Damiana, Dandelion, Devil's Claw, Elecampane, False Unicorn, Fennel, Hawthorn, Horsetail, Hydrangea, Juniper Berries, Lily-of-the-Valley, Marshmallow, Mullein, Nettle, Parsley, Queen of the Meadow, Saw Palmetto, and Uva Ursi.

EMETIC

An emetic is used to induce vomiting. Emetic herbs include: False Unicorn, Ipecac, Lobelia, and Mustard Seed.

EMMENAGOGUE

Herbs with emmenagogue properties help the body to promote and stimulate the menstrual flow. Some herbs which help with this situation are: Angelica, Aloe Vera, Black Cohosh, Blue Cohosh, Gentian, Ginger, Golden Seal, Horsetail, Juniper Berries, Mistletoe, Myrrh, Pennyroyal, and Saffron.

EMOLLIENT

This includes herbs used externally to help soften, soothe, and protect the skin. Some are: Almond Oil, Aloe Vera, Comfrey, Flaxseed, Fenugreek, Irish Moss, Linseed Oil, Marshmallow, Olive Oil, Slippery Elm, and Wheat Germ Oil.

EXPECTORANT

Expectorants help the body expel mucus from the lungs, nose and throat. Herbs used for this purpose include: Ainse Seed, Blue Cohosh, Blue Vervain, Comfrey Root, Elder Flowers, Elecampane Root, Ephedra, Flax Seed, Fennel, Fenugreek, Garlic, Horehound, Hyssop, Irish Moss, Licorice, Lobelia, Lungwort, Marshmallow, Mullein Leaves, Slippery Elm, Wild Cherry Bark, and Yerba Santa Leaves.

FEBRIFUGE

Herbs with this property help reduce fevers. Some are: Bilberry, Boneset, Borage, Brigham Tea, Buckthorn, Catnip, Chamomile, Elder Flowers, Fenugreek, Garlic, Gentian, Ginger, Hyssop, Pleurisy Root, Sarsaparilla, White Willow Bark, and Wormwood.

HEPATIC

These herbs help to strengthen, tone, and increase bile flow to promote normal liver function. Some herbs with hepatic properties are: Barberry Bark, Cascara Sagrada, Dandelion Root, Gentian, Golden Seal, Gravel Root, Horseradish, Liverwort, Mandrake Root, Mild Thistle, Olive Oil, Oregon Grape, Parsley, and Turkey Rhubarb.

LAXATIVE

Laxative herbs help produce a gentle, normal action of the bowels to relieve constipation. Herbs used for this purpose include: Boneset, Buckthorn Bark, Cascara Sagrada, Elder Flowers, Golden Seal, Mandrake Root, Oregon Grape Root, Psyllium, Senna Leaves, and Virginia Poke Root.

LITHOTRIPTIC

These are herbs which help dissolve and eliminate stones and gravel from the body. They include: Buchu, Butcher's Broom, Cascara Sagrada, Cornsilk, Dandelion, Devil's Claw, Gravel Root, Horsetail, Marshmallow, Parsley, Uva Ursi, and White Oak Bark.

NEPHRITIC

These are used in healing kidney problems. Herbs with nephritic properties include: Buchu Leaves, Couch Grass Root, Golden Seal, Horsetail, Hydrangea, Juniper Berries, Oregon Grape, Queen of the Meadow Root, and Virginia Poke Root.

NERVINE

Nervine herbs help soothe, calm and nourish the nervous system. Some of the nervine herbs are: Black Cohosh, Blue Vervain, Boneset, Catnip, Chamomile, Cramp Bark, Damiana, Gotu Kola, Hops, Lady's Slipper, Lemon Balm, Lobelia, Oatstraw, Passion Flower, Scullcap, Valerian Root, and Wood Betony.

OXYTOCIC

These are herbs which help stimulate uterine contractions to assist and induce a safe labor and delivery. Herbs with oxytocic properties are: Black Cohosh, Blue Cohosh, Pennyroyal, Red Raspberry, and Squawvine.

RUBERFACIENT

Herbs with ruberfacient properties help to increase the flow of blood to the surface of the skin to aid in healing in cases such as sprains and muscle soreness. Some herbs used for this purpose include: Camphor, Cayenne, Cloves, Eucalyptus, Garlic, Ginger, Horseradish, Mustard Seed, Peppermint Oil, Pine Oil, Stinging Nettle, and Thyme Oil.

SEDATIVE

Sedative herbs are used to relieve irritability and promote calm and tranquil feelings. Some are: Catnip, Chamomile, Cramp Bark, Dong Quai, Hawthorn, Hops, Kava Kava, Lady's Slipper, Lobelia, Passion Flower, Red Clover, Schizandra, Scullcap, St. John's Wort, Valerian, and Wood Betony.

SIALOGUGE

Herbs with this property help to promote the flow and secretion of saliva to aid in the digestion of starches. Some herbs include: Bayberry, Cayenne, Echinacea, Gentian, Ginger, Horseradish, Hydrangea, Licorice, Prickly Ash, Turkey Rhubarb, and Yerba Santa.

STIMULANT

These herbs help to increase the function of the body, energy levels, circulation, and help eliminate toxins. Herbs with stimulant properties are: Angelica, Boneset, Capsicum, Damiana, Devil's Claw, Echinacea, Elder Flower, Elcampane, Ephedra, False Unicorn, Garlic, Genitian, Ginger, Ginkgo, Ginseng, Ho-Shou-Wu, Linden Flowers, Milk Thistle, Prickley Ash Bark, Saffron, Sarsaparilla Root, and Suma.

TONIC

Tonic herbs are used to increase tone, energy, vigor and strength by nourishing the body. There are tonics for the liver, heart, nerves as well as all body system. Some tonic herbs include: Black Cohosh, Blue Cohosh, Blue Vervain, Cascara Sagrada, Cayenne, Chamomile, Damiana, Elcampane, Fenugreek, Gentian, Ginger, Ginkgo, Golden Seal, Hawthorn, Horsetail, Milk Thistle, Schizandra, and Suma. Some tonics used to nourish the organs, cells and tissues over a long period are: Alfalfa, Aloe Vera, Astragalus, Barley Greens, Blue-Green Algae, and Spirulina. Some tonics used to stimulate digestion include Dandelion, Endive, Gentian, Ginger, Gotu Kola, Golden Seal, and Peppermint.

VULNERARY

Herbs with vulnerary properties are used to help promote the healing of wounds, cuts and abrasions. Some used are: Aloe Vera, Black Walnut, Burdock, Cayenne, Fenugreek, Flaxseed, Garlic, Gentian, Golden Seal, Hops, Horsetail, Mullein, Oatstraw, Plantain Leaves, and Virginia Poke Root.

SINGLE HERBS

ALFALFA
(Medicago sativa)

Parts Used: The leaves and flowers
Properties: Nutrient, tonic, diuretic, and appetizer.
Body Parts Affected: Stomach, blood, spleen and pancreas.

Functions and Health Benefits:

Alfalfa was used anciently as a miracle herb. The Arabs called it the "Father of Herbs." (Al-Fal-Fa) It has been cultivated for over 2000 years. In 400 B.C., the Medes and the Persians invaded Greece and began cultivating Alfalfa in that region. It is known for its ability to survive even in harsh climates. The roots of the plant can reach as far as 66 feet into the subsoil. The Romans discovered that Alfalfa was excellent for their horses. Alfalfa was introduced to North America by the Spanish. The main uses of Alfalfa were to treat arthritis, boils, cancer, scurvy, urinary tract disorders, and bowel problems.

Modern scientific research has documented the health benefits of this useful herb. It has been found to be one of the most nutritious foods available. Alfalfa has been found to help build the blood in cases of anemia. It is also known to help with milk production in nursing mothers. It has also been researched and found to help lower cholesterol levels. (1) Alfalfa contains anti-bacterial and anti-fungal properties. The extracts produce anti-bacterial activity against Gram-positive bacteria. (2) It has been found to help in healing ulcers, arteriosclerosis, liver toxicity, arthritis, diabetes. (3) and in strengthening the capillaries and blood vessels.

Alfalfa is considered by herbalists to be beneficial for many problems, and some even recommend it for any ailment. It is used to remove poisons and the effects of toxins that may be in the body. It is also thought to neutralize the acidity of the body and break down carbon dioxide. Alfalfa is often used to treat water retention, infection, urinary and bowel problems, muscle spasms, cramps, and digestive problems.

Vitamin and Mineral Content:

Alfalfa contains valuable minerals and vitamins. It is thought to contain all the vitamins and minerals known to man. It also has high levels of chlorophyll, and it is thought to be balanced for complete absorption in the body. Alfalfa is high in vitamin A, which helps in the prevention of arthritis and is essential for healthy skin and mucous membranes. It is high in vitamin E, which is essential for a healthy heart. It is also high in vitamin D, which increases the absorption of calcium and phosphorus in the body. Alfalfa also contains vitamin K, which is necessary for blood clotting and may help prevent osteoporosis. It contains vitamin B12, which may help strengthen the nervous system. It is rich in calcium, phosphorus, iron, potassium, chlorine, sodium, silicon, magnesium, B1 and B2. It also is high in protein and contains eight of the essential amino acids.

ACIDITY	Fever (reduces)
Alcoholism	Gout
ALLERGIES	Heart Disease
ANEMIA	HEMORRHAGES
APPETITE STIMULANT	Hypertension
ARTHRITIS	Jaundice
ASTHMA	KIDNEYS (cleanses)
Bladder	Lactation
Blood Pressure (lowers)	NAUSEA
BLOOD PURIFIER	Nosebleeds
Body Building	PITUITARY GLAND
Boils	(strengthens)
Breath Odor	Teeth
Bursitis	TONIC
CANCER (prevention)	Toxemia
Cholesterol (lowers)	ULCERS, PEPTIC
DIABETES	Urinary Problems
Digestion	Weight gain/loss
Diuretic	Whooping Cough
FATIGUE	

ALOE VERA ————————
(Aloe vera)

Part Used: The leaves
Properties: Emollient, purgative, vulnerary, cholagogue, alterative, and tonic.
Body Parts Affected: Skin, stomach, colon, liver and uterus.

Functions and Health Benefits:

Aloe vera has been used for thousands of years to treat burns, heal wounds, treat ulcers, and relieve hemorrhoids. It is a member of the lily family, though it looks much like a cactus plant. Dioscorides, a Greek historian, recommended Aloe vera as a treatment for burns, kidney ailments and constipation. The ancient Egyptians were thought to have used Aloe vera in their embalming procedures. The plant thrives in warm climates.

Modern research has proven many of the benefits of Aloe vera. It is known to help promote healing when used externally in cases of wounds, frostbite and burns. (4) It has been used effectively for treating radiation burns. It is known to help increase movement in the intestines, relieve constipation, promote menstruation, and aid in digestion. It is also known to help with inflammation and ulcers. (5) It has been found to help in preventing the formation of kidney stones and to help reduce the size of the stone. (6) Aloe vera can help clean, soothe and relieve pain on contact. It penetrates through all three layers of the skin rapidly to promote healing. It contains salicylic acid and magnesium, which work together to produce an aspirin-like analgesic effect. It has also been used as a treatment for AIDS and may help prevent the virus from moving from one cell to the other.

Aloe vera can be used to help prevent scarring and to heal minor scars. It contains enzymes, saponins, hormones and amino acids which are absorbed through the skin. Aloe contains substances called uronic acids that are natural detoxicants and may take part in the healing process by stripping toxic materials of their harmful effects.

Vitamin and Mineral Content:

Aloe vera is high in vitamin C and selenium, which are among the antioxidants to help prevent diseases such as cancer and high blood pressure. It contains moderate amounts of sodium, which can help prevent calcium deposits in the joints. It may also help with diabetics, who often are lacking in sodium. It contains vitamin A, niacin, calcium, magnesium, phosphorus, potassium, iron, zinc, manganese and B-complex. Aloe vera contains trace amounts of copper, B2 and lecithin.

Abrasions	Jaundice
ACNE	Leg Ulcers
AIDS	Liver
ALLERGIES	POISON IVY AND OAK
Anemia	PSORIASIS
Asthma	RADIATION BURNS
Blood Cleansing	RINGWORM
Bruises	SCALDS
BURNS	SCAR TISSUE
Constipation	Sores
DEODORANT	SUNBURN
DIGESTION	Tapeworm
Heart	Tuberculosis
Heartburn	Ulcers (peptic)
HEMORRHOIDS	Varicose Veins
Inflammation	WOUNDS
INSECT BITES	Wrinkles

ANGELICA
(Angelica atropurpurea)

Part Used: The root
Properties: Stimulant, carminative, diaphoretic, emmenagogue, alterative, and tonic.
Body Parts Affected: Circulation, heart, stomach, intestines, spleen and lungs.

Functions and Health Benefits:

Anciently Angelica was used as a cure for the plague in Europe. Many benefited from its curative powers.

Modern scientific research has found Angelica to help stimulate and strengthen the immune system. It aids the stomach, spleen and intestines in their functions. (7) It is used for chronic bronchitis, asthma, lymph disorders, and menstruation problems. It helps to relax the nervous system and strengthen the immune system. (8) It has also successfully treated those suffering from nervous exhaustion. (9)

Angelica is often used to treat problems of the digestive system. It is used for digestion, heartburn, gas, colic, ulcers, and stomach cramps. It is known to be stimulating to the entire body and to improve mental well being. It is also used for toothaches, wounds, fevers, nervous headache, and general weakness.

Vitamin and Mineral Content:

Angelica contains vitamin E, calcium and some species contain vitamin B12.

APPETITE STIMULANT	GAS
Arthritis	HEARTBURN
Asthma	Hemorrhoids
Backaches	Inflammation
BRONCHIAL PROBLEMS	Liver
COLDS	Lung Disorders
COLIC	Menstrual Problems
COUGHS	Prostate Problems
Digestive Problems	RHEUMATISM
EPIDEMICS	Stomach Cramps
EXHAUSTION	TONIC
Fevers	Toothaches

BEE POLLEN

Part Used: Bee Pollen
Properties: Nutritive, and tonic.
Body Parts Affected: Whole body, immune system, and nerves.

Function and Health Benefits:

Ancient Greek marathon runners recognized the value of Bee Pollen and used it to increase their strength and endurance.

Modern scientific research has found Bee Pollen to contain properties beneficial to healing, revitalizing, and protecting against radiation therapy. It is a rich source of protein and carbohydrates and can be used as a food supplement. It can help athletes increase their stamina, endurance and athletic ability. (10) It may also help prevent plaque build up in the arteries.

Bee Pollen is considered a complete food because it contains every chemical substance needed to maintain life. It is a great supplement to build the immune system and provide energy to the body. It is thought to have the ability to correct body chemistry and eliminate unhealthy conditions. It is recommended for premature aging and as an immune system enhancer. Athletes often use this supplement to help increase their strength, endurance, and speed. It is also used to treat hay fevers, allergies, and asthma.

Vitamin and Mineral Content:

Bee Pollen contains essential fatty acids which are necessary for vital body functions. It contains 21 amino acids essential for life and health. It contains enzymes that are responsible for chemical reactions in the body. It contains all vitamins, minerals, and trace minerals. (11) It is considered to be a complete food.

ALLERGIES	HAY FEVER
Asthma	Hypoglycemia
Blood Pressure	IMMUNE BUILDER
Cancer	Indigestion
Depression	Liver Disease
ENDURANCE	LONGEVITY
ENERGY	Prostate Disorders
EXHAUSTION	Radiation
FATIGUE	Vitality

BILBERRY
(Vaccinium myrtillus)

Part Used: The fruit
Properties: Astringent, and febrifuge.
Body Systems Affected: Eyes, circulation, capillaries, and veins.

Functions and Health Benefits:

Bilberry has been used in Europe to treat fragile blood vessels related to high blood pressure. It is native to areas of northern Europe and Asia.

It has also been used to help with circulation in the body. (12) It can help to prevent strokes, heart attacks, and blindness. It contains essential antioxidants which are useful in preventing free radical damage. Bilberry is used in cases of diarrhea and other intestinal problems. (13) It helps nourish the pancreas in diabetes and aids healing in lung disorders such as chronic coughing, lung ailments, and TB. (14) The extract has been found to kill or inhibit the growth of fungus, yeast, and bacteria as well as protozoas such as Trichomonas vaginalis. (15)

Bilberry is known to be beneficial to the eyes and in strengthening the capillaries and small veins surrounding the eyes. It is also thought to help improve all capillaries, veins, and arteries, thus improving circulation to the feet, hands, brain, and heart. It also helps with varicose veins, arteriosclerosis, and blood clots.

Vitamin and Mineral Content:

It is rich in vitamin A, which helps the eyes, skin, veins, and cells in the body. Bilberry is high in vitamin C and bioflavonoids, which are necessary for healing and repairing the skin, bone, and cartilage. It may also clean and repair cholesterol build up. It contains manganese, which is necessary for proper nerve function. It is high in phosphorus, which helps with nerve and brain function. It contains iron, which is essential for healthy blood. The zinc in Bilberry helps with the eyes, liver, bones, prostate, semen and hair. It contains moderate amounts of magnesium, potassium, and selenium. It has trace amounts of calcium, sodium, and silicon.

Blood Thinner	Kidney Problems
BLOOD VESSELS	Light Sensitivity
COLD HANDS AND FEET	NIGHT BLINDNESS
DIABETES	Raynaud's Disease
Diarrhea	Scurvy
Dropsy	Thyroid
Immune System	VARICOSE VEINS
INFECTIONS	Water Retention

BLACK COHOSH
(Cimicifuga racemosa)

Part Used: The root
Properties: Nervine, emmenagogue, tonic, antispasmodic, alterative, diuretic, and expectorant.
Body Parts Affected: Uterus, nerves, lungs, and heart.

Functions and Health Benefits:

Black Cohosh was introduced by Dr. Young in 1831 and used as a cardiac tonic for a fatty heart, bronchitis, hysteria, and female problems. The Native Americans called Black Cohosh, Snakeroot, because of its ability to help with snake bites.

Modern research has revealed the benefits of Black Cohosh for equalizing circulation to help with high blood pressure and heart problems. (16) It can help with asthma, bronchitis, nervous conditions, irritability, TB, pleurisy, and tinnitus. (17) It has been used as an antidote for poisons, snake and insect bites. It has also been found to help with female complaints. (18)

Traditionally, Black Cohosh has been used for many different ailments such as hot flashes, excess mucus, yellow fever, spinal meningitis, nervousness, epilepsy, and hormone imbalance. It is also used to treat all types of inflammation.

Vitamin and Mineral Content:

Black Cohosh is rich in phosphorus, calcium and selenium. Phosphorus is necessary for brain and nerve function. It is needed each day to promote normal brain function. Calcium calms the nerves, builds bones, flesh and cartilage. Selenium is often lacking in the typical western diet. It is an antioxidant which helps protect the immune system. It contains moderate amounts of magnesium, potassium and iron. It also contains small amounts of vitamin K, F (fatty acids), sodium, silicon, manganese, zinc, vitamin A, C, niacin, B1, B2, and sulphur.

Arthritis	INSECT BITES
ASTHMA	Insomnia
BEE STINGS	Kidney Problems
Blood Cleanser	Liver Problems
Blood Pressure	Lumbago
BRONCHITIS	LUNGS
CHILDBIRTH	MALARIA
Cholera	MENOPAUSE
Convulsions	MENSTRUAL PROBLEMS
Coughs	Nervous Conditions
Cramps	Neuralgia
DIARRHEA	Pain
Digestive Problems	Rheumatism
EPILEPSY	Skin Problems
ESTROGEN DEFICIENCY	Smallpox
FEVERS	SNAKE BITES
Headaches	SPINAL MENINGITIS
Heart Problems	ST. VITUS DANCE
HORMONE IMBALANCE	TUBERCULOSIS
HOT FLASHES	Uterine Problems
INFLAMMATION	WHOOPING COUGH

BLACK WALNUT

(Juglans nigra)

Parts Used: The hulls and leaves
Properties: Antiseptic, astringent, vermicide, alterative, and anti syphilitic.
Body Parts Affected: Blood, intestines, skin, veins, and nerves.

Functions and Health Benefits:

Black Walnut has been used for centuries in Europe for different ailments such as skin ailments and constipation. Native Americans traditionally used it as a laxative. During the Civil War, Black Walnut was used as a remedy for diarrhea and dysentery.

Scientific research has found that it contains astringent properties healing to the skin and mucous membranes of the body. It cleans the blood and contains antiseptic properties. It is used for all skin problems including boils, eczema, herpes, and ringworm. (19) It is known to expel parasites and worms from the body. (20) It has been used for syphilis, TB, varicose veins, chronic infections of the intestines and urogenital organs.

Herbalists consider Black Walnut very useful for killing parasites, tapeworms, and ringworm. The brown stain found in the green husk of Black Walnut contains organic iodine, which has antiseptic and healing properties.

Vitamin and Mineral Content:

Black Walnut is high in organic iodine which is a potent antiseptic. It contains manganese, which is essential for healthy nerves, brain function, and cartilage. Magnesium found in Black Walnut helps prevent tooth decay, improve resistance to infection, and stimulate the glands and liver. It contains calcium, which is necessary for vitality, endurance, hearth rhythm and the nervous system. It also has silicon, which tones the entire system and promotes healthy skin. Black Walnut contains selenium, potassium, B15, iron, sodium, phosphorus, chlorine, B1, vitamin A, C, niacin, B2, B6, P and bioflavonoids.

Abscesses	Hemorrhoids
Acne	HERPES
Antiperspirant	INFECTIONS
ANTISEPTIC (external)	Liver
Asthma	Lupus
ATHLETE'S FOOT	MALARIA
Boils	Mouth sores
Cancer	PARASITES
CANDIDA ALBICANS	Poison Ivy
CANKER SORES	RASHES
Carbuncles	RINGWORM
COLD SORES	Scrofula
Colitis	Skin Diseases
DANDRUFF	TAPEWORM
Diarrhea	Teeth
Diphtheria	Tonsillitis
Dysentery	Tuberculosis
Eczema	Tumors
Eye Disease	Ulcers
Fevers	Varicose Veins
FUNGUS	WORMS
Gargle	Wounds
GUM DISEASE	

BLESSED THISTLE ———
(Cnicus benedictus)

Part Used: The herb
Properties: Bitter tonic, diaphoretic, emmenagogue, galactogogue, and alterative.
Body Parts Affected: Digestion, heart, blood, mammary glands, and uterus.

Functions and Health Benefits:

Herbalists in the past highly recommended this herb for female problems. Culpepper suggested Blessed Thistle for treating headaches, fevers and female difficulties. The Quinault tribe of Native Americans used the steeped whole plant, for birth control. It contains nutrients that help supply estrogen and balance other hormones in the body.

Modern research has shown that the extract of Blessed Thistle contains antibacterial and anti-yeast properties which can help with Candida albicans. (21) It also has been used to strengthen the stomach, spleen, intestine, liver and the nervous system. (22) It is also used to reduce fevers in childhood diseases, chicken pox, and measles.

Traditional uses of Blessed Thistle include digestive problems, headaches, stomach problems, heart conditions, circulation, liver problems, and internal cancer. It is sometimes taken in combination with Red Raspberry to stimulate milk production for nursing mothers.

Vitamin and Mineral Content:

Blessed Thistle is rich in vitamin A, which helps with digestion, assimilation of nutrients, and in maintaining normal glandular activity. It contains potassium, which aids in controlling normal weight and preventing germs from accumulating in the tissues. Selenium is also found in Blessed Thistle which protects against oxidation which is believed to help prevent cancer and boost heart function. It also contains high amounts of calcium, which assists in blood clotting, improving muscle tone and contractions, helps regulate the heart beat, and aids in nerve transmissions. Sodium is also found in this herb, which is a neutralizer of waster material and important in filtering toxins from the bloodstream through the lymphatic system. It also contains B-complex vitamins, magnesium, phosphorus, vitamin C, niacin and zinc.

ANGINA	HEADACHES
Arthritis	HEART
Birth Control	HORMONE BALANCE
BLOOD CIRCULATION	Jaundice
BLOOD PURIFIER	Kidneys
BREAST MILK	LACTATION
CANCER	Leucorrhea
CONSTIPATION	LIVER AILMENTS
Cramps	LUNGS
DIGESTION	MEMORY
Dropsy	MENSTRUATION
FEMALE PROBLEMS	Respiratory Infection
FEVERS	Senility
GALLBLADDER	Spleen
Gas	Worms

BLUE COHOSH ——————
(Caulophyllum thalictrodies)

Part Used: The rhizome
Properties: Anthelmintic, antispasmodic, emmenagogue, estrogenic, tonic, diuretic, alterative, and expectorant.
Body Parts Affected: Uterus, nerves, joints (muscular pain), and urinary tract.

Functions and Health Benefits:

Blue Cohosh was used by the Native Americans and early settlers to aid delivery in childbirth and to help reduce fevers. The dried root was an official entry in the *U.S. Pharmacopoeia* from 1882 to 1905.

Studies done in recent years have found Blue Cohosh to help with regulating menstrual cycles. (23) It also has been found to contain estrogenic and antispasmodic properties. (24) In addition, it may help during deliveries to make them easier. It has been reported to normalize the menstrual cycle when used along with pennyroyal. (25) It has helped with cases of toxemia, in promoting menses, and in balancing estrogen in deficiencies with excess progesterone. (26) It has also been found to be useful in reducing emotional and nervous tension. (27)

Herbalists have recommended Blue Cohosh for female problems such as irregular menstrual cycles, to promote menstruation, relieve cramps, to reduce inflammation of the uterus, to ease delivery, and to stop false labor pains. It has also been used as an antispasmodic and to ease muscle cramps.

Vitamin and Mineral Content:

Blue Cohosh has been found to be rich in iron, which is responsible for carrying oxygen from the lungs to all parts of the body. It also helps build the blood. It contains high amounts of manganese, which helps protect the lining of the heart, blood vessels, and urinary tract. Selenium (which may be lacking in the soil) is also found in Blue Cohosh, which helps prevent heart disease and auto-immune diseases and may be lacking in the soil. It contains vitamin E, which is essential to the reproductive system and is sometimes called the fertility vitamin. It also contains calcium, magnesium, phosphorus, potassium, silicon, vitamins B1 and B2 and trace amounts of vitamin A, C, niacin, sodium, chlorine, and zinc.

Bladder Infection	Heart Palpitations
Bronchitis	Hysteria
CHILDBIRTH	High Blood Pressure
Colic	LABOR
Convulsions	Leucorrhea
CRAMPS	MENSTRUATION
Diabetes	Mucus
Dropsy	Neuralgia
Edema	Spasms
EPILEPSY	UTERINE PROBLEMS
ESTROGEN	Vaginitis
FEMALE PROBLEMS	Whooping Cough

BLUE GREEN ALGAE
(Chloroplast membrane sulfolipids)

Part Used: The whole plant
Properties: Tonic, nutrient, and alterative.
Body Parts Affected: Whole body

Functions and Health Benefits:

Blue Green Algae is well known for its great nutritional value. Scientists at the National Cancer Institute have reported that Blue Green Algae may help protect against the AIDS virus. (28) It is rich in nutrients that help balance body chemistry and build resistance to viral diseases. It is known to increase the oxygen utilized by the body. Blue Green Algae has been found to help the body produce interferon, which helps the immune system. (29) It can help strengthen the immune system and is useful for growing children. It is excellent to use in cases of acute diseases such as colds, flu, and fevers.

Vitamin and Mineral Content:

It is rich in the essential amino acids: isoleucine, leucine, lysine, methionine, cystine, phenylalanine, tyrosine, and tryptophan. Amino acids are the raw materials of which the DNA(genetic coding material) in the body are constructed. They help protect the immune system. They provide material for bones, tissue, organs, hormones, neurotransmitters, enzymes, etc. Blue Green Algae is high in beta carotene, which is stored in the liver and used by the body as needed. It protects the lungs against air pollution. Vitamin C content is also high, which is an antioxidant needed on a daily basis by the body. It also has thiamine, riboflavin, and niacin which are components of the B-complex vitamins. It also contains choline, biotin, pantothenic acid, vitamin K, iodine, calcium, phosphorus, magnesium, potassium, copper, iron, manganese, zinc, and sodium.

AIDS	IMMUNE SYSTEM
Bones	INFECTIONS
CANCER	Liver
COLDS	Lungs
Fevers	Viruses
FLU	

BLUE VERVAIN
(Verbena hastata)

Part Used: The herb
Properties: Antispasmodic, nervine, diaphoretic, tonic, and expectorant.
Body Parts Affected: Circulation, lungs, nerves, spleen, liver and bowels.

Functions and Health Benefits:

The Chinese have used Blue Vervain for centuries for malaria, dysentery, and congestion. The Native Americans used Blue Vervain in treating nervous conditions as well as treating female problems. Dr. Shook recommended using it to treat all diseases of the spleen and liver. (30) It was used traditionally to restore circulation, menstrual problems, stomach problems, epilepsy, indigestion, dyspepsia, liver problems, and as a tonic for coughs due to colds.(31)

Modern research in Germany has found Blue Vervain to be beneficial for the nervous system, for pain relief, and as a tonic. It has also been found to help relieve pain and as an anti-inflammatory. (32)

Herbalists have recommended Blue Vervain for use as a natural tranquilizer and for all nervous conditions. It can help with fevers, upset stomach, colds, respiratory inflammation, mucus, and liver conditions. It is useful to use in liquid form for children to relieve colds, fevers, and other problems.

Vitamin and Mineral Content:

It contains moderate amounts of vitamins C and E, which are vital to a healthy immune system. Blue Vervain also contains calcium and manganese.

Ague	Headaches
ASTHMA	Hysteria
BLADDER	INDIGESTION
BOWELS	INSOMNIA
BRONCHITIS	Kidneys
Catarrh	Laxative
CIRCULATION	LIVER
COLDS	LUNG CONGESTION
COLON	Menstrual Problems
CONGESTION	Mucus
Constipation	NERVOUS CONDITIONS
CONVULSIONS	Pain
COUGHS	PNEUMONIA
Diarrhea	SEIZURES
Dysentery	Skin Diseases
Earaches	Sores
Epilepsy	SORE THROAT
Female Problems	Spleen
FEVERS	STOMACH
FLU	WORMS
Gallstones	

37

BONESET
(Eupatorium perfoliatum)

Part Used: The herb
Properties: Nervine, stimulant, antipyretic, and laxative.
Body Parts Affected: Stomach, liver, intestines, uterus, and circulation.

Functions and Health Benefits:

Boneset was listed in the *U.S. Pharmacopoeia* from 1820 through 1916 and in the *National Formulary* from 1926 through 1950. It has been used to restore strength in the stomach, spleen, and as a tonic for acute and chronic fevers. (33) Dr. Shook felt that Boneset was beneficial for every kind of fever man is subjected to. In addition, he felt that it had never failed in overcoming influenza. (34) Native Americans used this valuable herb for colds and flu. When taken cold, it acts as a tonic, and when taken warm, it has emetic diaphoretic properties. (35)

Research has shown that boneset contains antiseptic properties and promotes sweating to help in cases of colds and flu. It has also been shown to contain anti-viral properties and strengthens the immune system by enhancing the secretion of interferon. (36)

Traditionally, Boneset has been used for influenza, coughs and fevers. It has also been used to treat indigestion and pain.

Vitamin and Mineral Content:

Boneset contains moderate amounts of vitamin C, which strengthens the immune system and aids in healing. It also has calcium, which is calming to the nervous system and helps with healing. B-complex vitamins are in Boneset, which help build the blood and strengthen the nerves. Magnesium is also found which works with calcium to promote healthy nerves and strong bones. It contains potassium, which acts as an antiseptic, promotes healing, and helps heal lung disorders. It also helps regulate the acid and alkaline balance in the body.

Bronchitis	Mumps
Catarrh	PAIN
CHILLS	RHEUMATISM
COLDS	Rocky Mountain Spotted
COUGHS	Fever
FEVERS	Scarlet Fever
FLU	Sore Throat
Jaundice	Tonic
Liver Disorders	TYPHOID FEVER
MALARIA	Worms
Measles	YELLOW FEVER

BORAGE
(Borago officinalis)

Part Used: The leaves
Properties: Refrigerant, diaphoretic, febrifuge, aperient, and galactogogue.
Body Parts Affected: Lungs, heart, kidney, and bladder.

Functions and Health Benefits:

Ancient Celtic warriors often drank wine flavored with Borage before going to battle because of its reputation to encourage courage and strength. The Roman scholar Pliny thought this herb was useful for treating depression and lifting the spirits. John Gerard, the sixteenth-century herbalist, regarded Borage as an herb to comfort the heart and increase joy.

Borage is used to help clean toxins from the body and clear up inflammations. (37) Virgin Borage oil contains essential fatty acids especially a concentration of gamma linolenic acid (GLA). This fatty acid can account for as much as 26% of the oil's content, and it is the best known source of concentrated GLA. This plant is known to stimulate the adrenal glands to help the body during stressful times. (38) It promotes the activity of the kidneys to rid the body of catarrh. (39) It is also used to help restore vitality during the recovery of an illness.

Borage is often used to treat bronchitis because of its soothing effect and its ability to reduce inflammation. It is also known to help heal the mucous membranes of the mouth and throat. It helps stimulate the activity of the kidneys and adrenal glands.

Vitamin and Mineral Content:

Borage contains potassium, which is necessary for a strong heart. The potassium also helps prevent heart problems, acid stomach, calms the nerves, builds the blood, promotes wound healing, helps with iron utilization, and aids in insomnia.

Bladder	HEART
Blood Purifier	Insomnia
BRONCHITIS	Jaundice
CATARRH	LACTATION
Colds	Lungs
CONGESTION	Nerves
Digestion	Pleurisy
EYES (Inflammation)	RASHES
FEVERS	Ringworm

BURDOCK
(Arctium lappa)

Part Used: The root
Properties: Alterative, diaphoretic, diuretic, and demulcent.
Body Parts Affected: Blood, kidneys and liver.

Functions and Health Benefits:

Many Native America tribes used Burdock for skin ailments. The Chinese used it to lower blood sugar levels as well as to dispel wind and heat evils. Burdock was once widely used in cleansing remedies. It was a traditional blood purifier and used for indigestion.

Modern scientific research has uncovered diuretic properties and tumor inhibitors in Burdock in studies done on animals. (40) It has been found to contain antibiotic and anti-fungal properties. (41) It is beneficial for skin disorders, kidney problems, arthritis and gout. (42) Burdock Root has been used as a remedy for breast cancer, and ailments of the glands, intestines, knees, lips, liver, sinus, stomach, tongue and uterus in Chile, China, India, Canada, and Russia. (43)

Burdock is recommended for use during pregnancy and for female complaints because of its ability to aid in hormone balance and to prevent water retention. It is thought to be one of the best blood purifiers in the herbal kingdom. It is also used to promote kidney function. It contains high amounts of inulin, a form of starch, which is responsible for some of its healing properties and carbohydrate metabolism.

Vitamin and Mineral Content:

Burdock is rich in vitamin C and iron which help to purify the blood. It contains 12% protein needed for functions of the body. It contains 70% carbohydrate. It also has some vitamin A, P, B-complex, E, PABA and small amounts of sulphur, silicon, copper, iodine and zinc which are necessary for healthy blood.

ACNE	HEMORRHOIDS
ALLERGIES	HYPERGLYCEMIA
ARTHRITIS	HYPOGLYCEMIA
Asthma	Infection
Bladder Infections	Inflammation
BLOOD PURIFIER	KIDNEY PROBLEMS
Boils	LIVER PROBLEMS
Bronchitis	Lumbago
CANCER	LUNGS
Canker Sores	MEASLES
CATARRH	Nervousness
CHICKEN POX	Pneumonia
COLDS	POISON IVY/OAK
CONSTIPATION	PSORIASIS
Coughs	RHEUMATISM
Dandruff	SKIN DISORDERS
ECZEMA	TONSILLITIS
EDEMA	TUMORS
FEVERS	Ulcers
Gall Bladder	Wounds
Hay Fever	

BUTCHER'S BROOM ——
(Ruscus aculeatus)

Part Used: Rhizome
Properties: Aperient, deobstruant, diaphoretic, diuretic, and vasoconstriction.
Body Parts Affected: Circulation, veins, liver and kidneys.

Functions and Health Benefits:

Butcher's Broom was used in Europe and Greece over two thousand years ago for hemorrhoids, varicose veins, phlebitis, and thrombosis.

Recent studies have verified that this herb contains vasoconstrictive and anti-inflammatory properties. (44) Butcher's Broom is often used to treat varicose veins and hemorrhoids. (45) It is a useful preventative herb for circulatory problems and it increases circulation to the brain, arms and legs.

Butcher's Broom is useful for circulation problems. It has been used to treat thrombosis, arterioslcerosis, hemorrhoids, peripheral circulation problems, as a diuretic, and to lower cholesterol.

Vitamin and Mineral Content:

Butcher's Broom is high in iron which helps with the blood and veins, niacin which works to help the nervous system, and vitamin B1, which is essential to the nervous system and blood. It has zinc, which assists healing in the body and in the absorption of B-complex vitamins. It contains moderate amounts of calcium, potassium, manganese, selenium, and vitamin C. Small amounts of sodium, vitamin A and B2 are also found.

ARTERIOSCLEROSIS	INFLAMMATION
BLOOD CLOTS	Jaundice
Brain circulation	Leg Cramps
Dropsy	Menstrual Problems
Edema	Phlebitis
Headaches	STROKE (Prevention)
HEMORRHOIDS	THROMBOSIS
Jaundice	VARICOSE VEINS

CAPSICUM
(Capsicum frutescens)

Part Used: The fruit
Properties: Stimulant, astringent, carminative, antispasmodic, rubefacient, diaphoretic and tonic.
Body Parts Affected: Circulation, heart, intestines, spleen and lungs.

Functions and Health Benefits:

Capsicum was introduced as a natural, powerful stimulant by Dr. Samuel Thomson in the early 1800's. Subsequently, it was then introduced to England around 1840 by Dr. John Stevens. It was utilized as a chief ingredient in many of his formulas. It was used to sustain the natural heat of the system on which life depends. It was also valuable to prevent and rid the body of the effects of serious infectious disease.

Research has verified the benefits of this herb. It restores and stimulates the stomach and intestines. It also stimulates the heart and circulation. (46) Capsicum helps with cold hands and feet because of its effect of circulation. It is used to help clean and heal the stomach and digestive system. It is often found in combination with other herbs to improve their effectiveness and absorption. Capsicum is also thought to help lower serum cholesterol levels. (47) Studies indicate that capsicum has the ability to slow fat absorption in the small intestines and increase the metabolic rate and thermogenesis. It may promote the burning of fat in the body. (48) Capsicum has been used to control pain. (49)

Capsicum is often found in combination with other herbs to stimulate their action. It is considered to be a general stimulant. It helps to improve the function of the circulatory system and regulate the heart blood flow. It has also been used to help normalize blood pressure whether high or low.

Vitamin and Mineral Content:

Capsicum is rich in zinc, which is essential for hormonal glands, especially the prostate, mucous membranes, and healing broken bones. It is high in vitamins A, C, rutin, iron, calcium, and potassium. Vitamin A helps protect the tissues, improve resistance to diseases, including the eyes, respiratory and gastrointestinal tracts. Vitamin C and rutin strengthen the arteries, veins and capillaries. Capsicum also contains vitamin G, magnesium, phosphorus, sulphur, B-complex, sodium, and selenium.

Ague	Jaundice
Arteriosclerosis	KIDNEY PROBLEMS
ARTHRITIS	Lock Jaw
Asthma	LUNGS
BLEEDING	Mucus
Blood Purifier	Pain
BLOOD PRESSURE (high or low)	Pancreas
	PHLEBITIS
BRONCHITIS	Pyorrhea
Bruises	RHEUMATISM
Burns	SHOCK
CIRCULATION	Sinus Problems
COLDS	Skin Disorders
CONGESTION	SORE THROAT
DIABETES	Spasms
Digestive Problems	STOMACH
Eyes	STROKE
FATIGUE	Sunburn
Fevers	TUMORS
Gas	ULCERS
HEART	VARICOSE VEINS
Infection	Wounds

CASCARA SAGRADA ___
(Rhamnus purshiana)

Part Used: The bark
Properties: Laxative, hepatic, tonic and antispasmodic.
Body Parts Affected: Colon, stomach, liver, gallbladder, and pancreas.

Functions and Health Benefits:

Native Americans called Cascara Sagrada "sacred bark" and used it as a natural laxative. It was admitted to the *U.S. Pharmacopoeia* in 1877 and is still included as an official medicine.

Researchers have investigated the benefits of Cascara Sagrada. An element in the herb known as quinone emodin is being studied as it may be useful in treating lymphocytic leukemia and Walker carcinosarcoma tumor system. (50) It is used as a laxative and acts on the large intestine to increase the muscular activity in the colon. (51) It is used to replenish natural bowel movement without griping and to restore tone to the bowel. It can be used often and is not considered addictive.

Cascara Sagrada is thought to be one of the best herbs for chronic constipation. It enhances the peristaltic action in the intestines and increases secretions of the stomach, liver, and pancreas. It is also helpful in relieving hemorrhoids because of its non-irritating nature and softening action of stools.

Vitamin and Mineral Content:

Cascara Sagrada contains calcium, which calms the nerves and promotes growth. B-complex vitamins found in this herb help improve the tone of the intestinal tract and act as a nutritional stimulant. The potassium content helps the intestines and nerves function properly. Cascara Sagrada contains phosphorus, selenium, vitamin A, sodium, chlorine, magnesium, iron, niacin, and trace amounts of manganese, silicon and vitamin C.

BOWELS	Gout
Catarrh	HEMORRHOIDS
CONSTIPATION	Indigestion
Colitis	Insomnia
COLON	INTESTINES
Coughs	Jaundice
Croup	LIVER DISORDERS
Digestion	Nerves
Dyspepsia	Pituitary Gland
GALLBLADDER	Spleen
Gallstones	Stomach Problems
GAS	WORMS

CATNIP
(Nepeta cataria)

Part Used: The herb
Properties: Antispasmodic, diaphoretic, carminative, sedative and nervine.
Body Parts Affected: Lungs, liver, nerves and intestines.

Functions and Health Benefits:

Catnip tea has been used in Europe for centuries. Catnip was used by Native Americans for soothing colic in infants. It was used to induce sweating, cure colds and as a sedative. It was official in the *U.S. Pharmacopoeia* from 1842 to 1882 and in the *National Formulary* from 1916 to 1950.

Studies have proven the effectiveness of Catnip. It is valuable in calming the nerves, treating anemia, menstrual problems, and indigestion. (52) It also contains some antibiotic properties. (53) It acts as a mild tonic for colds, flu and fevers. It also helps stimulate the appetite.

Catnip has been used for many ailments including colic in infants, as a sedative, to treat fevers, insomnia, pain, convulsions, and restlessness. It is also used to improve circulation in the body and may also help regulate blood pressure.

Vitamin and Mineral Content:

It is rich in organic iron, which helps build the blood and nourishes glands and tissue. It is rich in selenium and vitamin E, which are antioxidants and help prevent tissue damage which may lead to serious diseases. It is high in vitamins A and C, which help protect and enhance the immune system. It is high in potassium and manganese and contains some magnesium, phosphorus, calcium, sodium, silicon and B-complex vitamins.

Anemia	Insanity
BRONCHITIS	INSOMNIA
CHICKEN POX	Kidneys
CIRCULATION	Liver
COLDS	Lung Congestion
COLIC	Menstruation
CONVULSIONS	Miscarriage (preventive)
Coughs	Morning Sickness
Cramps (menstrual)	Nerves
Cramps (muscular)	Nicotine Withdrawal
CROUP	Pain
DIARRHEA	Restlessness
DIGESTION	Shock
Fatigue	Skin Problems
FEVERS	Sores (external)
FLU	Spasms
GAS	Stomach (upset)
Headaches	Stress
Hemorrhoids	Vomiting
Hiccups	Worms
Infertility	

CHAMOMILE
(Anthemis nobilis)

Part Used: The flower
Properties: Nervine, antispasmodic, anodyne, carminative, diaphoretic, and tonic.
Body Parts Affected: Nerves, stomach, kidneys, liver, uterus and circulation.

Functions and Health Benefits:

The early Egyptians used Chamomile for its healing properties for ailments such as ague, and malarial chills. In the well known story of Peter Rabbit, his mother gives him Chamomile tea to calm his nerves. The European countries have used Chamomile for centuries. It is used for colic in infants and for vomiting.

Recent research has found Chamomile to contain properties which aid digestion and relieve indigestion. (54) It is also known to be a safe and mild sedative to induce sleep. (55) On animal studies, it was shown to have antihistiminic effects. (56) It has anti-ulcer and antibacterial properties. It can help cleanse the liver, promote natural hormones, increase mental alertness, and rejuvenate the texture of hair and skin.

Chamomile is one of the best known herbs around and can be useful to have on hand for emergencies. It is often used for colic, nervous conditions, menstrual cramps, as a sedative, for colitis, stomach troubles, and inflammation. Chamomile contains a natural hormone similar to thyroxine, which helps strengthen the hair and skin.

Vitamin and Mineral Content:

Chamomile is high in calcium and magnesium, which strengthen the nervous system and promote restful sleep. It also contains vitamins A, C and F, which strengthen the immune system. B-complex vitamins are also found, and they help the nervous system. Iron content in Chamomile is high and helps the blood. It contains silicon for strong bones and teeth, and selenium and zinc for the immune system. It also contains tryptophan, which works as a sedative to promote sleep.

ABSCESSES	FEVERS
Air Pollution	FLU
ALCOHOLISM	Gallstones
Anxiety	Gas
APPETITE STIMULANT	Headaches
Asthma	HYSTERIA
Bladder Problems	Indigestion
BRONCHITIS	INSOMNIA
Catarrh	Jaundice
Childhood Diseases	Kidneys
CIRCULATION	Measles
Colds	MENSTRUATION
COLIC	MUSCLE PAIN
Colitis	NERVOUSNESS
Constipation	Pain
Coughs	Spasms
CRAMPS (menstrual)	Stomach (upset)
Cramps (stomach)	Teething
Diarrhea	Throat
Dropsy	Tumors
Drug (withdrawal)	Typhoid
Eye (sore)	Ulcers (peptic)

DAMIANA
(Turnera aphrodisiaca)

Part Used: The leaves
Properties: Tonic, stimulant, aphrodisiac, diuretic, nervine, and aperient.
Body Parts Affected: Reproductive organs, nerves, and kidneys.

Functions and Health Benefits:

Indians of Northern Mexico used Damiana for nervous and muscular weaknesses. The ancient Mayans used this herb as an aphrodisiac. It has been used as a tonic for the nervous system and for sexual dysfunction.

Studies have concluded that Damiana has a beneficial affect on sexual debility and nervous tension. (57) It strengthens the nerves and brain. (58) It is also used for chronic fatigue and exhaustion, both mental and physical. (59) It is excellent when used in formulas with herbs such as ginseng, suma, sarsaparilla, and saw palmetto.

Traditional uses of Damiana include: nervousness, fatigue, hormone balance, female disorders, and for increasing sexual function. It is used most often for treating female disorders such as problems with menopause and for strengthening the reproductive organs. It has been found to help with infertility in both males and females by strengthening the egg in the female and increasing the sperm count in the male.

Vitamin and Mineral Content:

Damiana is high in calcium, which nourishes the nerves and silicon, which helps with calcium assimilation. It also is high in vitamin A and C, which are essential for healthy organs and the immune system. It is high in B-complex vitamins, which help build the blood, protect the nerves, tone muscles, and decrease cholesterol. It also contains potassium, protein, selenium, sodium, and zinc.

Asthma	FRIGIDITY
APHRODISIAC	Headaches
Brain (tonic)	HORMONE BALANCE
BRONCHITIS	HOT FLASHES
Constipation	MENOPAUSE
Cough	Nervousness
Depression	PARKINSON'S DISEASE
Energy	PMS
EMPHYSEMA	Prostate
Exhaustion	SEXUAL STIMULANT
FEMALE PROBLEMS	

DANDELION _____
(Taraxacum officinale)

Parts Used: The leaves and roots
Properties: Hepatic tonic, diuretic, stomachic, aperient, deobstruent, cholagogue, and depurative.
Body Parts Affected: Liver, kidneys, gallbladder, pancreas and blood.

Functions and Health Benefits:

This herb has a long history of use. The Chinese began mentioning Dandelion around the 7th century. Arabian physicians described it under the name of Tarakhshagun around the 10th century. Europeans have used Dandelion for at least 500 years.

Modern research has proven the validity of Dandelion. Studies in humans and laboratory animals have shown that its rhizomes and roots increases the flow of bile, which is beneficial for liver disorders, gallstones, jaundice, and the bile duct. (60) (61) It can help with arthritis as it stimulates the uric acid elimination from the body. It helps nourish and cleanse the blood, liver and spleen. It is also useful for treating anemia because it contains many nutrients. (62) Dandelion is also used to heal connective tissue and stop degeneration. (63) It is thought to have cancer and infection fighting potential. (64) Dandelion is considered a survival food because of its high protein, vitamin and mineral content.

Herbalists have long valued the curative powers of Dandelion. It is considered a great survival food. It promotes circulation, strengthens the arteries, restores gastric juices after severe vomiting, reduces cholesterol levels, and can help the liver. Dandelion is also used as a diuretic, for diabetes, and to purify the blood.

Vitamin and Mineral Content:

Dandelion has been found to contain all the nutritive salts which purify and balance the blood and destroy toxins in the blood. It is high in iron, which nourishes and strengthens the blood. It also contains high amounts of vitamins A and C, which strengthen the immune system and mucous membranes. It also contains magnesium, manganese, phosphorus, potassium, selenium, zinc, and B-complex vitamins. The roots contain inulin, which yields sub-variants of fructose and glucose.

ACNE	GALLBLADDER
Age Spots	Gas
ANEMIA	Gout
ARTHRITIS	Hemorrhage
ASTHMA	HEPATITIS
BLISTERS (external)	Indigestion
BLOOD CLEANSER	Infections
BLOOD PRESSURE	JAUNDICE
BLOOD PURIFIER	KIDNEYS
Bronchitis	LIVER
CHOLESTEROL	Metabolism
Constipation	Pancreas
Corns	PMS
Cramps	Psoriasis
Dermatitis	Rheumatism
Diabetes	Skin Problems
Eczema	Spleen
ENDURANCE	Stomach
FATIGUE	Ulcers
Female Organs	Warts
Fever	WEIGHT LOSS

DEVIL'S CLAW

(Harpagophytum procumbens)

Parts Used: The leaves and roots
Properties: Alterative, diuretic, discutient, lithotriptic, and stimulant.
Body Part Affected: Liver, stomach, kidneys, and joints.

Functions and Health Benefits:

Devil's Claw has been used in Africa for centuries without any harmful side effects. It has been used to help with joint pain, liver ailments, kidney disorders, arthritis, rheumatism, hardening of the arteries and stomach problems.

Research has indicated that Devil's Claw may help with gout and to relieve joint pain.(65) A German study found that the plant has anti-inflammatory properties comparable to anti arthritic phenylbutazine. (66) Another study showed that Devil's Claw taken as a tea may be beneficial in lowering cholesterol and fat levels. (67)

Devil's Claw has traditionally been used for arthritis, rheumatism, diabetes, arteriosclerosis, liver disorders, kidney and bladder problems. It is considered to be a great cleanser to remove impurities from the system.

Vitamin and Mineral Content:

Devil's Claw is very high in iron, which nourishes the blood and liver. It contains calcium and magnesium that work together to build the blood, calm nerves, clean the cells, and improve muscle tone. It also contains silicon, vitamins A and C, manganese, phosphorus, potassium, protein, selenium, sodium, and zinc.

ARTERIOSCLEROSIS	HEADACHES
ARTHRITIS	INFLAMMATION
BLADDER	KIDNEYS
BLOOD PURIFIER	LIVER
CHOLESTEROL	Malaria
DIABETES	POLLUTION
Gallbladder	RHEUMATISM
Gall Stones	STOMACH PROBLEMS
Gout	

DONG QUAI ———————
(Angelica sinensis)

Part Used: The root
Properties: Uterine tonic, antispasmodic, alterative, hypotensive, and sedative.
Body Parts Affected: Uterus, blood, muscles and nerves.

Functions and Health Benefits:

Dong Quai has been used by the Chinese since the beginning of time and was recorded in the Herbal of ShenNung. It was used as a tonic for all female problems.

Modern scientific research has shown that this herb is able to stimulate as well as inhibit uterine muscles. (68) Dong Quai is attributed with being able to increase energy and strengthen the system, while creating a sense of well being. It is used for all female complaints including: PMS, menopausal symptoms, cramps, backaches due to menstrual cramps, and hot flashes. It has also been used to improve digestion and assimilation, strengthen the nervous system, for stroke recovery, as a blood purifier, to dissolve blood clots, to improve circulation, stimulate production of interferon, and boost the immune system. Clinical research has proven Dong Quai to exhibit anti-tumor, anti fungal, imuuno-stimulant, and antibacterial properties. (69) Dong Quai has been proven to contain oestrogenic activity, which is responsible for female characteristics. (70)

Dong Quai has been used extensively for its ability to help with female disorders. It is also used to help during pregnancy to nourish the fetus in the womb. It has a tranquilizing effect on the central nervous system and nourishes the blood and brain cells. It helps to dissolve blood clots and increases circulation.

Vitamin and Mineral Content:

Pharmacological analysis has found Dong Quai to contain vitamin B12, nicotinic acid and vitamin E. Vitamin E is essential for the glands, heart and veins. B12 is important for the nervous system. and nourishes the blood. It is high in iron, which aids the blood and is important during the menstrual cycle. It contains vitamin A and C, which help the immune system. It also contains magnesium, manganese, phosphorus, potassium, B-complex vitamins, silicon, sodium, zinc and all essential minerals.

Abdominal pain	Hypoglycemia
ANEMIA	Insomnia
Angina	Laxative
Arthritis (pain)	Lumbago
Arteriosclerosis	Lungs
BLEEDING (internal)	MENOPAUSE
BLOOD PURIFIER	MENSTRUAL DISORDERS
Brain Nourisher	Metabolism
Bruises	MUSCLE SPASMS
CHILDBIRTH	NERVOUSNESS
Chills	Pain (reliever)
CIRCULATION	Plague
Cramps (menstrual)	Skin problems
Diabetes	Stomach
FEMALE GLANDS	Tonic
Headaches	Tumors
HOT FLASHES	UTERUS
Hypertension	

ECHINACEA
(Echinacea purpurea)

Part Used: The root
Properties: Alterative, antibiotic, carminative, demulcent, stimulant, and vulnerary.
Body Parts Affected: Blood, kidneys, lymph glands, and stomach.

Functions and Health Benefits:

Echinacea was used by the Native Americans for toothaches, snake bites, insect stings, and infections. Some individual tribes used Echinacea for headaches, swollen glands, and stomach cramps. Dr. John King in his medical journal in 1887 mentioned its benefits as a blood purifier and alterative.

Modern research has found Echinacea to be an effective alterative and blood purifier. Extracts of Echinacea root have been found to contain interferon-like properties. (71) Interferon is produced naturally in the body to prevent viral infections. Research has also found Echinacea to be effective in fighting tumor and infectious disease. (72) It has been found to effectively prevent the spread of infection. (73) German research has shown Echinacea to be useful in treating numerous allergies. A Russian study has shown this herb to help stimulate healing and blood clotting. (74)

Echinacea is used for many different ailments. It is used as a blood purifier against strep and staph infections. It is known to fight chemical toxic poisoning in the body. It has been used as a treatment for candida yeast infections and also has the ability to kill fungus. It is beneficial for blood poisoning, ulcers, tuberculosis, pyorrhea, childhood diseases, spinal meningitis and gangrene.

Vitamin and Mineral Content:

Echinacea contains vitamin A, which helps prevent against toxins in the body and air pollution. It also helps build resistance to germs and viruses. It helps protect the respiratory and circulatory systems. It also contains vitamin C, which promotes healing and aids in fighting infections. Calcium is also found which strengthens the bones. The vitamin E in Echinacea improves circulation and strengthens the heart. It helps protect the lining of the lungs against pollution and smoking by neutralizing free radicals which damage the cells. It also helps stimulate the immune system response. The iron content helps with the transport of oxygen to the blood. It helps build resistance to disease and improves energy levels. Echinacea contains iodine, which helps the thyroid gland to regulate metabolism, energy production and mental development. It contains potassium for nerve function, muscular contraction and kidney function. Its sulphur content helps dissolve acids in the body and improve circulation.

ACNE	Gingivitis
ANTIBIOTIC	GLANDS
ANTISEPTIC	Hemorrhage
Bites	INFECTIONS
BLOOD BUILDER	IMMUNE SYSTEM
BLOOD CLEANSER	Laryngitis
BLOOD POISONING	LYMPH GLANDS
BLOOD PURIFIER	MOUTH SORES
BOILS	MUCUS
Bronchitis	PERITONITIS
Cancer	PROSTATE
Catarrh	Pyorrhea
Carbuncles	SKIN DISORDERS
Digestion	Sore Throat
Diphtheria	Strep Throat
EAR INFECTION	Syphilis
Eczema	Typhoid Fever
Fevers	Tonsillitis
Flu	WOUNDS
Gangrene	

ELDER FLOWER
(Sambucus nigra)

Part Used: The flower
Properties: Diaphoretic, alterative, anti-inflammatory, laxative, and stimulant.
Body Parts Affected: Lungs, liver, circulation, blood, bowel, and skin.

Functions and Health Benefits:

In the *Anatomy of the Elder*, written in 1644, the Elder Flower is listed as a valuable plant for 70 different classes of diseases including rheumatism. Native Americans used this herb as a drink for rheumatism, neuralgia, sciatica, and back pain. Dr. Edward Shook considered Elder Flower to be one of the greatest and most versatile herbs in the treatment of disease. Elder Flower was found in the *U.S. Pharmacopoeia* from 1831 to 1905.

Research has found the properties of Elder Flower to be useful for acute diseases. It has been found to aid in the treatment of colds, flu, tonsillitis, laryngitis, rheumatic fever, and hay fever. (75)

It can help reduce a fever by increasing blood circulation and promoting sweating. Elder Flower is used for detoxifying the body at the cellular level. It also contains constituents known to act as a sedative and relieve pain. This herb works as an expectorant to relieve mucus and to reduce inflammation. It is used in herbal formulas. When combined with golden seal and yarrow, it is known to speed healing. It is combined with mullein to help heal lung congestion and asthma. It is also used as an eyewash along with eyebright and goldenseal.

Vitamin and Mineral Content:

Elder Flower contains Vitamin A, which is known to heal the lungs and is beneficial for all acute diseases. It contains vitamin C and bioflavonoids which work together in protecting against germs and viruses.

ALLERGIES	Gas
ASTHMA	HAY FEVER
Brain Inflammation	Hemorrhoids
BRONCHITIS	Inflammation
Cancer	Joints (swollen)
COLDS	Nerves
Digestive Problems	PNEUMONIA
Ear Infections	SINUS CONGESTION
Eye Infections	Skin Diseases
FEVERS	Ulcers
Flu	Wounds

ELECAMPANE
(Inula helenium)

Part Used: The root
Properties: Diuretic, tonic, diaphoretic, expectorant, alterative, antiseptic, astringent, and stimulant.
Body Parts Affected: Lungs, stomach, liver, and spleen.

Functions and Health Benefits:

Hippocrates stated that this herb was a stimulant to the uterus, kidneys, stomach and brain. The dried root was official in the *U.S. Pharmacopoeia* and listed as being beneficial for the respiratory organs, skin disease, digestion and liver problems. Dr. Edward Shook suggested using Elecampane for lung diseases such as catarrhal infections, tuberculosis, coughs, asthma, and to dissolve phlegm. (76)

Scientific research has found in clinical experiments that the extract of Elecampane contains a powerful antiseptic and bactericide which is particularly effective against tuberculosis. (77) Dr. Shook's studies had the same results! It has also been proven to be effective in lung problems, digestion, and liver disorders. Jethro Kloss has found it to be useful for coughs, asthma, and bronchitis. (78) It seems to strengthen, cleanse and tone the mucous membranes of the lungs and stomach.

Traditionally, Elecampane has been used to treat chest congestion and bronchial coughs. It helps to expel mucus and control excessive coughing and chest congestion. It helps control inflammation in the respiratory tract and soothe the tissue. It also contains antiseptic and anti-bacterial properties. ELECAMPANE has also been used to treat intestinal worms, edema, digestive problems, skin problems, tooth decay, and gum disorders. It is often found in combination with other herbs.

Vitamin and Mineral Content:

Elecampane contains calcium, which helps promote healthy blood, calm nerves, and increases resistance to infection. It can help prevent tuberculosis and aids in mineral metabolism. Potassium is also found, which protects the heart along with magnesium, prevents foreign material from accumulating in the tissues, promotes healing and aids in the resistance to disease. Sodium found in Elecampane aids digestion, helps alleviate congestion, purify the blood, eliminate bronchial phlegm, and dissolves toxins in the body.

Appetite	Digestion
Assimilation	EMPHYSEMA
Asthma	Female Problems
Bladder (catarrh)	LUNGS
BRONCHITIS (chronic)	Menstrual Problems
Catarrh	Phlegm
Colic	Poison (counteracts)
Consumption	Stomach
CONVULSIONS	Tuberculosis
COUGHS	Urinary Tract
Cramps	Whooping Cough
Diarrhea	Worms

EPHEDRA
(Ephedra sinensis)

Part Used: The whole herb
Properties: Stimulant, diaphoretic, expectorant, and astringent.
Body Parts Affected: Adrenal glands, circulatory and respiratory systems.

Functions and Health Benefits:

The Chinese have used Ephedra, known as Ma-haung, for centuries in formulas used to treat acute diseases such as colds, flu, bronchitis and pneumonia. Native Americans used the milder American species for its healthful properties to treat various ailments.

Recent studies with humans and laboratory animals have shown ephedrine (a component of ephedra) to be beneficial in promoting weight loss. Although ephedrine has an appetite-suppressing effect, its main mechanism for promoting weight loss appears to be found in its ability to increase the metabolic rate of adipose tissue. Its weight reducing effects are greatest in those who have a low basal metabolic rate. (79) Ma-Huang (Ephedra) is used in China as an excellent energy booster to replace caffeine drinks. It is free of caffeine, non-addicting, and non-toxic. Ephedrine is found in many over-the-counter cold and allergy medications. Ephedra is often used as a bronchiodilating agent, which helps relieve congestion from cods, flu, bronchitis, and asthma. (80) It is an excellent treatment for chronic and acute asthma.

Ephedra contains some of the same properties as adrenaline. It stimulates the nervous system and acts directly on the muscle cells. It is considered a bronchial dilator and decongestant.

Vitamin and Mineral Content:

It is high in vitamin A, which helps prevent lung disease, builds the immune system, and protects the mucous membranes and the skin. It is high in vitamin C, which is essential for preventing disease, protecting the immune system, strengthening the eyes, healing infection, and promoting normal adrenal and glandular function. Ephedra contains the B-complex vitamins, which promote a feeling of well-being, aid the immune system, improve nerve and digestive disorders. Iron is also found, which helps nourish the blood. Potassium helps maintain weight control, strengthens the heart, improves an acid stomach, and regulates the bowels. The selenium content helps protect the immune system. Silicon found in Ephedra is known to tone the body, protect against auto-intoxication and prevent cancer. It also contains sodium, which is known to help eliminate lung congestion, aid digestion, protect the kidneys and dissolve toxins in the body.

Arthritis	HAY FEVER
ASTHMA	HEADACHES
Bleeding (internal)	KIDNEYS
BLOOD PURIFIER	Menstruation
BRONCHITIS	Muscle Problems
BURSITIS	Nosebleeds
COLDS	Pain
Depression	Pneumonia
Diphtheria	SINUS
Drug Overdose	Skin Disorders
Fever	VENEREAL DISEASE

53

FALSE UNICORN ————
(Chamailirum luteum)

Part Used: The root
Properties: Stimulating tonic, diuretic, vermifuge, uterine tonic and emetic (large doses).
Body Parts Affected: Uterus, intestines, and kidneys.

Functions and Health Benefits:

False Unicorn was widely used by Native Americans for all disorders. The women chewed the root of the plant to prevent miscarriage. The tea was used as a tonic and as an anthelmintic by some early physicians. It was used for infertility problems. Dr. John Christopher recommended False Unicorn for all female problems.

Scientific research has shown that the steroidal saponins have a normalizing effect on the ovaries. (81) It has been shown to have oestrogenic activity and helps with female complaints. (82)

It has been used for both male and female problems associated with infertility. Sterility may be a problem and is often caused by unhealthy membranes in the uterus. False Unicorn can help restore health and muscle tone to the uterus. It is used for menopausal problems because of its effect on the uterus, headaches, and depression. It is also recommended as an overall tonic. It seems to help strengthen the mucous membranes and stabilizes a sensitive stomach. It is also a storing antiseptic and useful for getting rid of intestinal worms and parasites.

Vitamin and Mineral Content:

False Unicorn contains vitamin C, which aids the body in utilizing iron, which promotes normal glandular function. It also helps with preventing viral and bacterial infections. It contains copper, which is essential to the body in using iron, vitamin C and minerals. It also has sulphur, which is needed to combat bacterial infection and maintain oxygen balance for proper brain function. False Unicorn has zinc, which assists the body in absorbing B-complex vitamins, influences the hormonal system and all glands, including the prostate.

Appetite	KIDNEYS
Bright's Disease	MENOPAUSE
COLIC	MISCARRIAGE (prevents)
COUGHS	Nausea
Depression	Parasites
Digestion	PROSTATE
Dropsy	Sterility
Edema Enuresis	UTERUS
Headaches	Worms

FENNEL
(Foeniculum valgare)

Part Used: The seeds
Properties: Antispasmodic, carminative, diuretic, expectorant, stimulant, anti-inflammatory, and anti-microbial.
Body Parts Affected: Stomach, nerves, intestines, and eyes.

Functions and Health Benefits:

Fennel was used in ancient Egypt to aid digestion and prevent flatulence. In Italy, it was used to bring surgical patients out of anesthesia The ancient Greeks used it for weight reduction. Culpepper also recommended Fennel for losing weight.

Research has found the seeds to have estrogenic effects of the genital organs of female and male rats. (83) It has been found to promote the production of milk in nursing mothers. It is good for digestion, colic and other stomach complaints. It contains essential oils similar in composition to catnip and peppermint. (84)

Fennel is also used to expel phlegm from the throat, eliminate toxins from the body, and purify the blood. It is known to fortify the immune system and to be good for the eyes. Fennel also aids digestion, improves night vision, relieves gas, expels worms, improves the quality of milk in nursing mothers, and cleans the bladder and liver.

Vitamin and Mineral Content:

Fennel is high in calcium, which helps the nervous system, promote sleep, strengthens teeth and bones, builds the blood, strengthens the heart, and protects the lungs. It also contains magnesium, which is known to help the nervous system and protect against infections. It is high in phosphorus, which provides nutrients to the brain and nerves, promotes hormone secretion, aids in maintaining acid/alkaline balance, and fortifies the muscles. It also has vitamin A, C, B1, B2, niacin, and potassium.

Appetite Suppressant	INDIGESTION
Asthma	INTESTINAL PROBLEMS
Bronchitis	Kidneys
COLIC	Lactation
Congestion	Liver
Constipation	Lungs
Convulsions	Nervous Disorders
Coughs	SEDATIVE (for children)
Cramps	Stomach
DIGESTION	Spasms
GAS	WEIGHT REDUCTION
Gout	

FENUGREEK

(Trigonella foenum-graecum)

Part Used: The seeds
Properties: Demulcent, emollient, expectorant, aphrodisiac, astringent, galactogogue, and tonic.
Body Parts Affected: Lungs, stomach, intestinal system, and reproductive system.

Functions and Health Benefits:

Fenugreek was originally native to southwestern Asia and used for inflamed bowels and stomach problems. The ancient Greeks used Fenugreek for respiratory problems. Fenugreek was used in both the east and west and was thought of as one of the most effective medicinal herbs.

Studies using diabetics have found that Fenugreek seeds help reduce urinary glucose levels. The active ingredient seems to be the defatted portion of the seed, which has the alkaloid trogonelline, nicotinic acid and coumarin. (85) It contains choline and liptropic, which aid in dissolving cholesterol and lowering cholesterol levels.(86) It helps reduce mucus in cases of asthma, sinus and bronchial congestion. (87)

Fenugreek has a reputation of being able to dissolve hardened masses of accumulated mucus in the body. It is able to help in ridding the lungs of mucus and phlegm in the bronchial tubes. It also helps to expel waste through the lymphatic system. Fenugreek is known to contain antiseptic properties that help to kill infections in the lungs.

Vitamin and Mineral Content:

Fenugreek contains vitamins A and D, which are similar in composition to cod liver oil. It is high in protein, especially lysine and tryptophan. Lysine helps prevent infection, regulates pineal and mammary glands and aids the gall bladder. It is rich in iron to help the blood system. It also contains calcium, magnesium, phosphorus, potassium, selenium, silicon, and vitamin C. It contains small amounts of sodium, zinc, manganese, niacin, choline, and B-complex vitamins.

Abscesses	Gallbladder
ALLERGIES	GAS
Anemia	Heartburn
Asthma	Inflammation
Blood Poisoning	Lactation
Boils	LUNG INFECTIONS
Body Odor	MUCUS (dissolves)
Bowel lubricant	Sinus
BRONCHIAL CATARRH	SORE THROAT
Bronchitis	STOMACH
Cancer	Ulcers
CHOLESTEROL (dissolves)	Uterus
Eyes	Water Retention
Fever	

GARLIC ─────────────────
(Allium sativum)

Part Used: The bulb
Properties: Alterative, antibiotic, antispasmodic, diaphoretic, expectorant, and stimulant.
Body Parts Affected: Respiratory, circulation, stomach, nerves and sinus.

Functions and Health Benefits:

Garlic is well known for its health benefits. It was used by the ancient Hebrews, Greeks, Romans, and Egyptians. While building pyramids, the Egyptians ate garlic to increase their strength and endurance. (88) Hippocrates suggested it for the treatment of uterine cancer. Native Americans used Garlic to fight abdominal cancer. The Europeans used garlic during the plague years to provide immunity.

Research has discovered even more benefits of Garlic. Louis Pasteur found that Garlic contains antibiotic properties. Albert Schweitzer used Garlic when in Africa for treating amebic dysentery and as an antiseptic in preventing infections. Garlic is now known to be effective in inhibiting bacterial growth.(89). Garlic has been found to be effective in inhibiting the growth of many different strains of Mycobacterium. (90) Studies by Dr. Eric Block have found that Garlic will lower cholesterol, prevent blood clotting, protect the liver from drugs and toxins, kill parasites and worms, and protect the cells from free-radical and radiation damage. (91) Garlic contains anti-tumor properties and studies have shown it has the ability to inhibit the growth of cancer-causing nitrosamine. (92) The Russians consider garlic to be a natural antibiotic and consume it regularly. Several recent studies link garlic to lower incidence of cardiovascular disease. It has been found to reduce cholesterol and triglyceride levels in the blood, lower blood pressure, increase immunity, and reduce the blood's clotting ability. (93)

Garlic is often used to prevent disease and heal the body. It has the ability to stimulate the lymphatic system to rid the body of waste. It is nourishing for the body especially the heart, circulation, stomach, spleen and lungs. It has been used to, stimulate circulation and boosts the immune system to function more effectively. It may help prevent some forms of cancer, heart disease, strokes, and viral infections.

Vitamin and Mineral Content:

Garlic is high in phosphorus, which is essential for functions of the brain and nervous system, promotes hormone secretion, protects the heart and cells, and aids in acid/alkaline balance in the blood. Potassium is also found which may help prevent heart attacks, hypoglycemic blackouts, protects from germs accumulating in the tissues, strengthens the spleen and liver against disorders, and aids an acid stomach. It is high in sulphur, which protects the cells from a build-up of toxins, dissolves acids in the body, and improves circulation. Selenium is found in Garlic which helps protect the immune system. It contains vitamins A and C which are necessary for many functions of the body. It also contains calcium, magnesium, sodium, iron, manganese, and B-complex vitamins.

Acne	GAS
Allergies	HEART DISEASE
Arthritis	HIGH BLOOD PRESSURE
ASTHMA	Hypoglycemia
BLOOD POISONING	INFECTIONS
BLOOD PRESSURE	INFECTIOUS DISEASE
BLOOD PURIFIER	Insomnia
BRONCHITIS	Kidneys
CANCER	LIVER
CANDIDA	LUNGS
Childhood Diseases	Memory
CIRCULATION	Mucus
COLDS	PARASITES
COLITIS	Pneumonia
COUGHS	PROSTATE GLAND
Diabetes	RESPIRATORY
Diarrhea	PROBLEMS
DIGESTION	Rheumatism
Dropsy	Sinus
EAR INFECTIONS	STAPH AND STREP
Emphysema	INFECTIONS
FEVER	Ulcers
FLU	Warts
FUNGUS	Worms
Gallbladder	YEAST INFECTIONS

GENTIAN
(Gentiana lutea)

Part Used: The root
Properties: Febrifuge, emmenagogue, tonic, stomachic, antispasmodic, antiseptic, and vermifuge.
Body Parts Affected: Stomach, liver, blood, spleen, and circulation.

Functions and Health Benefits:

In Ancient Rome, Gentian was used as a stomach tonic and to aid in digestion. Gentian was an official drug in the *United States Pharmacopoeia* from 1820 to 1955 and was used as a gastric stimulant. At one time, it was used and acclaimed by medical science as being very beneficial for mankind.

Modern research by German scientists confirm that it is useful as a digestive aid. (94) Herbal bitters, including Gentian, are recommended as a treatment for indigestion. The bitter taste receptors in the tongue are known to stimulate the digestive processes. (95)

It is used to reduce fevers by cooling the system. Gentian contains a bitter principle, amarogentin, which stimulates the glands including the adrenals and the thyroid. It helps in the production of bile, which can have a positive effect on the liver and gallbladder. Gentian is also used to clean the bowels, stimulate the pancreas, stimulate circulation, aid in the digestive process, and help with female problems. It is considered a great herb for strengthening the entire body system and as a tonic when combined with other herbs.

Vitamin and Mineral Content:

Gentian is high in iron, which is essential to healthy blood and to preventing anemia and fatigue. It contains B-complex vitamins, which aid the nervous system and help maintain an overall feeling of well-being. It is high in inositol, which may help prevent multiple sclerosis, cerebral palsy, diabetes, muscular dystrophy, nerve disorders, and mental retardation. The niacin content is essential for preventing nervous disorders. Gentian also contains vitamin F, manganese, silicon, sulphur, and zinc.

Amenorrhea	Gas
Anemia	Gout
APPETITE STIMULANT	Heartburn
Blood Purifier	HYSTERIA
CIRCULATION	JAUNDICE
Colds	LIVER DISORDERS
Constipation	Nausea
Cramps	Spleen
Diarrhea	Stomach
DIGESTION	Urinary Tract
Dysentery	Vaginal Infections
Female Problems	Worm
Fevers	Wounds

GINGER
(Zingiber officinale)

Part Used: The root
Properties: Stimulant, carminative, tonic, diaphoretic, and diuretic.
Body Parts Affected: Circulation, stomach, intestines, lungs, spleen, and liver.

Functions and Health Benefits:

Ginger has been used medicinally for thousands of years. It was first used in the tropical Asian climates. The Greek historian, Dioscorides, recommended Ginger to stimulate the production of digestive juices and to combat chills and colds. The Chinese have used this herb for many ailments including colds, nausea, and indigestion. It is the Spaniards that are credited with introducing Ginger to America during the 16th century. Ginger was listed in the *U.S. Pharmacopoeia* from 1820 to 1873.

Recent studies are convincing concerning the value of Ginger. Ginger contains terpenses, which are chemically similar to those found in camphor and turpentine. Researchers claim that there are two natural antibiotics found in Ginger. It has been found to inhibit the growth of bacteria. (96) It has the ability to relieve dizziness and motion sickness, may help in preventing heart attacks, and contains anti-inflammatory agents. (97) In one study, powdered ginger was found to be more effective in treating motion sickness than some common over-the-counter treatments without causing drowsiness. (98)

Ginger is thought to have blood thinning properties and the ability to lower blood cholesterol levels. It is a blood stimulant and cleansing herb. It is also used for respiratory problems such as colds, sore throats, bronchitis, congestion, headaches, and pain. Ginger is also known to help with nausea, kidney problems, heart problems, fever, vomiting, cramps, and in herbal combinations to aid in the effectiveness of other herbs.

Vitamin and Mineral Content:

Ginger is high in potassium, which is important for the heart, in fighting germs, and as an antiseptic. It contains manganese, which builds resistance to disease, protects the lining of the heart, blood vessels and urinary passages. Silicon is also found, which tones the entire system, and promotes healthy skin, hair, teeth and nails. It also helps assimilate calcium. It contains vitamins A, C, B-complex, magnesium, phosphorus, sodium, iron and zinc.

Bowels	HEART
BRONCHITIS	Hemorrhage
CHILDHOOD DISEASES	INDIGESTION
CIRCULATION	Kidneys
COLDS	Menstrual Cramps
COLIC	MORNING SICKNESS
COLITIS	MOTION SICKNESS
Colon	NAUSEA
Coughs	Paralysis
CRAMPS	Perspiration (increases)
DIARRHEA	Sinus
DIGESTION	SORE THROAT
DIZZINESS	STOMACH
FATIGUE	Tonic
FEVERS	Toothache
FLU	VOMITING
GAS	WHOOPING COUGH
HEADACHE	

GINKGO
(Ginkgo biloba)

Part Used: The leaves
Properties: Adaptogen, alterative, antioxidant, stimulant, tonic and antiseptic.
Body Parts Affected: Brain, circulation, and whole body.

Functions and Health Benefits:

Ginkgo has been used in China for at least 5,000 years. The Ginkgo biloba tree is one of the oldest known and is a very hardy species. Its medicinal properties continue to help many in Asia today. It was used for arterial circulation problems, asthma, constriction of the blood vessels in diabetics, gangrene, angina, intermittent claudication and Raynaud's disease (a constriction of blood vessels in the fingers, toes, and tip of the nose).

Considerable research has been done in Europe on Ginkgo. It has been found to aid in arterial blood flow, senility, vertigo, tinnitus, depression, memory, and intermittent claudication. It has been used to improve electrical transmission in nerves and in supplying more oxygen and nutrition to the brain cells. (99) Ginkgo's effect on the brain and circulatory disorders seems very promising. Research has shown Ginkgo to be useful in treating irregular heartbeats. (100)

Ginkgo is often used to increase the blood flow to the brain improving memory problems such as in Alzheimer's, to prevent strokes, and to increase blood circulation through vaso-dilation. Because of the improved circulation, it is thought to improve ear conditions, help blood flow to the retina, aid in preventing muscular degeneration, reduce frequency of asthma attacks, and in helping transplant recipients avoid rejection.

Vitamin and Mineral Content:

Ginkgo is rich in bioflavonoids, which help protect against free radical damage, aid in enzyme regulation, protect the blood vessels and capillaries against plaque build up on the inner walls, and protect the liver from toxic damage.

Allergies	LONGEVITY
Alertness	Lung Conditions
ALZHEIMER'S	MEMORY
Anxiety	Mental Clarity
Arthritis	Mood Swings
Asthma	MUSCULAR
ATTENTION SPAN	DEGENERATION
Cancer	RAYNAUD'S DISEASE
CIRCULATION	Senility
Coughs	STROKE
Depression	Tinnitus
DIZZINESS	Toxic Shock Syndrome
Equilibrium	Varicose Veins
Eye Problems	Vascular Problems
Hearing	Vertigo
HEART PROBLEMS	

GINSENG

Siberian (Eleutherococcus)
Korean (Panax schin-seng)
Wild American (Panax quinquefolium)

Part Used: The root
Properties: Tonic, alterative, stimulant, and stomachic.
Body Parts Affected: Circulation, heart, brain, eyes, lungs, and spleen.

Functions and Health Benefits:

Ginseng is one of the oldest and most beneficial herbs in the world. In *Shen-Nung's Pharmacopoeia* (A.D. 206-220), it is rated the highest and most potent of herbs. It was used to increase vitality, invigorate the system, restore health and increase longevity.

Research has shown that the roots are effective against bronchitis and heart disease. (101) Ginseng has been found to reduce blood cholesterol, build the immune system, improve brain function and memory, increase physical stamina, stimulate the function of the endocrine glands and strengthen disorders of the central nervous system. (102)

Ginseng is stimulating on the entire body and helps overcome stress, increase longevity, combat fatigue, weakness, mental fatigue, improve brain cell function, and benefit the heart and circulation. It is also used to normalize blood pressure, reduce cholesterol levels, and to prevent arteriosclerosis. It is used to help protect the body against radiation and as an antidote to drugs and toxic chemicals.

Vitamin and Mineral Content:

Ginseng contains vitamin A, which is necessary for a healthy immune system, essential for mucous membranes, healthy eyes and skin, and to prevent and heal colds, flu, and fevers. It contains vitamin E, which is essential for a healthy heart and circulatory system. B-complex vitamins, thiamin, riboflavin, B12, and niacin, are important for maintaining healthy nerves, skin, hair, eyes, liver and muscle tone in the gastrointestinal tract. Ginseng also has calcium, iron, phosphorus, sodium, silicon, potassium, manganese, magnesium, and sulphur.

AGE SPOTS	HEMORRHAGE
Aging	HORMONE BALANCE
Anemia	Inflammation
Antidote (for some drugs)	Impotence
APPETITE (stimulant)	Insomnia
ASTHMA	Liver Disorders
Bleeding	LONGEVITY
Blood Diseases	Lungs
BLOOD PRESSURE	Menopause
Bronchitis	Menstruation
Cancer	Nausea
Concentration	Nervousness
DEPRESSION	Radiation Protection
Digestion	SEXUAL STIMULANT
Dyspepsia	STRESS
ENDURANCE	Ulcers
FATIGUE	Vitality
FEVERS	WEAKNESS

GOLDEN SEAL _____

(Hydrastis canadensis)

Parts Used: The rhizome and root
Properties: Alterative, antibiotic, antiseptic, emmenagogue, stomachic, tonic, and laxative.
Body Parts Affected: Stomach, intestines, spleen, liver, mucous membranes and eyes.

Functions and Health Benefits:

Native Americans used Golden Seal for a tonic, sore throats, and eye infections, ulcers and even arrow wounds. It was used as an insect repellent and as a pesticide for crops. It was also boiled in water and used externally for skin conditions. The dried root was official in the *U.S. Pharmacopoeia* from 1831 to 1842 and was re-admitted in 1863 to 1936.

Recent studies have found Golden Seal to be beneficial against viruses and infections. It contains the alkaloids hydrastine and hydrastinine that have strong astringent and antiseptic effects on mucous membranes. (103). It has been found to kill toxic bacteria in the intestinal tract such as giardiasis, found in streams in North America. (104) The antibiotic properties of Goldenseal are due to its alkaloid content including berberine which has been found to be effective against organisms such as Staphylococcus spp., Streptococcus, sp., Chlamydia spp., Salmonella typhi, Diplococcus pneumonia and Candida albicans. (105) It is also thought to help strengthen the immune system. (106) In England, some herbalists consider Golden Seal to be the "wonder remedy" for digestive problems.

Golden Seal has been used traditionally for many different conditions such as boosting the glandular system, for hormone imbalance, congestion, inflammation, female problems, infection, bronchitis, menstrual problems, catarrh of the bladder, gastritis, ulcers, bowel stimulation, antiseptic, and as an immune system builder. It is not recommended for those with low blood sugar or pregnant women.

Vitamin and Mineral Content:

It contains vitamins A and C which help in healing colds, flu and all acute and chronic diseases. B-complex vitamins are also found, which are necessary for the nervous system. Vitamin C and B12 have been shown to inhibit the formation of cancer in laboratory mice. (107) Golden Seal also has vitamins E, F, calcium, copper, potassium, phosphorus, manganese, iron, sodium, and zinc.

Allergies	GUM DISEASES
Asthma	Hay Fever
ANTIBIOTIC	Heart Trouble
ANTISEPTIC	HEMORRHAGE
Bladder	HEMORRHOIDS
Bowels	Herpes
Bright's Disease	INFECTIONS
BRONCHITIS	INFLAMMATION
Burns	INSULIN
Chicken Pox	INTESTINES
CIRCULATION	KIDNEYS
COLDS	LIVER DISORDERS
COLITIS	MENSTRUATION
COLON	MOUTH SORES
Constipation	MUCOUS MEMBRANES
COUGHS	Nausea
DIARRHEA	Nervous Disorders
Earaches	NOSEBLEEDS
Eczema	Ringworm
EYE INFECTIONS	Rhinitis
Fever	Skin Disorders
Flu	SORE THROAT
Gallbladder	Spleen
Gastritis	Stomach Problems
Glands	Tonsillitis
GONORRHEA	

GOTU KOLA ———————

(Hydrocotyle asiatica)

Part Used: The whole herb
Properties: Nervine, tonic, alterative, antispasmodic, and diuretic.
Body Parts Affected: Brain, nerves, circulation, heart, liver and kidneys.

Functions and Health Benefits:

Gotu Kola has been used in India and the islands of the Indian Ocean for centuries. It was used to treat leprosy, calm the nerves, increase mental and physical power, to stimulate and rejuvenate the brain, to prevent nervous disorders, mental fatigue and senility.

Studies have shown that the ingredient, asiaticoside, accelerates the healing of wounds. It is considered a blood cleanser and is also effective for diseases of the lungs as well as leprosy. (108) It stimulates the capillaries and helps to improve brain function, varicose veins, and hypertension.

Herbalists recommend Gotu Kola for rejuvenating the nervous system. It is used to improve circulation and enhance brain function. It is sometimes referred to as food for the brain because of its ability to energize brain function, treat mental problems, and increase memory function. It is thought to increase both physical and mental power. It is also useful because of its mild sedative effect, for balancing the hormones, to purify the blood, for strengthening the heart, to combat fatigue, and to normalize blood pressure.

Vitamin and Mineral Content:

Gotu Kola is rich in magnesium in an easily assimilated form. Experiments on children with magnesium deficiency are often found to have mental difficulties. It contains vitamins A, C and K, which protect the lungs from disease and protect the immune system against diseases such as cancer. Vitamin K is necessary for blood clotting and is helpful in healing colitis and celiac disease. It contains calcium, sodium, zinc, manganese, silicon, vitamins B1, B2, and niacin.

AGING	Menopause
ARTERIOSCLEROSIS	MENTAL PROBLEMS
Blood Purifier	NERVOUSNESS
BLOOD PRESSURE	Pituitary Gland
CIRCULATION	Psoriasis
Depression	Rheumatism
Dysentery	Schizophrenia
FATIGUE	Scrofula
Fevers	SENILITY
Headaches	Thyroid
HEART	TONIC
HYPOGLYCEMIA	Tonsillitis
Insomnia	Toxins
LEPROSY	Varicose Veins
Liver	Vitality
Longevity	Wounds
MEMORY	

GYMNEMA

(Gymnema sylvestre)

Parts Used: The leaves and roots.
Properties: Anti-periodic, stomachic, and diuretic.
Body Parts Affected: Pancreas, liver and blood.

Functions and Health Benefits:

Gymnema has been used in India for hundreds of years. It has been used in treating diabetics by Ayurvedic physicians. Gymnema sylvestre is known as gurmar, a Hindu name meaning "sugar destroyer."

Modern scientific research has confirmed that the active ingredient, gymnemic acid, blocks the taste of sugar as well as blocking sugar's absorption by the body. (109) It is also thought that Gymnema suppresses the taste of saccharin and cyclamate, two common artificial sweeteners. A study published in 1986, suggests that the extract of Gymnema can significantly increase liver and pancreatic function. (110) This is promising for diabetes, obesity, hypoglycemia, allergies, anemia and osteoporosis.

Gymnema is used to block the passages from which sugar is normally absorbed so the calories are not absorbed and blood sugar levels are not so drastically affected. It is thought to block the body's desire for sweets.

Allergies
Anemia
Cholesterol
DIABETES
Digestion
Hyperactivity
HYPOGLYCEMIA
Obesity
Weight Control

HAWTHORN BERRIES

(Crataegus oxycantha)

Parts Used: The berries and flowers
Properties: Cardiac tonic, antispasmodic, astringent, diuretic, and sedative.
Body Parts Affected: Heart, circulation, nerves and kidneys.

Functions and Health Benefits:

Hawthorn was used by the ancient Greeks for heart disease. It is thought that the crown of thorns placed on the head of Christ was made from the Hawthorn tree. Native Americans found it useful for rheumatism and heart problems.

Studies indicate the extract dilates blood vessels resulting in reduced peripheral resistance. It may also have a further cardioprotective effect that becomes pronounced after prolonged use. (111) Some experiments have determined that Hawthorn dilates the blood vessels, lowers blood pressure, and strengthens the heart. (112) Hawthorn is known as a tonic for heart problems. Hawthorn has been found useful in reducing blood pressure, lowering serum cholesterol levels, and preventing cholesterol deposits. (113)

It can feed and strengthen the heart and arteries. Hawthorn is used as a cardiac tonic and is thought to aid and improve conditions such as arteriosclerosis, angina, heart murmurs, heart valve defects, and cardiac weakness. It is also recommended for circulation, fatigue, cholesterol, insomnia, and high blood pressure. It is also an excellent food supplement for stressful situations.

Vitamin and Mineral Content:

Hawthorn is a nutritional herbal supplement. It is high in carotene (Vitamin A), which is helpful for the immune and nervous systems. It contains high amounts of vitamin C and bioflavonoids, which strengthen and feed the arteries. It contains B-complex vitamins, choline and inositol.

ANGINA	HEART WEAKNESS
ARRHYTHMIA	HIGH BLOOD PRESSURE
ARTERIOSCLEROSIS	Hypertension
Arthritis	HYPOGLYCEMIA
Blood Clots	Insomnia
BLOOD PRESSURE	Liver
Dropsy	LOW BLOOD PRESSURE
Edema	Rheumatism
HEART CONDITIONS	Sleeplessness
HEART PALPITATIONS	Stress
HEART VALVE	

HOPS
(Humulus lupulus)

Part Used: The flower
Properties: Nervine, sedative, stomachic, anodyne, antibiotic, carminative, cholagogue, and tonic.
Body Parts Affected: Nerves, stomach, blood, liver and gall bladder.

Functions and Health Benefits:

Culpepper suggested using Hops to open obstructions of the liver and spleen, cleanse the blood, loosen the belly, cleanse the veins from gravel and promote urine. The Romans used Hops as a food. Gerarde, a famous herbalist, recommended using the buds in salads. Native American tribes found Hops to be of value. The Mohicans used it as a sedative and for toothaches. The Menominee tribe used Hops as a cure-all. The lupulin found in Hops is described as a sedative and hypnotic drug and was recognized in the *U.S. Pharmacopoeia* from 1831 to 1916.

Studies indicate Hops as having sedative properties. It is known to be fast acting, soothing and calming on the nervous system. (114) Hops is one of the nervine herbs and aids in promoting sleep. (115)

Hops is best known for its sedative action and as one of the best nervine herbs. This herb is also thought to contain appetizer stimulant and tonic properties. It acts as a stimulant to the glands and muscles of the stomach in calming the hyper-excitability of the gastric nerves. It is also used for its antibiotic properties, which are beneficial for sore throats, bronchitis, infections, high fevers, delirium, toothaches, earaches, and pain.

Vitamin and Mineral Content:

It is very high in B-complex vitamins known for their calming effect on the nervous system. They also promote energy and aid in problems of depression, anxiety, nervousness, and memory. Hops is rich in potassium, which is necessary for nerve transmission, contraction of the muscles, and hormone secretion. Low levels of potassium have been found in people with high blood pressure. Hops also contains magnesium, zinc, copper, iodine, manganese, iron, sodium, and fluoride.

Alcoholism	Jaundice
Anxiety	Kidney Stones
APPETITE STIMULANT	Liver
Blood Cleanser	NERVOUSNESS
BRONCHITIS	Neuralgia
Coughs	PAIN
Cramps	Restlessness
DELIRIUM	Rheumatism
DIGESTION	SEXUAL DESIRE
Dizziness	(excessive)
Earaches	Skin Disorders
Female Problems	Sleeplessness
Fevers	Toothache
Gas	Ulcers
HEADACHES	Venereal Disease
HYPERACTIVITY	Water Retention
Hysteria	Whooping Cough
Indigestion	Worms
INSOMNIA	

HORSETAIL

(Equisetum arvense)

Part Used: The herb
Properties: Astringent, diuretic, lithotriptic, nutrient tonic, emmenagogue, galactogogue, and vulnerary.
Body Parts Affected: Bones, flesh, cartilage, digestion, kidneys, blood, heart and lungs.

Functions and Health Benefits:

The Native Americans used Horsetail, also known as Shavegrass, as a diuretic for kidney problems, cancer, and dropsy and to increase blood circulation. The Hopi tribe in New Mexico mixed Horsetail with corn meal as a mush and put it in their bread.

Recent studies in Europe have found silica, which is in Horsetail, to be essential for healing bones and keeping the arteries clean. They found that fractured or broken bones do not heal as well when high amounts of calcium are present and little or no silica. The silica in Horsetail seems to facilitate the use of calcium. Horsetail is known to have antibiotic properties and contributes to the overall healing process. (116) Horsetail is also thought to help with bleeding, urinary and prostate disorders, bed-wetting, skin problems, and lung disease. (117)

Horsetail is useful for urinary tract disorders, infections, to decrease bleeding, and for rheumatic conditions. It is also thought to strengthen the hair and nails, dissolve tumors, glandular disorders, and to aid in circulation.

Vitamin and Mineral Content:

Horsetail contains flavonoids essential for strengthening the capillaries and healing. The silicon content is high, which is an important component because of its ability to strengthen the bones, skin and cartilage. It also has cleansing properties and is beneficial for healthy blood cells and circulation. Vitamin E is also found which aids the arteries and heart. Horsetail contains pantothenic acid, PABA, manganese, sodium, iron and iodine.

ARTHRITIS	KIDNEY STONES
BLADDER PROBLEMS	Liver
CIRCULATION	Mucous Membranes
DIABETES	NAILS
Dropsy	NERVOUSNESS
Eyes	Neuralgia
Fingernails	OSTEOPOROSIS
Gas	Palsy
GLANDULAR DISORDERS	PARASITES
Gout	RHEUMATISM
HAIR	Skin Disorders
Heart	Tumors
Hemorrhage	Water Retention
Incontinence	Worms

HO-SHOU-WU
(Polygonum multiflorum)

Part Used: The root
Properties: Tonic, stimulant, diuretic, and vasodilator.
Body Parts Affected: Kidneys, liver, stomach, heart, and reproductive organs.

Functions and Health Benefits:

Ho-Shou-Wu is an herb valued and used by the Chinese for centuries. It is used to promote longevity for liver and spleen disorders, and to strengthen the heart. It is an herb to benefit the whole body.

Recent scientific research has found that Ho-Shou-Wu has properties to aid in lowering cholesterol, reducing inflammation, strengthening the heart, and has anti-viral activities. (118) It is considered an anti-toxic and nerve calming herb. (119)

It is also thought to be a tonic for the endocrine glands and will help improve health, stamina and resistance to disease. Ho-Shou-Wu is thought to be a cardio-vascular strengthener, and a tonic for the endocrine glands, liver and kidneys. It is used to help with premature graying of hair, backaches, pain of knee joints, neurasthenia, and bruises.

Vitamin and Mineral Content:

Ho-Shou-Wu is rich in selenium, which is useful in increasing the health of the immune system. It has magnesium, potassium, zinc and vitamin A, which are all important for a healthy body and mind. It also contains calcium, phosphorus, iron, manganese, B-complex vitamins, vitamin C, silicon and sodium.

Aging	Gout
Anemia	Hair (premature graying)
Arteriosclerosis	Heart Problems
Arthritis	Hypoglycemia
Backache	IMPOTENCY
Blood	INFERTILITY
Bones	Inflammation
Bruises	Knees
Cancer	Liver
Circulation	Menstrual Problems
Colds	MUSCLES
Constipation	NERVES
Diabetes	Spleen
Diarrhea	Tumors
Dizziness	Vertigo
FERTILITY	

HYDRANGEA
(Hydrangea arborescens)

Parts Used: The leaves and root
Properties: Cathartic, diuretic, tonic, nephritic, and antilithic.
Body Parts Affected: Kidneys, bladder, stomach, and colon.

Functions and Health Benefits:

The Native American tribe, the Cherokees, as well as the early American settlers used a decoction of Hydrangea with great success for calculous diseases. Dr. Edward E. Shook considered this herb very remarkable and thought that its curative powers were better than any other herb. He considered it a powerful solvent of stone and calculous deposits in the renal organs. It contains alkaloids that act like cortisone and has similar cleansing powers to that of chaparral.

Herbalists have found this herb to be gentle and effective as a remedy. It cleans toxins from the body by cleansing the kidneys. It can help stop infection and dissolve hard deposits in the veins and urinary organs. It contains alkaloids that act similar to cortisone without the side effects. It is thought to help with rheumatic conditions, to act as a diuretic, to help with bedwetting, and to treat lymphatic conditions.

Vitamin and Mineral Content:

It is high in calcium, which is essential for healthy arteries, urinary tract, and in preventing colon cancer. It contains potassium, which aids calcium in protecting the arteries. Potassium found in Hydrangea is also useful in protecting the kidneys against damage resulting from high blood pressure. It has organic sodium, which keeps calcium in the blood, helps prevent arthritis, thickening of the blood, hardening of the arteries, and excess mucus. Sulphur is also found, which works with the B-complex vitamins and is essential for protein absorption, eliminating acidosis and in protecting the heart muscles.

Arteriosclerosis	GOUT
ARTHRITIS	Inflammation
Backache	Kidney Problems
BLADDER INFECTIONS	KIDNEY STONES
BLADDER STONES	Pain
Calcium Deposits	Paralysis
Dropsy	RHEUMATISM
GALLSTONES	URINARY PROBLEMS
GONORRHEA	

HYSSOP
(Hyssopus officinalis)

Part Used: The whole herb
Properties: Expectorant, diaphoretic, stimulant, pectoral, and carminative.
Body Parts Affected: Lungs, stomach, circulation, bladder and colon.

Functions and Health Benefits:

In ancient Babylon, Hyssop tea was used to reduce fever sore throats, colds, lung infections and for eye infections. Hippocrates recommended Hyssop for pleurisy.

Hyssop is used most often for lung disorders such as bronchitis, chest congestion, hay fever, tuberculosis and asthma. It helps relax and expel phlegm from the lungs and relieve coughing. It helps promote sweating to expel toxins from the skin. It is a member of the mint family and is thought to aid in digestion and help relieve gas. (120) Hyssop has a history of use as a body purifier. It strengthens the immune system and works as a blood pressure regulator.

Asthma	Jaundice
Blood Pressure	Kidney Problems
Bronchitis	Lice (external)
Bruises	Liver Problems
CATARRH	LUNG AILMENTS
CONGESTION	Mucus
COUGHS	PHLEGM
Cuts	Rheumatism
Dropsy	Sore Throat
Ear Ailments	Spleen
Epilepsy	Tonic
Fevers	WHEEZING
Hoarseness	WORMS
Intestinal Mucus	

IRISH MOSS ——————
(Chondrus crispus)

Part Used: The whole herb
Properties: Demulcent, emollient, nutritive, and alterative.
Body Parts Affected: Lungs, stomach, kidneys, and skin.

Functions and Health Benefits:

Irish Moss, also known as "Carrageen Moss," is a seaweed first found in Ireland and used since the earliest days and is held in high esteem. In 1831, it was promoted by Dr. Todhunter in Ireland. It is high in iodine and considered a valuable food as well as a therapeutic agent. (121)

Studies done indicate a correlation between Irish Moss and an ability to reduce gastric secretions, high blood pressure, and ulcers. (122)

Irish Moss is valuable for treating lung problems, stomach conditions, and for strengthening the glandular system. It is beneficial for all chronic conditions because it is rich in vitamins and minerals to aid the body in healing itself. Because of its nutritional value, Irish Moss is beneficial for individuals recovering from illness. It is soothing to inflamed tissues and for lung and kidney ailments. Irish Moss is high in iodine, which aids the glandular system.

Vitamin and Mineral Content:

Irish Moss is high in iron which helps build the blood, which supplies strength to the body. It contains calcium for bones, teeth, cartilage and veins. Iodine found in Irish Moss helps the glands perform their functions. It is rich in sulphur, which is important for all cells in eliminating toxins. This herb contains 15 elements of the 18 which compose the human body. It is high in mucilage, which is soothing and healing for the mucous membranes. It also contains vitamins A, D, E, F, and K.

Bladder Problems	Parathyroid
BRONCHITIS	Pneumonia
Cancer	Radiation Poisoning
Catarrh	THYROID PROBLEMS
Coughs	Tuberculosis
Diarrhea	Tumors
GLANDS	Ulcers
GOITER	Varicose Veins
Intestinal Problems	Weight Reduction
LUNG PROBLEMS	

JUNIPER
(Juniperus species)

Part Used: The berries
Properties: Antispasmodic, diuretic, anodyne, aromatic, astringent, carminative, and stimulant.
Body Parts Affected: Stomach, intestines, bladder, kidneys, and uterus.

Functions and Health Benefits:

In ancient Greece, the berries were used as a diuretic. In Europe, the scent of Juniper Berries was used to help ward off the plague. Culpepper suggested using Juniper as an appetite stimulant. Native Americans used Juniper Berries as a survival food during the cold winter months. They would dry and ground the berries then make them into cakes. Some tribes roasted the berries, ground them and used them as a coffee substitute. Jethro Kloss recommended using the tea for kidney, prostate, bladder disorders, dropsy and for digestive diseases. (123) The berries and oil were listed in the *U.S. Pharmacopoeia* from 1820 to 1873 and in the *National Formulary* until 1960.

A recent study done using animals has found Juniper Berries to be an effective diuretic. (124) The berries are thought to stimulate the flow of urine and the filtration process. (125) Juniper Berries are often used for their diuretic properties.

Juniper Berries are often used to increase the flow or urine. They are beneficial for ridding the body of uric acid, which may crystallize in the kidneys. They are also used to dissolve kidney stones and sediment in the prostate. Juniper Berries are recommended for treating digestive problems and to cleanse the blood.

Vitamin and Mineral Content:

Juniper Berries are high in vitamin C which is known to be cleansing and healing on the entire urinary tract and can help dissolve excess mucus from the kidneys. This herb is high in potassium, which aids in protecting the kidneys from damage due to hypertension and other heart and artery diseases. It contains sulphur and copper.

Acne	Gout
ADRENAL GLANDS	Gums (bleeding)
Ague	Hay Fever
Allergies	HYPOGLYCEMIA
Arthritis	Incontinence
Arteriosclerosis	INFECTIONS
BEDWETTING	Insect Bites (poisonous)
BLADDER PROBLEMS	KIDNEY INFECTIONS
BLEEDING	KIDNEY STONES
Blood Cleanser	Mucus
Bursitis	Menstruation (regulates)
Catarrhal Inflammation	PANCREAS
COLDS	Prostate
Colic	Rheumatism
Coughs	Scurvy
Convulsions	Snakebites
Cramps	Sores
Cystic Fibrosis	Tuberculosis
DIABETES	Typhoid Fever
DROPSY	URIC ACID
Fungus	URINARY DISORDERS
Gas	WATER RETENTION
Gonorrhea	Worms

KAVA KAVA
(Piper methysticum)

Part Used: The root
Properties: Anodyne, antispasmodic, diuretic, sedative, and tonic.
Body Parts Affected: Nerves, liver and kidneys.

Functions and Health Benefits:

Polynesians used Kava Kava in their ceremonial drinks as a mild sedative, tonic, and stimulant. It is considered to be an important herb for pain relief. It is beneficial for insomnia and nervous conditions.

Research done has found Kava Kava to contain anticonvulsant and muscle relaxing properties in animal studies. (126)

This herb is recommended as a strong muscle relaxant. Kava Kava is used as an analgesic, sedative, for rheumatism, for insomnia, and to relax the body. It has antiseptic properties to help with bladder infections and may be applied directly to wounds.

Vitamin and Mineral Content:

Information is not available. It may contain calcium and magnesium because of its relaxing effects.

Anxiety	Pain
Asthma	Rheumatism
Bronchitis	Urinary Infections
Fatigue	Vaginitis
INSOMNIA	Venereal Disease
NERVOUSNESS	

KELP
(Fucus vesiculosus)

Part Used: The whole plant
Properties: Demulcent, nutritive, antibiotic, hypotensive, alterative, and diuretic.
Body Parts Affected: Glands (adrenal, pituitary, thyroid), nerves, brain, kidneys, and bladder.

Functions and Health Benefits:

Kelp is a principle source of natural iodine and is used extensively by the Japanese. The Polynesians also use kelp as a regular part of their diet. Dr. Bernard Russell, an English physician in 1750, used burned, dried kelp to treat his patients suffering from goiter. In 1862, it was used with success by Dr. C. Dupare to treat obesity.

The ocean water contains one of the richest sources of the vital life-sustaining mineral elements known to science. Kelp extracts assimilate the mineral elements from the ocean water and convert them into a usable form for man. This plant is thought to provide nourishment, enhance the immune system, aids in hormone balance, and restore strength.(127) Kelp may have antibiotic properties and work to kill infection present in the body. (128) Kelp has natural iodine to nourish the thyroid. The Japanese eat Kelp regularly in their diets and have an extremely low rate of thyroid disease. It helps increase energy through regulation of metabolism and may help reduce fat in the body. (129) Kelp is full of nutrients to nourish the entire body.

Traditionally, Kelp has been used for its rich abundance of iodine to treat thyroid disorders whether underactive or overactive. It is a great promoter of glandular health and regulates metabolism. It has a reputation of increasing the rate at which calories are burned. Kelp is used to rid the body of toxins and radioactive material by preventing their absorption. It promotes the growth of healthy tissue, skin, hair and nails. It is also able to improve the cardiovascular system, nervous system, mental alertness, and treat kidney, bladder, prostate, and uterine difficulties.

Vitamin and Mineral Content:

Kelp is rich in iodine for nourishing the glandular system including the thyroid. It contains calcium for the nervous system, bones and general health. Silicon is essential for calcium metabolism and is found in Kelp. The sulphur content helps rid the body of toxins. It contains phosphorus, iron, sodium, potassium, magnesium, chlorine, copper, zinc, and manganese. It is rich in the B-complex vitamins for the nervous system and over-all health. Kelp contains protein, essential fatty acids, fiber, carbohydrates and all the nutrients necessary for a healthy body.

Acne	Headaches
ADRENAL GLANDS	Heart Disorders
Anemia	High Blood Pressure
ARTERIES	Hypothyroidism
Arthritis	INFECTIONS
Asthma	Kidneys
Cancer	Morning Sickness
COLITIS	Nervous Disorders
COMPLEXION	OBESITY
Diabetes	Pancreas
Digestion	PITUITARY GLAND
ECZEMA	PREGNANCY
ENERGY	Prostate
FATIGUE	SKIN
FINGERNAILS	RADIATION POISONING
Gallbladder	THYROID
Gas	Tumors
Glands	Vitality
GOITER	Water Retention

LADY'S SLIPPER
(Cypripedium pubescens)

Part Used: The root
Properties: Nervine, antispasmodic, and sedative.
Body Parts Affected: Nerves, brain, and muscles.

Functions and Health Benefits:

Native American tribes used Lady's Slipper as a sedative and nerve medicine. The early settlers also found this herb valuable for insomnia and female problems. It was listed in the *U.S. Pharmacopoeia* from 1863 to 1916 as an antispasmodic and nerve medicine.

Lady's Slipper is used for all diseases of the nervous system. It may help with brain damage, epilepsy, stroke, cystic fibrosis, and muscular dystrophy. It is an excellent pain remedy for discomfort associated with muscular problems. It is often used as a nervine herb to calm the nerves, relieve stress, tension, insomnia and anxiety. Lady's Slipper is also used for fevers, headaches, depression, stomach ailments, and hyperactivity in children.

Vitamin and Mineral Content:

It is high in calcium, magnesium and B-complex vitamins, which are essential for normal brain and nerve function.

Abdominal Pain	INSOMNIA
Afterbirth Pain	Menstruation
Anxiety	Muscle Spasms
CHOREA	NERVOUSNESS
Colic	Neuralgia
Cramps	PAIN
Cystic Fibrosis	RESTLESSNESS
Epilepsy	Tremors
Headaches (nervous)	Typhoid Fever
HYSTERIA	

LICORICE

(Glycyrrhiza glabra)

Part Used: The root
Properties: Tonic, expectorant, demulcent, alterative, and aperient.
Body Parts Affected: Lungs, stomach, intestines, spleen, and liver.

Functions and Health Benefits:

Licorice was highly esteemed by the Egyptians, Romans, Greeks, and Chinese. It was used to quench thirst and as a sweetener in their drinks. The Chinese regard Licorice as a great detoxifier. It is often used in Chinese medicine and believed to increase strength and endurance as well as treat disorders such as female problems, fevers, infections, and colds it enhances the abilities of other herbs. It was introduced to the American continent by the English settlers. It was adopted by Native Americans and used with bitter herbs to disguise their taste. It is good for colds and lung congestion.

Scientific research has discovered that licorice does contain anti-inflammatory properties. (130) It has also been found to contain anti-allergic properties. (131) Licorice also has estrogenic properties. In one study, women who were not ovulating began to do so when given the extract of licorice. (132) Licorice has an estrogenic activity which helps the body to stimulate the production of estrogen if needed in the body. The properties in licorice (glycyrrhizin and glycyrrhetinic acid) stimulate the production of interferon in the body which helps protect the immune system. (133) Licorice may also be useful for protecting against and healing ulcers as well as a treatment for hepatitis. (134) It is also being studied as a therapy for Addison's disease, which involves inadequate adrenal function.

Licorice is a good source of the female hormone estrogen. It is often used to treat female problems. It may stimulate menstruation in females not experiencing normal ovulation. Licorice works as a mild laxative, to heal coughs and chest congestion, to stimulate adrenal function, to heal inflamed mucous membranes in the respiratory tract, and to restore energy.

Vitamin and Mineral Content:

Licorice contains vitamin E, which is necessary to strengthen and protect the glandular and immune systems. It has the B-complex vitamins, which aid in balancing hormones in both males and females. It contains biotin essential for the metabolism of carbohydrates and the synthesis of proteins. It is also being considered as a preventative agent for depression. It contains niacin, pantothenic acid, lecithin, manganese, iodine, and zinc.

Abscesses	Endurance
ADDISON'S DISEASE	ENERGY
ADRENAL GLAND	FATIGUE
Age Spots	FEMALE COMPLAINTS
Allergies	Fevers
Arteriosclerosis	Flu
Arthritis	Heart
Asthma	HOARSENESS
BLOOD CLEANSER	HYPERGLYCEMIA
Bronchitis	HYPOGLYCEMIA
Circulation	Impotency
COLDS	Liver
Constipation	LUNG PROBLEMS
COUGHS	Menopause
Cushing's Disease	Phlegm
DIABETES	SEXUAL STIMULANT
Dizziness	SORE THROAT
Dropsy	TONIC
DRUG WITHDRAWAL	Ulcers
EAR INFECTIONS	VITALITY
Emphysema	

LILY-OF-THE-VALLEY
(Convallaria majalis)

Parts Used: The flowers, leaves, and rhizome.
Properties: Diuretic, cardiac, tonic, laxative, and mucilaginous.
Body Parts Affected: Heart, brain, kidneys, and circulatory.

Functions and Health Benefits:

Dr. Edward Shook recommended Lily-Of-The-Valley as a valuable cardiac tonic. He said that it acts similar to digitalis without the cumulative effects of the drug. He also suggested it for slowing the action of the heart, increasing the heart contractions, as a diuretic, and as a remedy for dropsy involving a faulty heart. Culpepper, another well known herbalist, treated brain weakness and memory problems with this herb.

Scientific research has found that cardiac glycosides in Lily-Of-The-Valley are similar to the function of digitalis in its action on the heart. (135) In Europe, it is used extensively for apoplexy, convulsions, dropsy, epilepsy, heart ailments, palsy, and vertigo. It contains 20 cardiac glycosides.(136)

Lily-Of-The-Valley has been used to treat heart disorders much the same as digitalis but without the side effects. It can also help with water retention, which often accompanies heart problems. It can help to strengthen the heart and arteries.

Vitamin and Mineral Content:

Lily-Of-The-Valley contains potassium, which is effective in dissolving fibrous and catarrhal matter. The calcium content is essential for the heart. Iron is also found which strengthens the blood and helps slow the growth of varicose ulcers and veins, tumors, cancers, ulcerated gums and gangrene. It contains rutin, which helps strengthen the vascular system especially the capillaries.

ARRHYTHMIA
EDEMA
Epilepsy
HEART DISORDERS
WATER RETENTION

MARSHMALLOW
(Althaea officinalis)

Part Used: The root
Properties: Demulcent, diuretic, emollient, lithotriptic, alterative, nutritive, and vulnerary.
Body Parts Affected: Lungs, intestines, and kidneys.

Functions and Health Benefits:

The name althea is derived from the Greek altho, which means to cure. It has been used since ancient Egyptian times. From ancient time, the mallows have been known and used as food and medicine. (137) One of the herbs found in the grave of a Neanderthal man in a cave in Iraq was marshmallow. It was used anciently for irritated throats and intestinal tracts. (138) Europeans used Marshmallow for bronchitis, colds, and coughs because of its soothing and healing properties. Native Americans used it to treat snakebites and wounds.

Recent scientific research has found that the mucilaginous properties of althea root yield a soothing effect on the mucous membranes. (139)

Marshmallow helps to expel phlegm and relaxes the bronchial tubes while soothing and healing. It aids in healing lung ailments such as asthma and inflammation. It is also useful for sore throats, infections, diarrhea, dysentery, skin irritations and for coughs.

Vitamin and Mineral Content:

Marshmallow is rich in vitamin A, which accounts for its healing properties. It is rich in zinc which is also healing for wounds and broken bones and essential to the developing fetus. It contains high amounts of calcium, which aids in the formation of bones, flesh, and cartilage. It also contains iron, sodium, iodine, B-Complex, and pantothenic acid.

Allergies	Burns
ASTHMA	Catarrh
BEDWETTING	Constipation
BLADDER	Coughs
BLEEDING	Diabetes
BOILS	Diarrhea
Breast Problems	Dysentery
BRONCHITIS	EMPHYSEMA

Eyes (sore)
Gangrene
Glands
Gravel
Inflammation
Intestines
KIDNEYS
Lactation
Liver
LUNG CONGESTION

Mucous Membranes
NERVOUS CONDITIONS
PNEUMONIA
Skin Disorders
Sore Throat
Stomach Problems
URINARY PROBLEMS
WHOOPING COUGH
WOUNDS

MILK THISTLE ────────

(Silybum marianum)

Part Used: The seeds
Properties: Stimulant, alterative, and tonic.
Body Parts Affected: Liver, gallbladder, and
    stomach.

Functions and Health Benefits:

Milk Thistle was used in Europe as a well known remedy. A Roman named Pliny the Elder (A.D. 23-79) explains how the juice of Milk Thistle mixed with honey was used for carrying off bile. In 1597, Gerarde, an herbalist, said that Milk Thistle was one of the best remedies for melancholy (liver related) diseases.

Studies done recently indicate that Milk Thistle is beneficial for severe liver disorders such as hepatitis and cirrhosis, as well as general liver restoration, protection and strengthening. (140) The properties of Milk Thistle have been confirmed in animal studies to be a protection in liver disorders. (141)

Milk Thistle is thought to be an antioxidant with the ability to protect against free radical damage. It is especially healing on the liver, which is essential to a healthy immune system. It has traditionally been used to protect the kidneys, brain and other organs from damage due to toxins, to treat allergic reactions, reduce inflammation, and heal infections.

Vitamin and Mineral Content:

Milk Thistle is rich in bioflavonoids, which act in the body to increase membrane strength and reduce artery and vein permeability.

Alcoholism
Appetite Stimulant
Blood Pressure
Boils
Chemotherapy
CIRRHOSIS
Depression
Epilepsy
Fatty Deposits
Gas
Heartburn
Heart Disorders
Hemorrhage

HEPATITIS
Hypoglycemia
Indigestion
JAUNDICE
KIDNEYS
Lactation
LIVER
Menstruation
Radiation
Skin Diseases
Toxins
Varicose Veins

MULLEIN

(Verbascum thapsus)

Part Used: The leaves
Properties: Demulcent, expectorant, antispasmodic, antitussive, astringent, diuretic, and vulnerary.
Body Parts Affected: Lungs, glands, stomach, and lymphatics.

Functions and Health Benefits:

Discorides suggested using Mullein to treat eye problems, tonsillitis, coughs, stings, and toothaches. Mullein was introduced to America by the early European settlers. Native Americans used it to treat lung problems and some tribes smoked the leaves to treat asthma. They also made it into a syrup for coughs. Dr. Shook called Mullein a great herb in treating tuberculosis as well as other lung problems.

Modern research has found that the saponins, mucilage, and tannins contribute to the soothing topical effect of the plant. (142) These compounds are ideal for treating lung ailments, coughs, colds, asthma, whooping cough, and emphysema. (143) It is also suggested that mullein be used for pain, as a sleep aid, laxative, and to get rid of warts. (144)

Traditional uses of Mullein have been to relieve pain and to induce sleep. It has a calming effect on inflamed tissues and irritated nerves. Mullein helps control coughs, cramps and spasms. It can help loosen mucus from the respiratory and lymphatic systems. It nourishes as well as strengthens the lungs. The tea has been used for dropsy, sinusitis, swollen joints, and can be applied to mumps, tumors, and to treat a sore throat and tonsillitis.

Vitamin and Mineral Content:

Mullein is high in calcium and potassium, which are both necessary for the nervous system, healthy bones and healing the lungs. It is high in iron for rich blood and in sulphur for its healing properties. It also contains vitamins A, D, and B-complex.

ALLERGIES	JOINTS (swollen)
ASTHMA	LUNG PROBLEMS
BLEEDING (bowels and lungs)	LYMPHATIC CONGESTION
Bowel Problems	MUCOUS MEMBRANES
BRONCHITIS	Mumps
Bruises	Nephritis
COLDS	NERVOUSNESS
Constipation	PAIN RELIEVER
COUGHS	PLEURISY
CROUP	Pneumonia
Diaper Rash	PULMONARY DISEASE
DIARRHEA	SINUS CONGESTION
Dropsy	Skin Disorders
DYSENTERY	Sore Throat
EARACHES (oil)	Tonsillitis
EMPHYSEMA	Toothache
Eyes	Tumors
Female Disorders	TUBERCULOSIS
GLANDS	Venereal Disease
HAY FEVER	Ulcers
HEMORRHAGE	Warts
INSOMNIA	Wounds

MYRRH

(Balsamodendron myrrha) (Commiphora myrrha)

Part Used: The resin
Properties: Antiseptic, tonic, astringent, stimulant, expectorant, carminative, and emmenagogue.
Body Parts Affected: Stomach, lungs, liver, and the whole body.

Functions and Health Benefits:

Myrrh was valued anciently as a fragrance and healing agent. Ancient Egyptian women used the burned myrrh to rid their homes of fleas. The Chinese used Myrrh to heal wounds, for menstrual problems, bleeding, hemorrhoids and ulcerated sores. It is mentioned frequently throughout the Bible as in (Exodus 30:23) in the Old Testament. It is referred to in the preparation of the holy ointment. (Esther 2:15) Myrrh is used as a purification herb for women and in (Psalm 45:8) as a perfume.

Research has verified the use of Myrrh as an antiseptic. (145) Myrrh contains a compound known as silymarin, which protects the liver from chemical toxins and helps increase the function of the liver. (146)

Myrrh provides vitality and strength to the digestive system. It stimulates the flow of blood to the capillaries. It helps speed the healing of the mucous membranes including the gums, throat, stomach and intestines. It can be applied to sores and works as an antiseptic. It can help promote menstruation, aid digestion, heal sinus problems, soothe inflammation, and speed the healing process.

Vitamin and Mineral Content:

It is rich in minerals such as sodium, potassium, silicon, zinc and chlorine which purifies, cleanses, and expels waste from the system. These elements help assist the body in producing regular gastric juices or secretions. It helps regulate the correct balance of acid and alkaline in the blood.

Abrasions
ANTIBIOTIC
ANTISEPTIC
Arthritis
ASTHMA
Bad Breath
Boils
BRONCHITIS
Canker Sores
CATARRH
COLDS
COLITIS
COLON
Coughs
CUTS
Diarrhea
DIGESTION
Diphtheria
Eczema
EMPHYSEMA
GANGRENE
Gas
GUMS
Healing
HEMORRHOIDS
HERPES
HYPOGLYCEMIA
Indigestion
INFECTIONS
LUNG DISEASE
Menstrual Problems
MOUTH SORES
Nervous Conditions
Phlegm
PYORRHEA
Rheumatism
Scarlet Fever
SINUS PROBLEMS
SKIN SORES
STOMACH
Thyroid
TONSILLITIS
TOOTHACHE
Tuberculosis
Ulcers
Wounds
Yeast Infections

77

OATSTRAW ———————
(Avena sativa)

Parts Used: The stem
Properties: Nervine, tonic, anti-depressant, nutritive, demulcent and vulnerary.
Body Parts Affected: Nerves, uterus, stomach, lungs, and bones.

Functions and Health Benefits:

Oatstraw has been used as a valuable food for centuries. Oats were used in the Middle Ages as a food staple. Northern Europeans often used oats as a food source. The silica found in Oatstraw is of great value.

Oatstraw is found in many herbal calcium formulas. It is beneficial for depression, liver, kidneys, exhaustion, insomnia, to lower blood sugar levels, for skin conditions and many other ailments. Oatstraw is a powerful stimulant and is rich in nutrients to strengthen the body. It contains antiseptic properties and is an excellent tonic for the whole body. Oatstraw can help with physical fatigue, nervous conditions, depression, and colds.

Vitamin and Mineral Content:

Oatstraw is rich in silica, which is valuable for the nervous system, especially the nerve sheaths as well as for brain function, healthy bones, teeth, skin and cartilage. It is also rich in magnesium and phosphorus. About half of the magnesium found in the body is concentrated in the bones. It is essential for strong and healthy bones. A lack of magnesium has been linked to psychiatric problems. Phosphorus is also found in Oatstraw. It is the second most abundant mineral next to calcium. It also contributes to healthy bones and nerves. Phosphorus also contains vitamins A, B-complex, and E.

APPETITE	HEART
ARTHRITIS	INDIGESTION
BEDWETTING	INSOMNIA
Bladder	Kidneys
Boils	Liver
Bones	Lungs
Bursitis	NERVES
Constipation	Pancreas
Eyes	Paralysis
Fingernails	Rheumatism
Gallbladder	Skin Problems
Gout	URINARY TRACT
HAIR	Wounds

PAN PIEN LIEN ————

(Lobelia inflata)

Part Used: The herb
Properties: Antispasmodic, emetic, expectorant, nervine, stimulant, and alterative.
Body Parts Affected: Nerves, stomach, lungs, circulation and muscles.

Functions and Health Benefits:

Pan Pien Lien contains lobelia-like properties. Samuel Thomson introduced lobelia and called it the most powerful, certain, and harmless relaxant that has ever been discovered. He considered relaxation to be a big part of the healing process in the majority of diseases. Many doctors of his time agreed with this theory and used this herb in their treatments.

Scientific studies have found the ingredient lobeline to be effective as a smoking deterrent. Its action in treating lung problems is the stimulating effect it has on the adrenal glands to release hormones to relax the bronchial muscles. (147) It is considered useful for heart and lung conditions as both an expectorant and cardiac decongestant on one hand, and an antispasmodic relaxant on the other. Many similarities exist between the Chinese herb Tian nan Xing, tuber Arisaemae, and Lobelia. (148) Lobelia is beneficial for spasms, hysteria, convulsions, epilepsy, and nervous conditions. It is relaxing for croup's and coughs. It will expel phlegm from the lungs and is good for childhood diseases.

Vitamin and Mineral Content:

It contains sulphur which is needed and found mostly in the nervous system, brain and tissues. Sulphur also purifies and tones the system and cleans the fat that collects and holds toxins. Pan Pien Lien also contains iron and copper. Iron depends on copper for absorption. Iron increases the oxygen transported to the brain and muscles. It contains selenium, which is known to build the immune system and help prevent conditions such as cancer. Selenium helps prevent heart disease and arthritis. It contains sodium needed for digestion, and purifies the blood, halts fermentation and counteracts acidosis.

ALLERGIES	FEVERS
Angina	Hay Fever
ARTHRITIS	HEADACHES
ASTHMA	Heart
Bites	INSOMNIA
Blood Poisoning	LUNG PROBLEMS
BLOOD VESSELS	Mucous Membranes
BRONCHITIS	Nervousness
Bruises	PNEUMONIA
CANKER SORES	Rheumatic Fever
CATARRH	Rheumatism
CHILDHOOD	Respiratory System
COLDS	SEIZURES
Colic	SPASMS
CONGESTION	TEETHING
COUGHS	TOOTHACHES
CROUP	Tumors
EAR INFECTIONS	WHOOPING COUGH
EMPHYSEMA	WORMS
EPILEPSY	Wounds

PASSION FLOWER
(Passiflora incarnata)

Part Used: The herb
Properties: Antispasmodic, sedative, diaphoretic, anodyne, and nervine.
Body Parts Affected: Nerves, heart, and circulation.

Functions and Health Benefits:

Native Americans used Passion Flower as a tonic and a poultice for bruises and injuries. The Aztecs used it as a sedative and for pain. The juice was used for sore eyes and the crushed plant tops and leaves for treating hemorrhoids and skin eruptions. It was listed in the *National Formulary* from 1916 to 1936. Dr. R. Swinburne Clymer, M.D. referred to Passion Flower as the opium (non-poisonous and not dangerous) of the natural physician.

Research on Passion Flower has found it useful for insomnia, fatigue, spasms and nervous tension. (149) Some tests indicate the use of this herb for pain relief as well as for its sedative effects. (150) It contains anti-inflammatory properties which may be useful for those suffering from arthritis. (151)

Passion Flower is very soothing on the nervous system and for conditions such as insomnia, hysteria, anxiety, and hyperactivity. It is also useful for eye conditions such as inflammations, dimness of vision and eye irritations.

Vitamin and Mineral Content:

Passion Flower contains calcium and magnesium, both essential for the nervous system.

ALCOHOLISM	HIGH BLOOD PRESSURE
ANXIETY	Hysteria
ASTHMA (spasmodic)	INSOMNIA
Bronchitis	MENOPAUSE
Convulsions	Menstruation (painful)
Depression	Muscle Spasms
Diarrhea	NERVOUSNESS
Dysentery	NEURALGIA
Epilepsy	Pain
EYE INFECTIONS	Parkinson's Disease
Eye Strain	Restlessness
EYE TENSION	Seizures
FEVERS	Vision
HEADACHES	

PAU D'ARCO
(Tabebuia avellanedae)

Part Used: The inner bark
Properties: Analgesic, alterative, astringent, anti-fungal, and tonic.
Body Parts Affected: Circulation, stomach, nervous system, and the whole body.

Functions and Health Benefits:

In South America, this herb was known for its healing powers by the Callawaya tribe. They called the herb Taheebo and have been using it for over 1,000 years. In the Santo Andre Hospital in Rio de Janeiro, Brazil, Pau D'Arco has been used to treat cancer and other illnesses since the 1970's.

Scientific studies in the 1970's and 80's showed that lapachol, a component of Pau D'Arco, was effective against viral infections, parasites and cancers of all kind. (152)

Herbalists have used Pau D'Arco to treat many conditions and is effective as an immune system enhancer and can aid in treating conditions such as cancer, leukemia, tumors, and blood disorders. It is also used to treat the pain of arthritis, diabetes, candida, herpes, liver ailments, hypoglycemia, and assimilation of nutrients.

Vitamin and Mineral Content:

Pau D'Arco is rich in calcium and iron, which are both essential for a healthy body and mind. Calcium is effective in preventing disease and protecting the colon by forming an insoluble complex with free fatty acids, which can cause free radicals to multiply. Iron is necessary for healthy blood. Selenium in this herb helps protect the immune system against diseases such as cancer. It also contains vitamin C and zinc, which are antioxidants also protecting the immune system. Pau D'Arco contains magnesium, manganese, phosphorus, potassium, sodium, vitamin A and some B-complex vitamins.

AIDS	Diarrhea	Lupus
Allergies	ECZEMA	Nephritis
Anemia	Fevers	PAIN
Arthritis	Gastritis	PROSTATE
Asthma	Hemorrhages	Psoriasis
BLOOD PURIFIER	HERPES	RHEUMATISM
Bronchitis	HODGKIN'S DISEASE	Skin Disorders
CANCER	IMMUNE SYSTEM	TONIC
CANDIDA	Infections	TOXEMIA
Circulation	Intestines	TUMORS
Colitis	LEUKEMIA	Ulcers
Constipation	LIVER	Urinary Tract
DIABETES	Lungs	Venereal Disease

PEPPERMINT ─────────
(Mentha piperita)

Part Used: The leaves
Properties: Carminative, aromatic, diaphoretic, stimulant, and antispasmodic.
Body Parts Affected: Stomach, intestines, liver, muscles, and circulation.

Functions and Health Benefits:

The Romans used Peppermint as a stomach aid and to promote digestion. The Greeks also used this herb for many different ailments. Native Americans used Peppermint leaf tea as a carminative, to prevent vomiting, nausea, and fevers.

Modern research has found numerous volatile oils in Peppermint that possess antibacterial activity. (153) The oil of Peppermint is also thought to soothe gastrointestinal contractions and help relieve gas. (154).

Peppermint has been found to contain properties which stimulate the flow of bile and help settle the stomach after vomiting. It is beneficial for nausea, chills, colic, fevers, gas and diarrhea. It has a cleansing, soothing and relaxing effect on the body. Herbalists have long recommended the use of Peppermint for digestive problems. It is also used for convulsions in infants, to increase respiration, for colds and to strengthen the entire body.

Vitamin and Mineral Content:

It is rich in vitamin A, which is a protectant and healing agent for the organs and tissues of the body. Peppermint is rich in B-complex vitamins, which calm the nerves, protect against disease, promote a good appetite and digestion. It is high in calcium, magnesium, phosphorus, potassium, sodium, iron, selenium, manganese, vitamin C, silicon and zinc.

APPETITE	HEARTBURN
BOWELS SPASMS	Hysteria
Chills	Insomnia
Cholera	Menstruation
COLDS	Morning Sickness
COLIC	Motion Sickness
Constipation	Mouth Sores
Convulsions	NAUSEA
Cramps	NERVES
Depression	Neuralgia
DIGESTION	Shingles
Dizziness	SHOCKS
FEVER	Sore Throat
Flu	Stomach Spasms
GAS	Toothaches
HEADACHES	VOMITING
Heart	

PRICKLY ASH
(Xanthoxylum americanum)

Parts Used: The bark and berries
Properties: Stimulant, alterative, antispasmodic, anthelmintic, and astringent.
Body Parts Affected: Blood, circulation, stomach, spleen, and liver.

Functions and Health Benefits:

Prickly Ash was used by some Native American tribes for toothaches and infection. It was listed in the *U.S. Pharmacopoeia,* from 1829 to 1926 and in the *National Formulary,* from 1916 to 1947 and was listed as a treatment for rheumatism. Prickly Ash was used in the Southern states during cholera and typhus epidemics with great results. Samuel Thomson considered it a valuable remedy where stimulants are required, for rheumatism, cold hands and feet, ague and fever.

Extensive research has not been done, but some have shown promising results. It is stimulating for circulation and helps strengthen the heart and lungs. Prickly Ash can help in cases of impaired circulation such as cold extremities and joints. It can help with rheumatism, arthritis, lethargy, and in healing wounds. It is a very promising herb to enhance the immune system and relieve exhaustion. Its bitter and sweet qualities help heal deficiencies of the heart, lungs, spleen, and intestines. (155)

Arthritis	Gas
Asthma	Lethargy
Blood Purifier	Liver Problems
Cholera	MOUTH SORES
CIRCULATION	PARALYSIS
Colic	Rheumatism
Cramps	Scrofula
Digestion	Skin Diseases
Diarrhea	Syphilis
Dropsy	Thyroid
Female Problems	ULCERS
FEVERS	WOUNDS

PSYLLIUM
(Plantago ovata)

Part Used: The seeds
Properties: Demulcent and laxative
Body Parts Affected: Colon, stomach, liver and spleen.

Functions and Health Benefits:

Psyllium was used by Native Americans to treat abrasions, sprains, and as an eye wash. Anglo-Saxons considered this herb to be a strong healing agent. It was also used as a laxative to help with constipation.

Research has found Psyllium to be beneficial for lowering cholesterol and for strengthening the heart. Studies have also indicated Psyllium to be useful for treating irritable bowel syndrome. (156) It has also been suggested as a help for diabetics. It produces copious mucilage to soothe and heal the large intestines and clean the colon. It does not irritate the delicate mucous membranes of the intestines but works to strengthen and restore the tissues. Jethro Kloss suggested using Psyllium in cases of colitis and anal ulcers. (157)

It can help prevent auto-intoxication and help with any disease by protecting the colon and preventing toxins from being absorbed into the blood. Psyllium also works as a lubricant on the intestinal tract.

Vitamin and Mineral Content:

Psyllium contains aucubine, enzymes, fats, glycosides, mucilage, and protein.

COLITIS	Gonorrhea
COLON	Hemorrhage
CONSTIPATION	Intestinal Tract
Cystitis	Irritable Bowel Syndrome
Diarrhea	Ulcers
DIVERTICULITIS	Urinary Tract
Dysentery	

QUEEN OF THE MEADOW _
(Eupatorium purpureum)

Part Used: The leaves
Properties: Diuretic, astringent, tonic, nervine, stimulant, and stone solvent.
Body Parts Affected: Kidneys, bladder, nerves, and joints.

Functions and Health Benefits:

Queen of the Meadow is also known as gravel root. It was used by Native Americans, who called it, Joe-Pye weed, after a medicine man who used it to treat typhus. The Iroquois and Cherokees used Queen of the Meadow as a diuretic, as a burn poultice and for ailments of the genitourinary tract.

Studies done have found it to be effective for arthritis, rheumatism and gout, due to uric acid build-up. (158) A European species related to this herb has been studied and found to contain immunostimulant properties, which help against viral infections. (159)

Herbalists have used this herb in formulas for gravel and stones of the kidneys and bladder. Queen of the Meadow is used for urinary disorders. It helps with water retention and joint pain caused by uric acid deposits. It is used for Bright's disease, rheumatism, gout, dropsy, cystitis, backache, strains, sprains, and pulled ligaments and tendons.

Vitamin and Mineral Content:

It contains vitamin A necessary for strong and healthy mucous membranes. It also has vitamin D, which works with calcium in preventing inorganic mineral deposits in the joints.

BLADDER INFECTIONS	Menstruation
BURSITIS	Nervous Conditions
Childbirth	NEURALGIA
Diabetes	Prostate
DROPSY	RHEUMATISM
Edema	RINGWORM
GALLSTONES	Typhus
GOUT	URINARY PROBLEMS
Headaches	WATER RETENTION
KIDNEY INFECTIONS	

RED CLOVER
(Trifolium pratense)

Part Used: The flowers
Properties: Alterative, antispasmodic, nutritive, antibiotic, sedative, stimulant, tonic, and vulnerary.
Body Parts Affected: Blood, nerves, lungs, liver, and lymph.

Functions and Health Benefits:

The use of Red Clover probably originated in Europe and was used as an expectorant and a diuretic. Native Americans used Red Clover as an infusion gargle for sore throats, whooping cough and asthma. They used it on children because of its mild nature in treating wasting diseases.

Studies indicate that Red Clover contains some antibiotic properties beneficial against bacteria including the one which causes tuberculosis. (160)
It has been used for treating cancer, bronchitis, nervous conditions, spasms and toxins in the body. Herbalists consider it to be a blood cleanser and recommend this mild herb in formulas when using a cleansing program.

It is used mixed with honey and water as a cough syrup. It is a mild sedative, and useful for spasmodic conditions, for bronchitis, wheezing and fatigue.

Vitamin and Mineral Content:

Red Clover is rich in vitamins and minerals. It is high in vitamin A, which protects the mucous membranes and helps protect the cell membranes against oxidation and viral infections. It is high in iron, which helps with oxygen and hemoglobin. B-complex vitamins are found in Red Clover, which help the nervous system. It also has vitamin C necessary for the immune system and disease prevention. It is high in selenium, which is important and may be lacking in the diet. It also contains manganese, sodium, magnesium, calcium, and copper.

ACNE	Leprosy
AIDS	LEUKEMIA
Arthritis	LIVER CONDITIONS
ATHLETE'S FOOT	Lymphatic System
Bladder	Muscle Cramps
BLOOD PURIFIER	NERVOUS CONDITIONS
BLOOD CLEANSER	PSORIASIS
Boils	Rheumatism
BRONCHITIS	SKIN DISORDERS
Burns	Sores
CANCER	SPASMS
Childhood Diseases	Syphilis
Colds	TOXINS
Constipation	TUMORS
Coughs	Ulcers
Digestion	Urinary Tract
Eyewash	Vaginal Irritations
Flu	Whooping Cough
Gallbladder	Wounds

RED RASPBERRY
(Rubus idaeus)

Part Used: The leaves
Properties: Astringent, analgesic, antispasmodic, alterative, tonic, stimulant, homeostatic, and antiseptic..
Body Parts Affected: Liver, spleen, blood, and genitourinary.

Functions and Health Benefits:

A famous herbalist in England, Henry Box, praised Red Raspberry as the best gift God ever gave to women. He said, "if the pains of childbirth are premature, it will make all quiet. If the mother is weak, it will abundantly strengthen her, cleanse her and enrich her milk." (161) It is excellent for a safe and easy childbirth. Gerard recommended Red Raspberry for a weak stomach.

Scientific research has proven the value of Red Raspberry. One of the properties discovered, fragarine, was found to have a relaxing effect on the pelvic and uterine muscles. (162) It also contains tannins, which are effective for nausea, vomiting, and diarrhea. Other studies indicate that Red Raspberry contains anti-viral properties to help fight viral diseases such as herpes and the flu. (163)

Red Raspberry has traditionally been used for women especially during pregnancy to strengthen the uterus, prevent nausea, prevent hemorrhage, reduce pain during childbirth, and to enrich colostrum found in breast milk. It is a wonderful herb for treating children for conditions such as colds, diarrhea, colic, fever, and other childhood diseases.

Vitamin and Mineral Content:

Red Raspberry is high in calcium, which may help relax the uterine muscles. It is rich in iron to strengthen the blood and protects against toxemia and provides nourishment to the fetus. It contains essential minerals required during pregnancy and menstrual periods. It contains vitamins A, C, D, G, F, and B-complex all of which are vital for a healthy body.

AFTER BIRTH PAINS	Lactation
BOWEL PROBLEMS	Leucorrhea
Breast Feeding	Measles
Bronchitis	MENSTRUATION
Canker Sores	MISCARRIAGE
CHILDBIRTH	MORNING SICKNESS
Cholera	MOUTH SORES
Colds	MUCOUS MEMBRANES
Constipation	NAUSEA
Coughs	Nervous Conditions
Diabetes	PREGNANCY
DIARRHEA	Prostate
Digestion	Rheumatism
Dysentery	Sore Throat
Eyewash	Stomach
FEMALE ORGANS	Teething
FEVERS	Ulcers
FLU	Urinary Problems
HEART	Uterus (prolapsed)
Hemorrhoids	VOMITING
Indigestion	Wounds
LABOR PAINS	

ROSE HIPS
(Rosa species)

Part Used: The fruit
Properties: Nutritive, stomachic, astringent, antiseptic, and antispasmodic.
Body Parts Affected: Blood, nerves, heart, kidneys, and colon.

Functions and Health Benefits:

Native Americans used this herb rich in vitamin C as a food because it was available all year round. Scurvy was uncommon among them because of its vitamin C content. Swiss herbalist, Father Kunzle, recommended the use of Rose Hips to expel kidney stones. It was used often as a survival food.

Modern research has recognized the value of Rose Hips for its vitamin C content and compounds which act as astringents. (164)

Rose Hips are useful for all acute diseases such as childhood diseases, colds, flu, and fevers. It is also useful for preventing and healing infections. Rose Hips can help fill the body's need for vitamin C, which must be replaced daily.

Vitamin and Mineral Content:

Rose Hips is high in vitamin C and bioflavonoids needed daily to protect the immune system against pollution, germs, and viruses. It also has vitamin A essential for healthy eyes, mucous membranes, lungs, stomach, and organs. It contains vitamin E necessary for a healthy heart and blood vessels. It is rich in B-complex vitamins important for the nervous system, stomach, and the immune system. It contains iron, calcium, sodium, potassium, sulphur, and silica.

ADRENAL GLANDS	EXHAUSTION
Arteriosclerosis	FEVERS
Bites	FLU
Bruises	HEADACHES
Bladder	Heart
BLOOD PURIFIER	Hemorrhoids
CANCER	INFECTIONS
CIRCULATION	Kidneys
COLDS	Mouth Sores
Colic	NERVOUSNESS
Coughs	PMS
Cramps	Psoriasis
Diarrhea	SORE THROAT
Dizziness	SORES
Earaches	Stings
Emphysema	STRESS

SAFFRON _____
(Crocus sativus)

Part Used: The flowers
Properties: Emmenagogue, stimulant, carminative, antispasmodic, tonic, aphrodisiac, and alterative.
Body Parts Affected: Heart, liver, kidney, and spleen.

Functions and Health Benefits:

The Greeks and Chinese used Saffron as a royal dye for its yellow color. The wealthy Romans used Saffron to perfume their homes. It was used medicinally and as a spice in Europe during the 4th to 18th centuries. Culpepper recommended using Saffron for the heart, brain and lungs. He also suggested it for acute diseases such as pestilence, smallpox and measles, and for female obstructions and hysteric depression. It was listed in the *Materia Medica and Pharmacology* by Culbreth in 1917 as being a diaphoretic, carminative, emmenagogue, anodyne; to promote exanthematous eruptions in measles, etc., and to treat dysmenorrhea, and conjunctivitis.

Research done on Saffron suggests the ingredient crocetin may have the potential to act as an anti-cancer agent. It also shows promise in oxygen utilization. (165) In Valencia, Spain, Saffron is eaten daily and little heart disease exists among the people. Evidence points to the fact that Saffron provides more oxygen to the veins and heart. (166)

Saffron is soothing to the stomach and colon. It may help reduce cholesterol levels by neutralizing uric acid buildup in the system. It may also help to prevent heart disease. It can help with digestion, as a blood purifier, to reduce inflammation, to treat arthritis, gout, bursitis, and kidney stones, hypoglycemia, chest congestion, to improve circulation, and to promote energy.

Vitamin and Mineral Content:

Saffron contains vitamin A, which protects the epithelial cells that are in constant contact with the environment such as the eyes, mouth, digestive tract, lungs, and urinary and reproductive tracts. It contains vitamin B-12, which is usually not found in plants. It is needed to produce genetic building blocks such as DNA and RNA. It helps prevent memory loss, irritability, confusion, anemia, difficulty in swallowing and digestive problems. It also contains potassium, calcium, phosphorus and sodium.

Arthritis	LIVER DISORDERS
Bronchitis	MEASLES
Cancer	Menstruation
Colds	PERSPIRATION
Conjunctivitis	PHLEGM
Coughs	PSORIASIS
DIGESTION	RHEUMATISM
FEVERS	SCARLET FEVER
Gas	Skin Diseases
GOUT	STOMACH (acid)
Headaches	Tuberculosis
Heartburn	Ulcers
Hyperglycemia	Uterine Hemorrhages
Hypoglycemia	Water Retention
Insomnia	Whooping Cough
Jaundice	

ST. JOHN'S WORT
(Hypericum perforatum)

Part Used: The herb
Properties: Alterative, antispasmodic, astringent, diuretic, nervine, sedative, and vulnerary.
Body Parts Affected: Stomach, liver, blood, kidneys, and nerves.

Functions and Health Benefits:

Nicholas Culpepper mentioned St. John's Wort in his book, *The Complete Herbal*, published in 1649. He suggested it for conditions such as tertian and quartan agues (fevers that occur every 3 to 4 days, may refer to malaria), alexipharmic (an antidote or defensive remedy against poison, venom, or infection), worms, injuries, bruises, open obstructions, dissolves swelling, and sciatica. It was used in Europe on the Crusade battlefields to treat war injuries.

St. John's Wort is used in Europe and Russia and is currently officially listed in the pharmacopoeias in many Eastern European countries. (167) Studies have found that it contains diuretic properties, strengthens the capillaries, dilates coronary arteries, prevents tumors, helps diarrhea and viruses, and kills germs. It also has anti-fungal properties and is effective for nervous disorders. (168) St. John's Wort is currently being studied as a treatment against HIV infection. It has been shown in studies to contain anti-HIV activity. (169) It is a very promising herb for the immune system and to protect the circulatory system.

Traditionally St. John's Wort has been used to rid the chest and lungs of mucus and in conditions such as bronchitis. It is used to treat nervous conditions such as neuralgia, anxiety, and nervous tension. It can help relieve pain, reduce swelling, treat abscesses and insect bites, and for rheumatism. It is an excellent blood purifier.

Vitamin and Mineral Content:

St. John's Wort contains bioflavonoids including rutin, quercetin, and hyperoside, which may explain its effect on the arteries and capillaries.

AFTERBIRTH PAINS	Hemorrhaging
Anemia	Hysteria
Anxiety	Insomnia
Appetite	Jaundice
BEDWETTING	LUNG CONGESTION
Bites	Melancholy
Bleeding	Menopause
Blood Purifier	MENSTRUATION
Boils	Nervous Conditions
BRONCHITIS	Palsy
CANCER	Skin Problems
Coughs	Spasms
Depression	TUMORS
Diarrhea	Ulcers
Dysentery	URINATION
Gallbladder	UTERUS
Gout	Worms
Headaches	Wounds
Heart	

SAW PALMETTO
(Serenoa repens)

Part Used: The fruit
Properties: Diuretic, tonic, antiseptic, sedative, and aphrodisiac.
Body Parts Affected: Kidneys, spleen, reproductive tract, urinary tract, and lungs.

Functions and Health Benefits:

Native American tribes in the south used Saw Palmetto for sore eyes. The dried root was used to lower high blood pressure and the crushed root was applied to sore breasts in women. John Lloyd, an early American botanist noticed that animals eating the berries were fat and healthy. (170) It was listed in the *U.S. Pharmacopoeia,* from 1910 to 1916, and the *National Formulary,* from 1926 to 1950 as being a diuretic, sedative, expectorant, and an analgesic recommended for neuralgia. It has also been known in folk history as an aphrodisiac and sexual stimulant. It was used to treat urination problems and inflammation of the bladder and prostate enlargement. (171)

Research has shown that Saw Palmetto has diuretic properties and is effective in treating an enlarged prostate. (172) Preliminary evidence suggests that it may aid those suffering from thyroid deficiency. (173)

Saw Palmetto has been used to treat conditions of the genito-urinary system. It is also used as an antiseptic, for excessive mucus in the head and sinuses, and for both male and female reproductive organs.

Vitamin and Mineral Content:

Saw Palmetto contains vitamin A, essential for healthy lungs, reproductive organs and the immune system. It is also known as an antioxidant and can protect against immune related illnesses such as cancer.

Alcoholism	Mucus
Asthma	IMPOTENCY
Bladder	Infertility
BREAST ENLARGEMENT	Kidneys
Bright's Disease	Lung Congestion
Bronchitis	Nerves
Catarrh	Neuralgia
Colds	Obesity
Diabetes	PROSTATE
DIGESTION	REPRODUCTIVE ORGANS
GLANDS	Sore Throat
Frigidity	Urinary Tract
HORMONE REGULATION	Whooping Cough

SCHIZANDRA
(Schizandra chinensis)

Part Used: The berries
Properties: Astringent, tonic, and sedative.
Body Parts Affected: Heart, kidneys, and lungs.

Functions and Health Benefits:

Schizandra grows wild in northern China. It has been used as a natural medicine for thousands of years and prescribed by physicians in that region. In the 16th century, it was listed in a book on pharmacy written by Li Schizheng. It was used to increase energy, replenish and nourish the viscera (internal abdominal organs such as intestines and lungs), improve vision, boost muscular activity, and soothe both coughs and digestive upsets.

Scientific studies have found that Schizandra is an antibacterial, stimulant, and protects the liver against toxins. It also has been found to help allergies, depression and fatigue in mice. In addition, it protects against the effects of alcohol and pentobatbital in mice. (174) Other studies have found this herb to have a mild regenerative effect on the liver. It was used in China to treat infectious hepatitis. (175)

Schizandra is an adaptogen herb, and it helps the body heal itself. It can help increase energy in the cells of the brain, muscles, liver, kidney, glands, nerves and the entire body. It stimulates the immune system and protects against free radical damage, radiation, the effects of sugar, boosts stamina, normalizes blood sugar and blood pressure and protects against infections.

Vitamin and Mineral Content:

Schizandra is high in vitamin C, which helps protect against allergies and toxins. It is high in magnesium, which is lacking when stress is present in the body and may lead to a magnesium deficiency in the heart. Studies indicate that low levels of magnesium may lead to abnormal cell development, which could lead to cancer. Phosphorus is also found in Schizandra, which nourishes the brain and nervous system. It also contains iron, potassium, calcium, manganese, selenium, silicon, and sodium, which are all important for strengthening and nourishing the body.

Aging	Hepatitis
Anxiety	IMPOTENCY
Arteriosclerosis	Infections
Asthma	Insomnia
Blood Pressure	Kidneys
Coughs	Lung Problems
DIABETES	MENTAL ALERTNESS
Diarrhea	Motion Sickness
Digestion	NERVOUS DISORDERS
Edema	Radiation
ENERGY	STRESS
FATIGUE	Tonic
Gastritis	Uterine Problems
Heart Palpitations	Vision

SCULLCAP
(Scutellaria lateriflora)

Part Used: The herb
Properties: Nervine, antipyretic, antispasmodic, sedative, and tonic.
Body Parts Affected: Nerves, stomach and kidneys.

Functions and Health Benefits:

Scullcap was used by the Cherokee tribe as an emmenagogue and was used historically as an anticonvulsant. Chinese physicians have used an Asian Scullcap (S. Baikalensis) as a tranquilizer/sedative and to treat convulsions. (176) In 1772, it was considered a cure for rabies by some physicians. It was later recommended by Eclectic physicians for insomnia, nervousness, malaria, and convulsions. It was officially listed in the *U.S. Pharmacopoeia*, from 1863 to 1916, and in the *National Formulary*, from 1916 to 1947.

Research done in Europe and Russia has proven the benefits of Scullcap as a tranquilizer. (177) It is used and prescribed widely in Europe. Studies in Japan using animals showed that Scullcap could increase levels of good cholesterol and may suggest it as a heart disease and stroke preventative. (178)

Scullcap may treat a variety of conditions including pain, anxiety, high blood pressure and epilepsy. It is well known for its ability to calm the nerves and help with all nervous system conditions. It has also been used to treat infertility, fatigue, inflamed tissues, digestion, coughs, and headaches.

Vitamin and Mineral Content:

Scullcap contains calcium, which acts as a natural pain killer, calms the nervous system, increases resistance to infections, and decreases acidity levels to promote a balance in the body.

Potassium is necessary for the muscles to contract, to reduce hypoglycemic blackouts, help prevent germs from accumulating in the tissues, aids in insomnia, and help motor nerve function. It also has magnesium, which may calm the nerves, improve resistance to infections, and strengthen the nervous system. Scullcap contains vitamin C, which acts as a detoxifying agent and combats viruses and germs in the body. It also contains vitamin E, which enables the body to utilize oxygen more efficiently, improves circulation, reduces uric acid and prevents sterility. It also has iron and zinc.

Alcoholism	INFERTILITY
ANXIETY	Insanity
BLOOD PRESSURE	INSOMNIA
Childhood Diseases	NERVES
Circulation	Neuralgia
CONVULSIONS	Pain
Coughing	Palsy
Delirium	Parkinson's Disease
Drug Withdrawal	Poisonous Bites
EPILEPSY	Rabies
Fevers	RESTLESSNESS
Fits	Rheumatism
Hangover	Rickets
Headaches	Spasms
HIGH BLOOD PRESSURE	Spinal Meningitis
Hydrophobia	St. Vitus Dance
Hypertension	Thyroid
Hysteria	Tremors
Hypoglycemia	Urinary Tract

SENNA

(Cassia acutifolia)

Parts Used: The leaves and pods.
Properties: Laxative, vermifuge, cathartic, and
   purgative.
Body Parts Affected: Intestines

Functions and Health Benefits:

American Senna has been widely used for its laxative effect. Native Americans used it as a drink to reduce fevers, for sore throats, and as a laxative. It was official in *U.S. Pharmacopoeia* from 1820 to 1882. The Chinese were aware of Senna (Fan xia ye) in Chinese medicine. Senna and other laxatives were used since prehistoric time for colonic and menstrual obstructions. (179) Senna is found along the Nile River and was used in Arab medicine as an effective and safe laxative. Culpepper claimed that Senna cleaned the stomach, purged melancholy and phlegm from the head, brain, lungs, heart, liver and spleen.

Many believe that a clean colon can prevent autointoxication and may be an underlying cause of many diseases. Senna is usually combined with other herbs for better results. It has been used throughout history and is still used throughout the world.

Vitamin and Mineral Content:

Senna is rich in calcium and magnesium to help balance the acid/alkaline in the body and nourish the nervous system. It contains sodium, which is essential for digestion, stopping fermentation and purifying the blood. It is high in iron to build the blood and zinc, which acts as an antioxidant. Senna contains silicon to support calcium absorption. It also contains vitamins A, C and B-complex necessary for a healthy liver and colon. It contains moderate amounts of potassium, selenium, and manganese.

Acne	JAUNDICE
Bad Breath	Menstruation
Bilousness	Obesity
Colic	Rheumatism
CONSTIPATION	Skin Diseases
Gallstones	WORMS
Gout	

SLIPPERY ELM

(Ulmus fulva)

Part Used: The inner bark
Properties: Demulcent, emollient, nutritive, astringent, and expectorant.
Body Parts Affected: Lungs, stomach, and nutritive for the entire body.

Functions and Health Benefits:

Slippery Elm was known by Native Americans as a valuable survival food. It was used for colds, coughs, sore throats, wounds, as a poultice to bring boils to a head, and for bowel complaints. Dr. Shook called it one of the most valuable remedies in herbal practice for its abundant mucilage, strengthening and healing qualities. (180)

Studies done on Slippery Elm have found it to be an excellent demulcent and beneficial for diarrhea, coughs, stomach problems, colitis, and lung problems. (181) The bark of Slippery Elm contains mucilage, which swells in water and can be applied to wounds or taken internally to soothe and heal. (182)

It contains as much nutrition as oatmeal and forms a wholesome and sustaining food for young children and invalids. Slippery Elm has been used mainly to treat gastrointestinal problems such as stomach and intestinal ulcers, soothing the stomach and colon, digestion, acidity, and to lubricate the bowels. It was used for asthma, bronchitis, colitis, colon problems, and all lung problems.

Vitamin and Mineral Content:

Slippery Elm contains vitamins A, F, K and P, which are all important for building and toning the stomach, lungs and colon. It contains iron, sodium, calcium, selenium, iodine, copper, zinc, potassium and phosphorus.

ABSCESSES	Flu
Appendicitis	Hemorrhoids
ASTHMA	Herpes
Bladder Problems	Inflammation
Boils	Kidneys
BRONCHITIS	Laxative
BURNS	LUNGS
Cancer	Pain
COLITIS	Phlegm
COLON	Pneumonia
CONSTIPATION	Sore Throat
COUGHS	Sores
Croup	Syphilis
DIAPER RASH	Tuberculosis
DIARRHEA	Tumors
DIGESTION	Ulcers
Diphtheria	Urinary Problems
Dysentery	Vaginal Irritations
Eczema	Warts
Eyes	Worms
Female Problems	Wounds
Fevers	Whooping Cough

SUMA
(Pfaffia paniculata)

Parts Used: The bark and root
Properties: Tonic, nutrient, stimulant, and adaptation.
Body Systems Affected: Blood, liver, spleen, and glands.

Functions and Health Benefits:

Suma is found in the rain forests of Brazil. It has an ancient reputation among herbalists, shamans and physicians in Brazil and is used as a tonic, food, wound healer, anti-diabetic and an aphrodisiac. Suma has been used as a source of energy, a rejuvenator, a treatment for serious diseases, and for almost all illnesses. It is reported to be more powerful than ginseng.(183) Suma is thought to be valuable in treating diabetes, joint diseases, osteomyelitis, elevated blood cholesterol, uric acid build-up and a range of cancers. Suma has been found to stimulate the production of estrogen without stimulating an excess.(184) A professor, Nobushige Nishimoto, researched Suma in Japan and found that the root contains pfaffic acid, capable of inhibiting certain types of cancerous cells. He also reported that Suma has properties that combat anemia, bronchitis, cholesterol, diabetes, fatigue, stress and other infirmities. (185)

Suma has been used traditionally to strengthen the immune system and to treat immune related diseases such as cancer, leukemia, Hodgkin's disease, and diabetes. It enhances energy in the body and promotes longevity. It may also help relieve stress on the body, protect against viral infections, restore sexual function and promote the healing of wounds.

Vitamin and Mineral Content:

Suma contains some B-complex vitamins, minerals and amino acids. It is an adaptogenic plant, which contains essential nutrients such as iron, magnesium and germanium. Germanium is a natural mineral found to have anti-cancer properties. It helps promote a healthy flow of oxygen to the cells. It contains allantoin known to promote wound-healing.

Anemia	Hot Flashes
Arthritis	Hypoglycemia
Bronchitis	IMMUNE SYSTEM
CANCER	Joint Diseases
CHOLESTEROL	Menopause
CIRCULATION	Osteomyelitis
Colds	Osteoporosis
DEGENERATIVE	Skin Problems
DISEASES	STRESS
DIABETES	Strokes
Emotional Swings	TONIC
Energy	Tumors
FATIGUE	VITALITY
Heart	Wounds
HORMONE BALANCE	

TEA TREE OIL
(Meleleuca alternifolia)

Part Used: The oil of the leaves
Properties: Disinfectant, germicide, fungicide, bactericide, antiseptic, and mild anesthetic.
Body Parts Affected: Skin and blood.

Functions and Health Benefits:

Tea Tree Oil was discovered by Captain James Cook in 1770 while on an expedition to Australia with a botanist, Sir John Banks, who collected samples of the leaves and took them to England for further studies. The Aborigines were known to chew on the leaves. It was used as a medicinal agent for cuts, burns, bites and many skin ailments.

Research done in the 1950's and early 1960's found that Tea Tree Oil is a germicide and fungicide with additional characteristics of dissolving pus and debris. (186) Recent studies have found it effective for thrush, vaginal infections of candida albicans, staph infections, athlete's foot, hair and scalp problems, mouth sores, muscle and joint pain, pain, and boils. (187)

Vitamin and Mineral Content:

Research has found that Tea Tree Oil is a very complex substance containing 48 different compounds. All these work together synergistically to produce the maximum healing power. These compounds consist mainly of terpinenes, cymones, pinenes, terpineols, cinerol, sesquiterpenes, and sesquiterpene alcohols.

Athlete's Foot	JOINT PAIN
BOILS	Mouth Sores
Bruises	Muscle Pain
Burns	SKIN DISORDERS
CANDIDA	STAPH INFECTION
Fungus	STREP INFECTION
INFECTIONS	Thrush
Insect Bites	

UVA URSI

(Arctostaphylos uva-ursi)

Part Used: The leaves
Properties: Astringent, antiseptic, diuretic, alterative, and tonic.
Body Parts Affected: Kidneys, spleen, and urinary tract.

Functions and Health Benefits:

A Roman physician, Galen, used Uva Ursi's leaves to treat wounds and to stop bleeding. (188) It has been used by the Chinese for more than 1,000 years as a diuretic and antiseptic for the urinary tract. Native Americans knew the value of Uva Ursi also known as Bearberry. They drank the tea of the steeped leaves to strengthen and heal bladder and kidney problems and women's disorders. Uva Ursi was admitted to the *London Pharmacopoeia* in 1763, and the *U.S. Pharmacopoeia* in 1820 until 1963. Dr. Edward E. Shook used it for its diuretic action for diseases of the bladder and kidneys.

Uva Ursi has been studied and been found to contain allantoin, a substance found to be healing and soothing to irritated tissues. Experiments by Rumanian scientists in 1980 found it to contain anti-trichomonal, anti viral, and antibacterial properties. (189)

Herbalist have recommended Uva Ursi for strengthening the urinary system, and preventing and treating bladder and kidney infections. It can help increase the flow of urine. It helps to reduce inflammation, aids with diabetes, arthritis, and hemorrhaging.

Vitamin and Mineral Content:

Uva Ursi contains iron and some trace minerals, which enable the blood to carry oxygen from the lungs to the rest of the body. Manganese content is found and needed for the nervous system, brain, and strong bones. Vitamin A is known for its healing powers. It works with the other properties of Uva Ursi for healing the urinary tract.

Arthritis	Infection
Bedwetting	KIDNEY INFECTIONS
BLADDER	Liver
INFECTIONS	Lung Congestion
Bright's Disease	Menstruation
Bronchitis	NEPHRITIS
CYSTITIS	Pancreas
DIABETES	Prostate
Diarrhea	Rheumatism
Digestion	SPLEEN
Dysentery	URETHRITIS
Female Problems	Uric Acid
Fevers	Urinary Disorders
Gallstones	Uterus
GONORRHEA	Vaginal Discharge
Gravel	Venereal Disease
Hemorrhoids	Water Retention

VALERIAN
(Valeriana officinalis)

Part Used: The root
Properties: Antiseptic, nervine, stimulant, carminative, diuretic, and tonic.
Body Parts Affected: Nerves, brain, liver, and heart.

Functions and Health Benefits:

Galen, a Greek physician, prescribed Valerian as a decongestant. The ancient Greeks also used it for digestion, nausea, and urinary tract disorders. John Gerard, an herbalist in 1597, recommended this herb for chest congestion, convulsions, bruises and falls. Native Americans used Valerian for healing wounds. Samuel Thomson recommended using Valerian as a tranquilizer. It was accepted in the *U.S. Pharmacopoeia* as a tranquilizer in 1820 until 1942 and in the *National Formulary* until 1950.

Studies done have identified some of the properties of Valerian. It has been found to act as a relaxant and is effective for insomnia. (190) The active ingredients in the herb are responsible for relaxing the smooth muscle tissue and depressing the central nervous system. (191)

Valerian is beneficial for the heart, lungs, liver, stomach as well as the nerves and the brain. It may also help with epilepsy, hysteria, migraines, and eliminating worms. It is a strong nervine herb which produces a calming effect to aid individuals suffering from insomnia, anxiety, muscle spasms, and nervous tension. It is usually recommended for short term use.

Vitamin and Mineral Content:

Valerian is rich in calcium, which accounts for its ability to strengthen the spine, nerves and brain. It is high in magnesium, which works with calcium for healthy bones and the nervous system. It is high in selenium, which strengthens the body against immune related disorders. Manganese is also found which is needed along with calcium for strong nerves and bones. The niacin content helps prevent cholesterol build-up, irritability, depression, loss of memory and weakness. Valerian also contains potassium, iron, sodium, zinc, silicon, vitamins A and C.

AFTERBIRTH PAINS
Alcoholism
Arthritis (pain)
Bladder
BLOOD PRESSURE
Bronchial Spasms
Colds
Constipation
CONVULSIONS
Coughs
Cramps
Digestion
Drug Addiction
Epilepsy
Fatigue
Fever
Gas

Headache
HEART PALPITATIONS
HIGH BLOOD PRESSURE
HYPOCHONDRIA
HYSTERIA
Insomnia
Measles
Menstruation
MUSCLE SPASMS
NERVOUS CONDITIONS
PAIN
Palsy
Restlessness
Stomach
Stress
Ulcers
Worms

WHITE OAK BARK
(Quercus alba)

Part Used: The bark
Properties: Astringent, antiseptic, and diuretic.
Body Parts Affected: Skin, kidneys, and gastro-intestinal tract.

Functions and Health Benefits:

Native Americans used White Oak Bark as a poultice for gangrene. The Iroquois used it as an astringent, the Penobscotts for bleeding piles, the Houmas crushed the roots and mixed them with whiskey for a liniment to rub on rheumatic parts, the Ojibwas scraped the root bark and inner bark and boiled them for a decoction for diarrhea, the Meskwakis drank the tea to expel phlegm from the lungs, and the Menominees used the bark as an infusion for treating hemorrhoids. The inner bark was listed in the *U.S. Pharmacopoeia* from 1820 to 1916.

Research has found that White Oak Bark has astringent and antiseptic properties. (192)

The clotting and shrinking action of this herb is very useful to tighten gums in loose teeth and pyorrhea as well as any gum infection. It has been used for excess stomach mucus which causes common complaints of sinus congestion and post-nasal drip. The stomach is strengthened for better absorption and secretion thus improving metabolism. It has been used to treat diarrhea, external and internal bleeding, varicose veins, hemorrhoids, and excess mucus. It is used to treat inflamed areas of the skin, mucous membranes, stomach and intestines. It aids the stomach by increasing the internal absorption and secretion and improving metabolism.

Vitamin and Mineral Content:

White Oak Bark is rich in calcium, which is involved in blood clotting along with the astringent properties which make it healing and nourishing. Calcium is responsible for helping regulate contraction and relaxation of the muscles and also for the absorption of vitamin B-12. It is high in manganese, which is important for the immune system. It also contains selenium, which is an essential mineral found to protect against immune related diseases including cancer. It also contains iodine and sulphur.

Bites (insect and snake)	Liver
Bladder	MENSTRUAL PROBLEMS
BLEEDING (internal and external)	MOUTH SORES
Bruises	Nausea
Cancer	Prostate
Canker Sores	Pyorrhea
Dental Problems	SKIN IRRITATIONS
Diarrhea	Spleen
Enema	TEETH
Fevers	THRUSH
Gallstones	Tonsillitis
Gangrene	Tumors
Gingivitis	ULCERS
Glandular Swelling	Uterus
Goiter	Vaginal Problems
Gums	VARICOSE VEINS
HEMORRHOIDS	Venereal Disease
Indigestion	Vomiting
Jaundice	WORMS
Kidneys	Wounds

WILD YAM

(Dioscorea villosa)

Part Used: The root
Properties: Antispasmodic, cholagogue, diaphoretic, and anti-inflammatory.
Body Parts Affected: Muscles, joints, uterus, liver and gall bladder.

Functions and Health Benefits:

Wild Yam was used by Native Americans as a root decoction to relieve the pains of childbirth and to treat muscular rheumatism. The Aztecs used Wild Yam to treat skin disorders such as scabies and as a poultice for boils. The Mexican yam is a source of testosterone. Jethro Kloss in his book says that Wild Yam combined with ginger can help in preventing miscarriage. (193)

Studies on animals suggest that the Wild Yam contains steroid-like properties which inhibit inflammation. (194)

Wild Yam relaxes the muscular fiber, soothes the nerves and relieves pain, especially on the uterus. It is often used to balance hormones to treat nausea in pregnant women and to aid in preventing miscarriage, cramps and general pains during pregnancy. It is a blood cleanser and helps strengthen the liver, reduces cholesterol levels, and lower blood pressure. It helps relieve pain associated with gallstones, relaxes muscular fiber and soothes the nervous system.

Vitamin and Mineral Content:

Wild Yam contains vitamin A and zinc, which are both healing and protect against cell damage. It contains iron, manganese, calcium, magnesium, phosphorus, potassium, selenium, vitamin C, sodium, silicon and some B-Complex vitamins.

Abdominal Pain
ARTHRITIS
ASTHMA (spasmodic)
Blood Purifier
Boils
BOWEL SPASMS
Bronchitis
Catarrh
Cholera
COLIC
GAS
Hiccough
Inflammation
Intestines
Jaundice
LIVER
MENSTRUAL CRAMPS
MORNING SICKNESS
MUSCLE PAIN
Nausea
Nervousness
Pain
Rheumatism
SPASMS
Stomach
Ulcers
Whooping Cough

WOOD BETONY
(Betonica officinalis)

Part Used: The herb
Properties: Nervine, alterative, aromatic, hepatic, parasiticide, and analgesic.
Body Parts Affected: Nerves, liver, spleen, and gallbladder.

Functions and Health Benefits:

An ancient herbalist, Antonius Musa, who was the Roman physician to Caesar Augustus wrote a book devoted to the value of Betony. He suggested it for preserving the liver and bodies of men from epidemic diseases, digestion of meat, weak stomachs, and belching. In 1611, a German pharmacist, Schroeder, said that Wood Betony could help with almost any ailment.

Research has found Wood Betony to have hypotensive properties and is a relaxing nervine herb. (195) More research needs to be done but it is useful for pain relief, as a relaxant, catarrh, fatigue, as a brain enhancer, and a general tonic.

Traditional uses of Wood Betony include nervous disorders, as a sedative, head and facial pain, blood purifier, strengthens the liver, gentle laxative, and indigestion.

Vitamin and Mineral Content:

Wood Betony contains magnesium which along with calcium soothes the nerves. Low levels are associated with mental disturbances such as depression, schizophrenia and insomnia. It also contains manganese which is important for thyroid function and vital to the nerves and brain. Phosphorus is found, which is important for every chemical reaction in the body as well as in strengthening the bones, nerve impulses, hormone secretions and protein synthesis.

Anemia	HYSTERIA
Arthritis	Indigestion
Asthma	Insanity
Bladder	Insomnia
Bleeding (internal)	JAUNDICE
Blood Purifier	Kidneys
Bronchitis	LIVER
Colds	Lung Congestion
Colic	Menstruation
Convulsions	Muscle Spasms
Consumption	NERVOUSNESS
DELIRIUM	Neuralgia
Diarrhea	Pain
Digestion	Parasites
Dropsy	PARKINSON'S DISEASE
Epilepsy	Rheumatism
Fainting	Stomach Cramps
FEVERS	Ulcers
Gout	Varicose Veins
HEADACHES	WORMS
Heartburn	Wounds
Heart	

WORMWOOD ―――――――

(Artemisia absinthium)

Parts Used: The herb and leaves
Properties: Tonic, stomachic, febrifuge, and anthelmintic.
Body Parts Affected: Liver, gallbladder, stomach and intestines.

Functions and Health Benefits:

European Wormwood was used in medicine since ancient times. It was used against worms by Dioscorides and Pliny. It was mentioned by Tragus in *Brunfels' Herbal*, in 1531, imported to Italy, and mentioned as having its most positive effect upon roundworms. It was used in Germany as a wine flavoring. Edward E. Shook, M.D. mentions it as being of great value in melancholia, yellow jaundice and dropsy. Herbalists value Wormwood as a stimulant to promote sweating and improve digestion. It can expel worms and improve liver function.

Research has been done on its anti-malarial properties. No recent research has been done on the anti-parasitic effects of Wormwood.

It has been used for poor circulation, rheumatism, fevers, colds, and jaundice. Herbalists have also recommended Wormwood for indigestion, stomach acidity, and constipation. It has also been used to expel worms, promote menstruation, stimulate uterine circulation, menstrual cramps, and as an insect repellent. It is usually recommended to be used for only short periods of time and is not for children.

Vitamin and Mineral Content:

Wormwood contains B-complex vitamins necessary for liver health, eliminating toxins and estrogen activity. It also has vitamin C, which is necessary for physical and mental stress and needed by the adrenal glands to synthesize hormones. It also contains manganese, calcium, potassium and sodium.

Appetite
Blood Circulation
CONSTIPATION
CRAMPS (menstrual)
DEBILITY
Diarrhea
DIGESTION
Dropsy
Earaches
Female Disorders
FEVER
Gallbladder
Gout
Indigestion
INFLAMMATION (GI tract)
Insect Repellent

JAUNDICE
Kidneys
LIVER PROBLEMS
MENSTRUATION
   (promotes)
Morning Sickness
Nausea
Neuralgia
Obesity
Poisons
Rheumatism
STOMACH PROBLEMS
Swelling
Tonic
WORMS

YARROW
(Achillea millefolium)

Part Used: The flower
Properties: Astringent, antiseptic, diaphoretic, homeostatic, diuretic, and stimulant.
Body Parts Affected: Circulation, liver and lungs.

Functions and Health Benefits:

Yarrow was used anciently by the Greeks and named after the legendary warrior Achilles. It was used in the old world for menstrual problems, indigestion, hemorrhoids, and wounds. Culpepper, a 17th century English herbalist, suggested Yarrow for wounds. The Paiutes used it as a tea for a weak stomach. It was used by some Native American tribes for swelling, earaches, bruises, and abrasions. Yarrow was listed in the *U.S. Pharmacopoeia* from 1863 to 1882 and recommended for promoting menstruation and for its stimulant properties. Yarrow has been used for just about every ailment in its history and has proven healing properties.

Research has found Yarrow extract to contain slight antibiotic properties. (196) Yarrow has also demonstrated some anti-spasmodic properties. (197) A volatile oil in Yarrow known as azulene and related compounds have been shown in studies to have anti-inflammatory properties. (198) The properties of each species, the age and environment may contain different chemical components.

Yarrow acts as a blood cleanser, is good for colds, fevers, flu, lung disorders, nose bleeds, and perspiration. It also helps regulate and improve the function of the liver. It tones the mucous membranes of the stomach and bowels and aids the glandular system.

Vitamin and Mineral Content:

Yarrow contains vitamin A, which is useful for healing, lung protection, the immune system, skin disorders, colds, flu and fevers. Vitamin E is also found, which heals and protects the heart and circulatory system. It contains vitamin F, an essential fatty acid necessary for all body membranes, including the brain cells, and they are the basis for the production of the prostaglandins, a hormone like substances produced in the cells. Yarrow also contains manganese, potassium, iodine, and iron.

Abrasions	Hair Loss
Ague	Headaches
Appetite	Hemorrhoids
Bladder	Hysteria
BLOOD PURIFIER	Jaundice
Blood Pressure	LUNGS (hemorrhage)
BOWELS (hemorrhage)	Malaria
Bright's Disease	MEASLES
Bronchitis	Menstrual Bleeding
Bruises	Mucous Membranes
Burns	NOSE BLEEDS
Cancer	PERSPIRATION
CATARRH	(obstructed)
Chicken Pox	Pleurisy
COLDS	Pneumonia
Cramps	Rheumatism
Cuts	Skin Problems
Diarrhea (infants)	Smallpox
Epilepsy	Stomach Problems
Female Disorders	SWEATING (promotes)
FEVERS	Typhoid Fever
FLU	Ulcers
Gas	Urinary Problems

YELLOW DOCK
(Rumex crispus)

Part Used: The root
Properties: Alterative, astringent, antibiotic, cholagogue, laxative, and nutrient.
Body Parts Affected: Blood, skin, spleen, liver, and gallbladder.

Functions and Health Benefits:

Yellow Dock was a favorite herb among Native Americans for a variety of ailments including scrofula, eruptive diseases, and infections of the eyes, ears and skin. Many herbalists have used Yellow Dock for blood and glandular problems including cancer, leprosy, and lung and bowel bleeding. Yellow Dock was listed in the *U.S. Pharmacopoeia* from 1863 until 1905.

It has been found to be a good alterative, especially for chronic skin problems. It is useful for leprosy, psoriasis and cancer. (199)

Modern herbalists recommend Yellow Dock for anemia, as a blood purifier, for liver congestion, and skin problems. It is also considered beneficial for toxemia, infections, lymph congestion, ulcers and wounds. It is considered one of the best blood builders in the herbal kingdom.

Vitamin and Mineral Content:

Yellow Dock is rich in organic iron, which is essential for cleaning and nourishing the blood. It also contains vitamins A and C, which are both important antioxidants for protecting against auto-immune diseases. It is also high in manganese which may be responsible for many functions in the body. It also has magnesium, phosphorus, selenium, and some B-complex vitamins.

Acne	Hay fever
ANEMIA	Hemorrhoids (external)
Arthritis	Hepatitis
Bladder	HIVES
Blood Disorders	Jaundice
BLOOD PURIFIER	Leprosy
Bowels (bleeding)	Leukemia
Bronchitis	LIVER CONGESTION
CANCER	Lymphatic System
Constipation	RHEUMATISM
COUGHS	Scurvy
Dysentery	SKIN PROBLEMS
Dyspepsia	Spleen
Ear Infections	Stomach Problems
Eczema	Thyroid Gland
Energy	Tumors
EYELIDS (ulcerated)	Ulcers
Fatigue	Varicose Veins
Fevers	Venereal Disease
Gallbladder	Vitality

YUCCA
(Yucca glauca)

Part Used: The root
Properties: Antibacterial, astringent, tonic, and aperient.
Body Parts Affected: Blood, digestive system, skin, liver, spleen and gallbladder.

Functions and Health Benefits:

Native Americans used Yucca for arthritis and rheumatism. The Hopi tribe in northern Arizona used Yucca for childbirth, and as a laxative. It was also used for skin disorders, to stop bleeding, and as a poultice for breaks, sprains and for rheumatism.

Studies have shown that Yucca contains non-toxic steroid saponins which are similar to cortisone. These properties are useful in cases of arthritis, rheumatism, high blood pressure, and high cholesterol levels in the blood. (200)

Yucca contains saponins that improve the body's ability to produce a natural cortisone to help with inflammation, healing and pain. Herbalists often recommend Yucca for arthritis and rheumatism. It is also used for intestinal problems and to aid digestion.

Vitamin and Mineral Content:

Yucca contains calcium, which is easily assimilated to help nourish and clean the joints. It contains sodium, zinc and selenium, which are all necessary for healing. It also has magnesium, phosphorus, potassium, iron, manganese, silicon, vitamins A, C and niacin.

Addison's Disease	Gallbladder
ARTHRITIS	Gonorrhea
BLOOD PURIFIER	Gout
Bursitis	Inflammation
Cancer	Liver
CHOLESTEROL	RHEUMATISM
Colitis	Skin Disorders
Dandruff	Venereal Disease

REFERENCES

SINGLE HERBS

Alfalfa

1. Weiner, Michael A. Ph.D. and Janet A. Weiner. *Herbs That Heal.* Mill Valley, CA: Quantum Books, 1994, p 59.

2. Duke, James. *Handbook of Medicinal Herbs.* Boca Raton, Florida: CRC Press, Inc. 1985, p 299.

3. Weiner, Michael A. Ph. D. and Janet A. Weiner. *Herbs That Heal.* Mill Valley, CA: Quantum Books, 1994, p 59.

Aloe vera

4. Weiner, Michael A. Ph. D. and Janet A. Weiner. *Herbs That Heal.* Mill Valley, CA: Quantum Books, 1994, p 61.

5. Duke, James. *Handbook of Medicinal Herbs.* Boca Raton, Florida: CRC Press, Inc. 1985, p 31.

6. Murray, Michael, N.D. and Joseph Pizzorno, N.D. *Encyclopedia of Natural Medicine.* Rocklin, CA: Prima Publishing, 1991, p 406.

Angelica

7. Holmes, Peter. *The Energetics of Western Herbs.* Boulder: Artemis Press, 1989, p 275.

8. Holmes, Peter. *The Energetics of Western Herbs.* Boulder: Artemis Press, 1989, p 276.

9. Montagna, Joseph F. *The People's Desk Reference.* Lake Oswego, OR: Quest For Truth Publishing, Inc., 1979, p 719.

Bee Pollen

10. Weiner, Michael A. Ph. D. and Janet A. Weiner. *Herbs That Heal.* Mill Valley, CA: Quantum Books, 1994, p 80.

11. Weiner, Michael A. Ph. D. and Janet A. Weiner. *Herbs That Heal.* Mill Valley, CA: Quantum Books, 1994, p 80.

Bilberry

12. McCaleb, Rob. "Bilberry, Health From Head to Toe." *Better Nutrition For Today's Living.* June, 1991.

13. Weiss, Rudolf Fritz MD. *Herbal Medicine.* Beaconsfield, England: Beaconsfield Publishers LTD, 1988, p102.

14. Holmes, Peter. *The Energetics of Western Herbs.* Boulder: Artemis Press, 1989, p 84.

15. Weiner, Michael A. Ph. D. and Janet A. Weiner. *Herbs That Heal.* Mill Valley, CA: Quantum Books, 1994, p 84.

Black Cohosh

16. Duke, James. *Handbook of Medicinal Herbs.* Boca Raton, Florida: CRC Press, Inc. 1985, p 120.

17. Holmes, Peter. *The Energetics of Western Herbs.* Boulder: Artemis Press, 1989, p 436.

18. Murray, Michael, N.D. and Joseph Pizzorno, N.D. *Encyclopedia of Natural Medicine.* Rocklin, CA: Prima Publishing, 1991, p 462.

Black Walnut

19. Mowrey, Daniel B. *The Scientific Validation of Herbs.* New Canaan, Connecticut: Keats Publishing, Inc., 1986, p 230.

20. Holmes, Peter. *The Energetics of Western Herbs.* Boulder: Artemis Press, 1989, p 416.

Blessed Thistle

21. Weiner, Michael A. Ph. D. and Janet A. Weiner. *Herbs That Heal.* Mill Valley, CA: Quantum Books, 1994, p 87.

22. Holmes, Peter. *The Energetics of Western Herbs.* Boulder: Artemis Press, 1989, p 278.

Blue Cohosh

23. Duke, James. *Handbook of Medicinal Herbs.* Boca Raton, Florida: CRC Press, Inc. 1985, p 108.

24. Duke, James. *Handbook of Medicinal Herbs.* Boca Raton, Florida: CRC Press, Inc. 1985, p 108.

25. "Blue Cohosh." *The Lawrence Review of Natural Products.* St Louis: Facts and Comparisons, Oct. 1992.

26. Holmes, Peter. *The Energetics of Western Herbs.* Boulder: Artemis Press, 1989, p 638.

27. Holmes, Peter. *The Energetics of Western Herbs.* Boulder: Artemis Press, 1989, p 638.

Blue Green Algae

28. Weiner, Michael A. Ph. D. and Janet A. Weiner. *Herbs That Heal.* Mill Valley, CA: Quantum Books, 1994, p 296.

29. Weiner, Michael A. Ph. D. and Janet A. Weiner. *Herbs That Heal.* Mill Valley, CA: Quantum Books, 1994, p 296.

Blue Vervain

30. Shook, Edward E. *Advanced Treatise In Herboloby.* Lakemont, Georgia: CSA Press, 1978, 276.

31. Meyer, Joseph E. *The Herbalist.* Glenwood, Illinois: Meyer Books, 1918, p 22.

32. Mowrey, Daniel B. *The Scientific Validation of Herbs.* New Canaan, Connecticut: Keats Publishing, Inc., 1986, p 120.

Boneset

33. Holmes, Peter. *The Energetics of Western Herbs.* Boulder: Artemis Press, 1989, p 131.

34. Shook, Edward E. *Advanced Treatise In Herboloby.* Lakemont, Georgia: CSA Press, 1978, 285.

35. Hutchens, Alma R. *Indian Herbology of North America.* Ontario, Canada: Merco, 1969, pp 60-61.

36. Murray, Michael, N.D. and Joseph Pizzorno, N.D. *Encyclopedia of Natural Medicine.* Rocklin, CA: Prima Publishing, 1991, p 61.

Borage

37. Murray, Michael, N.D. and Joseph Pizzorno, N.D. *Encyclopedia of Natural Medicine.* Rocklin, CA: Prima Publishing, 1991, p 391.

38. Ody, Penelope. *The Complete Medicinal Herbal.* London: Dorling Kindersley, 1993, p 41.

39. Tenney, Louise. *Today's Herbal Health*. Provo, Utah: Woodland Books, 1992, p 36.

Burdock

40. Weiner, Michael A. Ph. D. and Janet A. Weiner. *Herbs That Heal*. Mill Valley, CA: Quantum Books, 1994, p 101.

41. Mowrey, Daniel B. *The Scientific Validation of Herbs*. New Canaan, Connecticut: Keats Publishing, Inc., 1986, p 58.

42. Mowrey, Daniel B. *The Scientific Validation of Herbs*. New Canaan, Connecticut: Keats Publishing, Inc., 1986, p 3.

43. Duke, James. *Handbook of Medicinal Herbs*. Boca Raton, Florida: CRC Press, Inc. 1985, p 53.

Butcher's Broom

44. Weiner, Michael A. Ph. D. and Janet A. Weiner. *Herbs That Heal*. Mill Valley, CA: Quantum Books, 1994, p 102.

45. Murray, Michael, N.D. and Joseph Pizzorno, N.D. *Encyclopedia of Natural Medicine*. Rocklin, CA: Prima Publishing, 1991, p 538.

Capsicum

46. Holmes, Peter. *The Energetics of Western Herbs*. Boulder: Artemis Press, 1989, p 322.

47. Mowrey, Daniel B. *The Scientific Validation of Herbs*. New Canaan, Connecticut: Keats Publishing, Inc., 1986, p 40.

48. Hobbs, Christopher. "Cayenne, This Popular Herb is Hot." *Let's Live*. Apr. 1994, p 55.

49. Murray, Michael, N.D. and Joseph Pizzorno, N.D. *Encyclopedia of Natural Medicine*. Rocklin, CA: Prima Publishing, 1991, p 419.

Cascara Sagrada

50. Duke, James. *Handbook of Medicinal Herbs*. Boca Raton, Florida: CRC Press, Inc. 1985, p 404.

51. Murray, Michael, N.D. and Joseph Pizzorno, N.D. *Encyclopedia of Natural Medicine*. Rocklin, CA: Prima Publishing, 1991, p 235.

Catnip

52. Weiner, Michael A. Ph. D. and Janet A. Weiner. *Herbs That Heal*. Mill Valley, CA: Quantum Books, 1994, p 107.

53. Mowrey, Daniel B. *The Scientific Validation of Herbs*. New Canaan, Connecticut: Keats Publishing, Inc., 1986, p 76.

Chamomile

54. Murray, Michael, N.D. and Joseph Pizzorno, N.D. *Encyclopedia of Natural Medicine*. Rocklin, CA: Prima Publishing, 1991, p 55.

55. Murray, Michael, N.D. and Joseph Pizzorno, N.D. *Encyclopedia of Natural Medicine*. Rocklin, CA: Prima Publishing, 1991, p 393.

56. "Chamomile." *The Lawrence Review of Natural Products*. St. Louis: Facts and Comparisons, Mar 1991.

Damiana

57. Hutchens, Alma R. *Indian Herboloby of North America*. Ontario, Canada: Merco, 1969, p 108.

58. Holmes, Peter. *The Energetics of Western Herbs*. Boulder: Artemis Press, 1989, p 300.

59. Holmes, Peter. *The Energetics of Western Herbs*. Boulder: Artemis Press, 1989, p 300.

Dandelion

60. Weiner, Michael A. Ph. D. and Janet A. Weiner. *Herbs That Heal*. Mill Valley, CA: Quantum Books, 1994, p 139.

61. Murray, Michael, N.D. and Joseph Pizzorno, N.D. *Encyclopedia of Natural Medicine*. Rocklin, CA: Prima Publishing, 1991, p 353.

62. Murray, Michael, N.D. and Joseph Pizzorno, N.D. *Encyclopedia of Natural Medicine*. Rocklin, CA: Prima Publishing, 1991, p 141.

63. Holmes, Peter. *The Energetics of Western Herbs*. Boulder: Artemis Press, 1989, p 581.

64. Mowrey, Daniel B. *The Scientific Validation of Herbs*. New Canaan, Connecticut: Keats Publishing, Inc., 1986, p 249.

Devil's Claw

65. Murray, Michael, N.D. and Joseph Pizzorno, N.D. *Encyclopedia of Natural Medicine*. Rocklin, CA: Prima Publishing, 1991, p 339.

66. Duke, James. *Handbook of Medicinal Herbs*. Boca Raton, Florida: CRC Press, Inc. 1985, p 222.

67. Weiner, Michael A. Ph. D. and Janet A. Weiner. *Herbs That Heal*. Mill Valley, CA: Quantum Books, 1994, p 140.

Dong Quai

68. Weiner, Michael A. Ph. D. and Janet A. Weiner. *Herbs That Heal*. Mill Valley, CA: Quantum Books, 1994, p 63.

69. Weiner, Michael A. Ph. D. and Janet A. Weiner. *Herbs That Heal*. Mill Valley, CA: Quantum Books, 1994, p 63.

70. Murray, Michael, N.D. and Joseph Pizzorno, N.D. *Encyclopedia of Natural Medicine*. Rocklin, CA: Prima Publishing, 1991, p 462.

Echinacea

71. Murray, Michael, N.D. *The Healing Power of Herbs*. Rocklin, CA: Prima Publishing, 1992, p 88.

72. "Echinacea." *The Lawrence Review of Natural Products*. St. Louis: Facts and Comparisons, Jan. 1990.

73. Mowrey, Daniel B. *The Scientific Validation of Herbs*. New Canaan, Connecticut: Keats Publishing, Inc., 1986, p 119.

74. Mowrey, Daniel B. *The Scientific Validation of Herbs*. New Canaan, Connecticut: Keats Publishing, Inc., 1986, p 250.

Elder Flower

75. Holmes, Peter. *The Energetics of Western Herbs*. Boulder: Artemis Press, 1989, pp 121, 122.

Elecampane

76. Shook, Edward E. *Advanced Treatise In Herbology.* Lakemont, Georgia: CSA Press, 1978, pp 292, 293.

77. Weiner, Michael A. Ph. D. and Janet A. Weiner. *Herbs That Heal.* Mill Valley, CA: Quantum Books, 1994, p 144.

78. Kloss, Jethro. *Back to Eden.* Loma Linda, CA: Back to Eden Books, 1971, p 238.

Ephedra

79. Murray, Michael, N.D. *The Healing Power of Herbs.* Rocklin, CA: Prima Publishing, 1992, p 143.

80. Weiner, Michael A. Ph. D. and Janet A. Weiner. *Herbs That Heal.* Mill Valley, CA: Quantum Books, 1994, p 146.

False Unicorn

81. Weiner, Michael A. Ph. D. and Janet A. Weiner. *Herbs That Heal.* Mill Valley, CA: Quantum Books, 1994, p 151.

82. Murray, Michael, N.D. and Joseph Pizzorno, N.D. *Encyclopedia of Natural Medicine.* Rocklin, CA: Prima Publishing, 1991, p 462.

Fennel

83. "Fennel." *The Lawrence Review of Natural Products.* St. Louis: Facts and Comparisons, Mar 1988.

84. Mowrey, Daniel B. *The Scientific Validation of Herbs.* New Canaan, Connecticut: Keats Publishing, Inc., 1986, p 76.

Fenugreek

85. Murray, Michael, N.D. and Joseph Pizzorno, N.D. *Encyclopedia of Natural Medicine.* Rocklin, CA: Prima Publishing, 1991, p 282.

86. Weiner, Michael A. Ph. D. and Janet A. Weiner. *Herbs That Heal.* Mill Valley, CA: Quantum Books, 1994, p 153.

87. Balch, James F. MD and Phyllis A. Balch, C.N.C. *Prescription for Nutritional Healing.* Garden City Park, N.Y.: Avery Publishing Group Inc., 1990, p 52.

Garlic

88. Balch, James F. MD and Phyllis A. Balch, C.N.C. *Prescription for Nutritional Healing.* Garden City Park, N.Y.: Avery Publishing Group Inc., 1990, p 42.

89. Mowrey, Daniel B. *The Scientific Validation of Herbs.* New Canaan, Connecticut: Keats Publishing, Inc., 1986, pp 122, 123.

90. "Garlic." *The Lawrence Review of Natural Products.* St. Louis: Facts and Comparisons, Apr 1994.

91. Weiner, Michael A. Ph. D. and Janet A. Weiner. *Herbs That Heal.* Mill Valley, CA: Quantum Books, 1994, p 160.

92. Weiner, Michael A. Ph. D. and Janet A. Weiner. *Herbs That Heal.* Mill Valley, CA: Quantum Books, 1994, p 160.

93. *Reader's Digest Family Guide to Natural Medicine.* Pleasantville, N.Y.: The Reader's Digest Association, Inc., 1993, p 308.

Gentian

94. Weiner, Michael A. Ph. D. and Janet A. Weiner. *Herbs That Heal*. Mill Valley, CA: Quantum Books, 1994, p 162.

95. Murray, Michael, N.D. and Joseph Pizzorno, N.D. *Encyclopedia of Natural Medicine*. Rocklin, CA: Prima Publishing, 1991, p 55.

Ginger

96. "Ginger." *The Lawrence Review of Natural Products*. St. Louis: Facts and Comparisons, Nov 1991.

97. Weiner, Michael A. Ph. D. and Janet A. Weiner. *Herbs That Heal*. Mill Valley, CA: Quantum Books, 1994, pp 163, 164.

98. *Reader's Digest Family Guide to Natural Medicine*. Pleasantville, N.Y.: The Reader's Digest Association, Inc., 1993, 308.

Ginkgo biloba

99. Braly, James MD. "A Scientific Herb for the Symptoms of Aging." *Doctor's Best*. Laguna Hills, CA.

100. Ody, Penelope. *The Complete Medicinal Herbal*. London: Dorling Kindersley, 1993, p 64

Ginseng

101. Duke, James. *Handbook of Medicinal Herbs*. Boca Raton, Florida: CRC Press, Inc. 1985, p 174.

102. Carr, Ann et. al. *Rodale's Illustrated Encyclopedia of Herbs*. Emmaus, Pennsylvania: Rodale Press, 1987, pp 227-229.

Golden Seal

103. Weiner, Michael A. Ph. D. and Janet A. Weiner. *Herbs That Heal*. Mill Valley, CA: Quantum Books, 1994, p 174.

104. Mowrey, Daniel B. *The Scientific Validation of Herbs*. New Canaan, Connecticut: Keats Publishing, Inc., 1986, p 257.

105. Murray, Michael, N.D. and Joseph Pizzorno, N.D. *Encyclopedia of Natural Medicine*. Rocklin, CA: Prima Publishing, 1991, p 67.

106. Murray, Michael, N.D. and Joseph Pizzorno, N.D. *Encyclopedia of Natural Medicine*. Rocklin, CA: Prima Publishing, 1991, p 116.

107. Lieberman, Shari and Nancy Bruning. *The Real Vitamin and Mineral Book*. Garden City Park, N.Y.: Avery Publishing Group, Inc. 1990, p 98.

Gotu Kola

108. Weiner, Michael A. Ph. D. and Janet A. Weiner. *Herbs That Heal*. Mill Valley, CA: Quantum Books, 1994, p 175.

Gymnema sylvestre

109. Kamen, Betty. "Gymnema Extract." *Let's Live*. Sep. 1989, pp 40, 41.

110. *Journal of Ethmopharmacology*. 1986, pp 143-146.

Hawthorn

111. "Hawthorn." *The Lawrence Review of Natural Products*. St. Louis: Facts and Comparisons, May 1987.

112. *Reader's Digest Family Guide to Natural Medicine*. Pleasantville, N.Y.: The Reader's Digest Association, Inc., 1993, p 311.

113. Murray, Michael, N.D. and Joseph Pizzorno, N.D. *Encyclopedia of Natural Medicine*. Rocklin, CA: Prima Publishing, 1991, p 383.

Hops

114. Mowrey, Daniel B. *The Scientific Validation of Herbs*. New Canaan, Connecticut: Keats Publishing, Inc., 1986, p 217.

115. Murray, Michael, N.D. and Joseph Pizzorno, N.D. *Encyclopedia of Natural Medicine*. Rocklin, CA: Prima Publishing, 1991, p 393.

Horsetail

116. Mowrey, Daniel B. *The Scientific Validation of Herbs*. New Canaan, Connecticut: Keats Publishing, Inc., 1986, p 32.

117. Ody, Penelope. *The Complete Medicinal Herbal*. London: Dorling Kindersley, 1993, p 55.

Ho-Shou-Wu

118. Weiner, Michael A. Ph. D. and Janet A. Weiner. *Herbs That Heal*. Mill Valley, CA: Quantum Books, 1994, p 157.

119. Mowrey, Daniel B. *The Scientific Validation of Herbs*. New Canaan, Connecticut: Keats Publishing, Inc., 1986, p 289.

Hyssop

120. *Reader's Digest Family Guide to Natural Medicine*. Pleasantville, N.Y.: The Reader's Digest Association, Inc., 1993, p 313.

Irish Moss

121. Shook, Edward E. *Advanced Treatise In Herbology*. Lakemont, Georgia: CSA Press, 1978, p 150.

122. Mowrey, Daniel B. *The Scientific Validation of Herbs*. New Canaan, Connecticut: Keats Publishing, Inc., 1986, p 260.

Juniper Berries

123. Kloss, Jethro. *Back to Eden*. Loma Linda, CA: Back to Eden Books, 1971, pp 251, 252.

124. Weiner, Michael A. Ph. D. and Janet A. Weiner. *Herbs That Heal*. Mill Valley, CA: Quantum Books, 1994, p 205

125. Mowrey, Daniel B. The Scientific Validation of Herbs. New Canaan, Connecticut: Keats Publishing, Inc., 1986, p 83.

Kava Kava

126. "Kava Kava." *The Lawrence Review of Natural Products*. St. Louis: Facts and Comparisons, May 1987.

Kelp

127. Holmes, Peter. *The Energetics of Western Herbs*. Boulder: Artemis Press, 1989, p 366.

128. Mowrey, Daniel B. *The Scientific Validation of Herbs*. New Canaan, Connecticut: Keats Publishing, Inc., 1986, p 123.

129. Mowrey, Daniel B. *The Scientific Validation of Herbs*. New Canaan, Connecticut: Keats Publishing, Inc., 1986, p 268.

Licorice

130. "Licorice." *The Lawrence Review of Natural Products*. St. Louis: Facts and Comparisons, June 1989.

131. Murray, Michael, N.D. *The Healing Power of Herbs*. Rocklin, CA: Prima Publishing, 1992, p 160.

132. Mowrey, Daniel B. *The Scientific Validation of Herbs*. New Canaan, Connecticut: Keats Publishing, Inc., 1986, p 109.

133. "Licorice." *The Lawrence Review of Natural Products*. St. Louis: Facts and Comparisons, June 1989.

134. *Reader's Digest Family Guide to Natural Medicine*. Pleasantville, N.Y.: The Reader's Digest Association, Inc., 1993, p 315.

Lily of the Valley

135. Weiner, Michael A. Ph. D. and Janet A. Weiner. *Herbs That Heal*. Mill Valley, CA: Quantum Books, 1994, p 214.

136. Duke, James. *Handbook of Medicinal Herbs*. Boca Raton, Florida: CRC Press, Inc. 1985, p 142.

Marshmallow

137. Shook, Edward E. *Advanced Treatise In Herbology*. Lakemont, Georgia: CSA Press, 1978, p 127.

138. Griggs, Barbara. *Green Pharmacy*. Rochester, Vermont: Healing Arts Press, 1981, pp 5, 16.

139. "Marshmallow." *The Lawrence Review of Natural Products*. St. Louis: Facts and Comparisons, Dec 1991.

Milk Thistle

140. Foster, Steven. "Milk Thistle." *Nutrition News*. Vol. XII, No. 10, 1989.

141. Weiss, Rudolf Fritz MD. *Herbal Medicine*. Beaconsfield, England: Beaconsfield Publishers LTD, 1988, pp 82, 83.

Mullein

142. "Mullein." *The Lawrence Review of Natural Products*. St. Louis: Facts and Comparisons, Sep 1989.

143. Mowrey, Daniel B. *The Scientific Validation of Herbs*. New Canaan, Connecticut: Keats Publishing, Inc., 1986, p 241.

144. Balch, James F. MD and Phyllis A. Balch, C.N.C. *Prescription for Nutritional Healing*. Garden City Park, N.Y.: Avery Publishing Group Inc., 1990, p 56.

Myrrh

145. Mowrey, Daniel B. *The Scientific Validation of Herbs*. New Canaan, Connecticut: Keats Publishing, Inc., 1986, p 273.

146. *Reader's Digest Family Guide to Natural Medicine.* Pleasantville, N.Y.: The Reader's Digest Association, Inc., 1993, p 316.

Pan Pien Lien

147. Murray, Michael, N.D. *The Healing Power of Herbs.* Rocklin, CA: Prima Publishing, 1992, pp 138, 139.

148. Holmes, Peter. *The Energetics of Western Herbs.* Boulder: Artemis Press, 1989, p 429.

Passion Flower

149. Holmes, Peter. *The Energetics of Western Herbs.* Boulder: Artemis Press, 1989, p 656.

150. Mowrey, Daniel B. *The Scientific Validation of Herbs.* New Canaan, Connecticut: Keats Publishing, Inc., 1986, p 110.

151. *Reader's Digest Family Guide to Natural Medicine.* Pleasantville, N.Y.: The Reader's Digest Association, Inc., 1993, p 319.

Pau D'Arco

152. Murray, Michael, N.D. *The Healing Power of Herbs.* Rocklin, CA: Prima Publishing, 1992, p 99.

Peppermint

153. "Peppermint." *The Lawrence Review of Natural Products.* St. Louis: Facts and Comparisons, Jul 1990.

154. Murray, Michael, N.D. and Joseph Pizzorno, N.D. *Encyclopedia of Natural Medicine.* Rocklin, CA: Prima Publishing, 1991, p 399.

Prickly Ash

155. Holmes, Peter. *The Energetics of Western Herbs.* Boulder: Artemis Press, 1989, p 334.

Psyllium

156. Weiner, Michael A. Ph. D. and Janet A. Weiner. *Herbs That Heal.* Mill Valley, CA: Quantum Books, 1994, p 271.

157. Kloss, Jethro. *Back to Eden.* Loma Linda, CA: Back to Eden Books, 1971, p 299.

Queen of the Meadow

158. Mowrey, Daniel B. *The Scientific Validation of Herbs.* New Canaan, Connecticut: Keats Publishing, Inc., 1986, p 4.

159. Ody, Penelope. *The Complete Medicinal Herbal.* London: Dorling Kindersley, 1993, p 57.

Red Clover

160. Mowrey, Daniel B. *The Scientific Validation of Herbs.* New Canaan, Connecticut: Keats Publishing, Inc., 1986, p 54.

Red Raspberry

161. Christopher, John R. "Red Raspberry." *Herbalist Magazine.* Vol. 1 No. 4, 1976, p 129.

162. Challem, Jack Joseph and Renate Lewin-Challem. *What Herbs Are All About.* New Canaan, Connecticut: Keats Publishing, 1980, pp 110, 111.

163. Weiner, Michael A. Ph. D. and Janet A. Weiner. *Herbs That Heal*. Mill Valley, CA: Quantum Books, 1994, p 276.

Rose Hips

164. Weiner, Michael A. Ph. D. and Janet A. Weiner. *Herbs That Heal*. Mill Valley, CA: Quantum Books, 1994, p 281.

Saffron

165. "Saffron." *The Lawrence Review of Natural Products*. St. Louis: Facts and Comparisons, Apr 1993.

166. "Saffron." *The Lawrence Review of Natural Products*. St. Louis: Facts and Comparisons, Apr 1993.

St. John's Wort

167. Hobbs, Christopher. "St. John's Wort." *Herbalgram*. Fall/Winter, 1988, p 31.

168. Hobbs, Christopher. "St. John's Wort." *Herbalgram*. Fall/Winter, 1988, p 27.

169. *Reader's Digest Family Guide to Natural Medicine*. Pleasantville, N.Y.: The Reader's Digest Association, Inc., 1993, p 323.

Saw Palmetto

170. Ritchason, Jack. *The Little Herb Encyclopedia*. Pleasant Grove, Ut: Woodland Books, 1994, p 213.

171. Weiner, Michael A. Ph. D. and Janet A. Weiner. *Herbs That Heal*. Mill Valley, CA: Quantum Books, 1994, p 290.

172. Murray, Michael, N.D. and Joseph Pizzorno, N.D. *Encyclopedia of Natural Medicine*. Rocklin, CA: Prima Publishing, 1991, p 484.

173. Weiner, Michael A. Ph. D. and Janet A. Weiner. *Herbs That Heal*. Mill Valley, CA: Quantum Books, 1994, p 291.

Schizandra

174. Weiner, Michael A. Ph. D. and Janet A. Weiner. *Herbs That Heal*. Mill Valley, CA: Quantum Books, 1994, pp 292, 293.

175. Schechter, Steve, ND. "Schizandra." *Let's Live*. Sept 1994, p 76.

Scullcap

176. Castleman, Michael. *The Healing Herbs*. Emmaus, Pennsylvania: Rodale Press, 1991, p 339.

177. Mowrey, Daniel B. *The Scientific Validation of Herbs*. New Canaan, Connecticut: Keats Publishing, Inc., 1986, p 225.

178. Castleman, Michael. *The Healing Herbs*. Emmaus, Pennsylvania: Rodale Press, 1991, p 339.

Senna

179. Balch, James F. MD and Phyllis A. Balch, C.N.C. *Prescription for Nutritional Healing*. Garden City Park, N.Y.: Avery Publishing Group Inc., 1990, p 180.

Slippery Elm

180. Shook, Edward E. *Advanced Treatise In Herbology.* Lakemont, Georgia: CSA Press, 1978, p 163.

181. Shook, Edward E. *Advanced Treatise In Herbology.* Lakemont, Georgia: CSA Press, 1978, p 384.

182. *Reader's Digest Family Guide to Natural Medicine.* Pleasantville, N.Y.: The Reader's Digest Association, Inc., 1993, p 323.

Suma

183. Balch, James F. MD and Phyllis A. Balch, C.N.C. *Prescription for Nutritional Healing.* Garden City Park, N.Y.: Avery Publishing Group Inc., 1990, p 58.

184. Pitchford, Paul. *Healing With Whole Herbs.* Berkeley, CA: North Atlantic Books, 1993, p 182.

185. Murray, Frank. "Suma Lauded." *Better Nutrition.* June 1987, p 17.

Tea Tree Oil

186. Olsen, Cynthia B. *Australian Tea Tree Oil.* Pagosa Springs, CO: Kali Press, 1991.

187. Balch, James F. MD and Phyllis A. Balch, C.N.C. *Prescription for Nutritional Healing.* Garden City Park, N.Y.: Avery Publishing Group Inc., 1990, pp 681, 682.

Uva Ursi

188. Castleman, Michael. *The Healing Herbs.* Emmaus, Pennsylvania: Rodale Press, 1991, p 358.

189. Weiner, Michael A. Ph. D. and Janet A. Weiner. *Herbs That Heal.* Mill Valley, CA: Quantum Books, 1994, pp 78, 79.

Valerian

190. Murray, Michael, N.D. *The Healing Power of Herbs.* Rocklin, CA: Prima Publishing, 1992, p 196.

191. *Reader's Digest Family Guide to Natural Medicine.* Pleasantville, N.Y.: The Reader's Digest Association, Inc., 1993, p 325.

White Oak

192. Weiner, Michael A. Ph. D. and Janet A. Weiner. *Herbs That Heal.* Mill Valley, CA: Quantum Books, 1994, p 247.

Wild Yam

193. Kloss, Jethro. *Back to Eden.* Loma Linda, CA: Back to Eden Books, 1971, p 329.

194. Weiner, Michael A. Ph. D. and Janet A. Weiner. *Herbs That Heal.* Mill Valley, CA: Quantum Books, 1994, p 339.

Wood Betony

195. Mowrey, Daniel B. *The Scientific Validation of Herbs.* New Canaan, Connecticut: Keats Publishing, Inc., 1986, p 193.

Yarrow

196. "Yarrow" *The Lawrence Review of Natural Products.* St. Louis: Facts and Comparisons, Dec. 1987.

197. *Reader's Digest Family Guide to Natural Medicine*. Pleasantville, N.Y.: The Reader's Digest Association, Inc., 1993, p 327.

198. Carr, Anna, et. al. *Rodale's Illustrated Encyclopedia of Herbs*. Emmaus, Pennsylvania: Rodale Press, 1987, p 517.

Yellow Dock

199. Mowrey, Daniel B. *The Scientific Validation of Herbs*. New Canaan, Connecticut: Keats Publishing, Inc., 1986, p 250.

Yucca

200. Spencer, Mike. "Yucca, New Hope For Arthritics." *Let's Live*. Feb 1975.

HEALTH MAINTENANCE

HEALTH MAINTENANCE IN THE MODERN AGE

Even in this advanced technological age, there is something vital missing from people's lives. This is shown in the increase in chronic diseases such as cancers, even among children; the rampant prevalence of cardiovascular disease, as well as autoimmune disorders and other serious ailments.

Benjamin Franklin once quipped: *"Health is Wealth."* How true this is! When you feel good and your body is functioning properly, you have the steady nerves and the energy to accomplish your daily tasks. For people who do not have this treasure, much of life is devoted to a search for that which is truly meaningful...good health. A lifestyle which embraces healthful practices such as stress control, exercise, proper rest, and a nutritious diet, along with herbal supplements has changed countless lives in a positive way. Herbs are natural and act as catalysts to work *with the body*. These gifts from nature can help the body correct imbalances and assist in the healing process.

Herbs can do a better job if the body is kept as free as possible from toxins. We are exposed to toxins everyday from many sources: tap water, the air we breathe, the preservatives and additives in food, even stress can cause harmful substances to form in our bodies. Many nutritionists recommend a *cleanse* before embarking upon a strengthening program in which herbs are taken.

WHAT IS A CLEANSE AND WHY IS IT IMPORTANT?

Basically, a cleanse is just that—a method of treatment in which toxins are eliminated from the body. The body will first try to expel wastes from the intestinal tract and the kidneys. When those areas are free from accumulations, then the liver is able to cleanse and do a better job of filtering toxins from the blood via the hepatic artery. Next, the blood is cleansed, thereby allowing nutrients to be more accessible to the cells and tissues.

Why is it so important to first cleanse the intestinal tract? Of course, we all know that wastes are expelled through this area, but did you know that digestion and assimilation also take place? Nutrients are actually absorbed through the special membranes that line the small intestine. They are then distributed throughout the body to perform the function of fortifying the cells and tissues. However, if the intestinal membrane is coated with years worth of rubbery, hardened accumulations of toxins caused by hard fats, coal-tar based preservatives, etc. these nutrients will be barred from entrance.

In what other ways can the intestinal tract become an impermeable barrier to absorption? In his book "Death Begins in the Colon," Sir Jason Winters writes, "Let's say that you have a perfect bowel, and on a perfect diet. Once in awhile you may ingest something that is harmful. In order to protect itself, the body causes mucus to be formed in the colon long before the harmful food or substance reaches there. The substance reaches the colon several hours later. The mucus has been prepared by the body and is lining the colon so it will not be absorbed when it gets there, so it literally coats the poison. Then later it breaks down and will be discharged from the colon with no harmful effect. Nature's protective mechanism functioned properly, so no harm was done.

"Now, let's say that you ingest mucus-forming foods, which are usually low in fiber. The mucus is secreted maybe five times in a day to protect against toxins from the food you eat and drink. If you do this every day of your life, the mucus lining of the bowel thickens, especially, if you eat white flour products, meat, milk, fried products and other denatured foods. It will be like glue sticking to the colon walls. Nature tries to help, but if forced to work continuously day after day, year after year, the colon will accumulate layers of mucus, like rings of a tree." (*"Death Begins in the Colon,"* by Sir. Jason Winters).

You can compare this process to making tea with a tea strainer. After the nutritious herbs are steeped, the nutrient-laden water is strained into a container. Now, if that tea strainer were lined with clay, what would happen? None of the water could pass through and you would not receive any benefits of the herbs. Interestingly, one study revealed that after cooked food is eaten, white blood cells increase in the intestinal tract in a response to the toxic condition produced there. It has been found that a diet in raw foods does not provoke this occurrence.

It is vital to cleanse the intestinal tract first, because if you try to cleanse the liver or blood first, they would be recontaminated over and over from the toxic intestinal and urinary tracts. If the kidneys and intestines are clogged, then the body will try to eliminate toxins on its own, through the skin. Many skin ailments can be eradicated through utilizing a combination of cleansing and a healthful diet. A conclusion by a medical doctor, after a statistical analysis of 900 patients, stated that "intestinal toxemia is an important causative factor in the production of many skin diseases." (Schwartz, H.J. "Association of Intestinal Indigestion with Various Dermatoses," *Archives of Dermatology and Syphiology*, Vol. 13, 1926, p 674).

It is universally accepted in the wholistic health world that all disease starts in the intestinal tract and that every organ is only as clean as the bowel. Dr. Bernard Jensen, renowned nutritionist has said, "I know this, if you have arthritis you will never get over it until your bowel is right. I don't care what disease you mention, there is a chemical relation to that disease. And the chemical relation should be taken care of first through the bowel." Dr. Jensen has worked with thousands of patients, and helped them through proper colon management.

CONSTIPATION

Simple Constipation

There are three kinds of constipation. The first is *simple constipation*. This occurs when fecal matters remain in the intestines for more than 24 hours. Some would have us believe that three days to a week is normal. However, this is unhealthy. The normal time to eliminate is every six waking hours, or after each full meal. If the bowels do not move every day, constipation does exist. Simple constipation can turn into chronic constipation if the evacuation of the bowel content is not complete for more than a week. This is usually caused by a low-fiber diet, irregular meals, lack of exercise, and neglecting nature's urges to eliminate.

Cumulative Constipation

The second type of constipation is *cumulative constipation*. This is the most common form and it is almost always confined to the lower part of the colon. It is caused by a lazy lower bowel. Straining can cause injury to the colon walls and the ileocecal valve. It can also promote hemorrhoids (both internal and external), varicose veins, lower back pain and many other ailments.

Latent Constipation

The third kind of constipation is *latent constipation*. In this condition, the bowels move regularly, or at least daily. The person has no idea that constipation exists. However, the symptoms are numerous. They include headaches, bad breath, appendicitis and colitis. This is caused by advanced putrefaction because of long retention and incomplete evacuation of wastes. Some people can have more than one type of constipation and this is referred to as *mixed constipation*. (Kellogg, M.D., John Harvey, *Colon Hygiene*, 1916, pp 195-200.)

Acute and Chronic Disease

An acute disease is a short-term ailment like a cold or flu. It is actually nature's way of initiating a cleanse on its own. When a person has a "runny nose", diarrhea, vomiting, etc., nature is purging the body of toxins. To help nature along, go on a short fast and use herbs and juices to heal. A chronic disease, such as arthritis, is more deep-seated and requires long-term and intensive effort by the body to root out the accumulations. You should cleanse, then give the body a rest, and cleanse again, over and over until results are experienced. Sometimes this can take six months to a year. *(For detailed information on how to go on a cleanse please refer to Louise Tenney's Nutritional Guide with Food Combining, pages 4-6).*

Proper Diet

A high (complex) carbohydrate and low-protein diet is the best one for healthful colon maintenance. Complex carbohydrates are primarily found in grains, beans, legumes, and vegetables. If a diet is high in protein, especially meats, then the bacteria which inhabit the intestinal tract will be "proteolytic" or protein splitting and *putrefactive* or protein decomposing. The proteolytic bacteria can change the amino acids in the proteins to powerful poisons in the intestinal tract. Some of these poisons are known as phenol, indole and skatole. (Robbins, S.L.: *Pathologic Basis of Disease,* 1st ed., W.B. Saunders Co., Philadelphia, 1974, p 520. Korenchevsy, V.: *"Autointoxications and Processes of Aging,"* Texas Rep. Biology and Medicine, Vol. 26, 1956, p 106).

The greatest misunderstanding and confusion in the field of nutrition is the failure to properly understand the symptoms and changes which are connected with a better nutritional program.

What happens when foods introduced in the diet are higher quality than what one is used to? When you change from less meat to more grains, beans, fruit, vegetables, nuts, seeds, sprouts, and juices, the body begins to discard the existing excess materials and tissues to make room for the new, cleaner and healthier tissue.

The higher quality of food we learn to add to our diet, the quicker we can expect to recover from disease. We need to learn the proper combination of food, with the most easily digested food eaten first, the more complex one second, the most concentrated ones last. As we get older, we need less food.

Headaches are probably the most common symptom when toxic stimulants such as coffee, tea, soft drinks, cakes, cookies, chocolate, and all sweet junk food are suddenly stopped. This is due to the discarding of toxin by the body when they are removed from the tissues and transported through the bloodstream. Before the toxins are eliminated, they will irritate different parts of the body such as the head and, besides headaches, can also cause depression. They can even stimulate colds, which is nature's way of cleansing the body. The depressive letdown is caused by the slower action of the heart. However, usually within three days (but maybe longer), the heart begins to beat regularly, the symptoms vanish, and then a person feels stronger and has more energy.

One of the main things to realize is not to abandon the improved diet until you have given it a chance. If you go off of it too soon, you may want to return to the old diet because it did not provoke any symptoms. You can fail if you do not give your body a chance to adjust and complete its first recuperative phase. If you wait a little longer, you will feel better than ever before.

After about the first ten days or so, the energies which are primarily contained in the muscles and the skin begin to move to the vital internal organs and will start the reconstruction process. This will produce less energy in the muscles which makes us feel temporarily weak. This is a time when you need to rest. In fact, a change of diet or a fast should only be undertaken when you have the time to rest and relax. The body is using its energies to detoxify the cells.

As one continues to eat higher quality of food, the body begins a process called retracing. This happens when the body is ready to get rid of the toxins. It removes excess bile from the liver and gallbladder and sends it to the intestines to be eliminated. The arteries, veins and capillaries begin to move "sludge" and eliminate it. The deposits in the joints begin to clean. The wastes caused by drugs, preservatives, aspirin, sleeping pills, and fatty accumulations are discarded more rapidly than the new tissue is being renewed. This is the phase when you notice weight loss.

The next phase is known as stabilization. This is the period of time when the amount of waste material being discarded daily is equal to the amount of tissue which is being formed and replaced by the newer, more nourishing food. This phase is followed after awhile by the *anabolic* phase. This is when weight increases, even though the new diet is lower in calories than the old one. New tissues are now being formed faster. This is due to the improved assimilation made possible by the discontinuance of wrong food combining. Weight is maintained and increased energy is experienced.

While cleansing, we will experience symptoms that we have suppressed in the past, such as colds we have not let run a full course. Rashes or eruptions may occur as poisons, like harmful drugs, are eliminated through the skin. If we understand this, we won't go to the doctor for drugs to stop it. This process means that the skin is becoming more active and alive. It is throwing off toxins more rapidly. These discarded toxins are saving us from more serious disease, which would inevitably result the longer we kept the toxins in our bodies. This elimination may save us from liver damage, kidney disorders, blood disease, arthritis, heart and nerve degenerations and maybe even cancer. We should not try to stop these constructive actions of the body with drugs because the symptoms are part of the healing process. If we understand how the body works, we can be patient and let nature take its course.

Herbs: When to take them

The strengthening effects of herbs are more beneficial if they are taken at the right time. A general rule to follow is: strong herbs are taken during acute diseases and mild herbs are taken between acute attacks and for chronic conditions.

Some herbs show a specific action for certain organs or body systems. They work as specific tonics or nutrients for the part of the body involved...such as Hawthorn Berry for the heart, Eyebright for the eyes, Scullcap for the nerves or Cascara Sagrada for the colon. Herbs are especially useful when a tendency toward illness is recognized but has not manifested itself in a disease crisis. Using herbs to prevent a disease and building up the body systems, is the most beneficial way to take them.

Acute disease: Herbs can be taken every half hour or more frequently if they are required—such as in cases of acute diseases like colds, flu, asthma, bronchitis or vomiting.

Colon, Kidneys, or Reproductive Organs: Herbs should be taken before meals. Food should be light and easy on digestion.

Digestive Problems: Herbs that benefit the stomach, spleen, liver, or small intestine work better when taken with meals. They can be taken 20 minutes before meals if you take encapsulated herbs with a glass of water. They can also be taken right after eating.

Insomnia: Herbs for insomnia should be taken one hour before going to sleep. The body as well as the mind needs time to relax.

Lungs, Heart, or Brain: Herbs for these areas of the body should be taken after meals.

Metabolism: To increase metabolism, herbs should be taken between meals. Dieting is more beneficial if you use herbs for weight loss between meals.

Mucus: To eliminate mucus, take herbs first thing in the morning. At night, your body is experiencing a mini-cleanse, therefore herbs such as Fenugreek help further the cleanse.

Purgatives: These herbs cleanse the colon and cells. They are best taken in the evening before going to bed. (This has to be adjusted for those who work outside of the home).

Digestion

The assimilation of herbs and food is dependent upon proper digestion. Raw foods contain the enzymes necessary to digest those foods. Conversely, cooked foods are robbed of these catalysts and put a burden upon the digestive tract.

Other factors also are detrimental to digestion.

- Drinking liquid with meals dilutes the gastric juices and reduces the ability of the body to completely break down foods. This can cause upset stomach, "sour" stomach and gas, as well as putrefaction. It is suggested that you drink any beverage at least one half hour before a meal.

- Overeating taxes the digestion and also depletes the body of energy. There is no physiological process which requires more effort by the body than that of digestion.

The body relies upon a full spectrum of vitamins, minerals, enzymes and other nutrients to help it operate at maximum efficiency. A lack of even one element can cause an imbalance and reduction in vitality. An excellent source of fatty acids is salmon Omega-3 oil. The special fatty acids in this oil have shown to help with blood pressure, arthritis, cholesterol and triglyceride levels, eczema, psoriasis and arteriosclerosis.

Fiber is an important component for digestion, as it helps cleanse the walls of the colon. It is best if you take it before breakfast in a glass of juice. Drink immediately after stirring. A light fruit breakfast is advised, but for those who require a more substantial start in the morning because of physical labor, thermos-cooked whole grains (oats, cracked wheat, brown rice) are a good choice. Lunch should be the main meal of the day with a hearty green salad, whole grains and occasional lean meats. Dinner should be light because the body stops digesting during sleep, and minimum calories are expended by the body during this period of time. It should be eaten at least three hours before retiring to bed.

Cleansing the Body...inside and out

The human body accumulates toxins and excess mucus as the years go by. This condition is the result of eating the wrong combinations of foods or junk foods and impaired digestion/ elimination. Stress can imbalance the body so that it cannot spontaneously rid itself of poisons. Parasites and germs thrive in this type of environment which further strains the immune capabilities of the body. Relaxation and periodic cleanses are the keys to wellness. A load of debris inside the cells, tissues and organs of the body puts a drag on energy levels and after a proper cleanse, many individuals report a marked surge in vitality.

It is suggested that a person prepares for a cleanse four weeks in advance by going on partial fasts. The first week a person could eliminate salt and meat from their diet. During this time, they can begin taking an herbal cleansing tea formula once daily, just before bedtime. The second week they should eliminate all sugars and white flour products from the diet and continue taking the tea.

Many people are addicted to salt, meat and sugar without realizing it. These individuals may experience a type of withdrawal such as intense cravings for these things. To help alleviate cravings for salt, a person could add herbal seasonings to foods. Onions, basil, rosemary, etc. could be used, or one of several commercial salt substitutes which contains combinations of savory herbs and spices. Vegetarian patties which contain vegetables, nuts and grains, could minimize cravings for meat. Fresh fruit is an excellent food to eat when sugar cravings become an annoyance.

The third week the tea should continue to be

taken, and if extra help is needed to flush toxins from the intestinal tract, a lower bowel formula could be added.

The following are different types of cleanses that may be employed after the four-week preparatory period. (Each cleanse is normally followed for a 24-hour duration unless otherwise noted). During a cleanse, eliminate all chemicals such as food additives, non-prescription drugs, nicotine, alcohol and caffeine.

Cleanse #1
Transitional Cleanse (prepares the body for a more intense cleanse)

Breakfast
Drink an 8-10 ounce glass of fresh fruit juice with a fiber and herbal formula stirred briskly into it. Then (approximately 30 minutes later) eat all the fruit you want...such as apples, berries, pears, peaches, etc., but no bananas, as they do not have laxative properties.

Lunch
Eat a main dish with millet or brown rice or baked potato, with a fresh green salad.

Dinner
Eat lightly steamed vegetables of your choice with a large vegetable salad.

*Please note: If you still become hungry, you may increase portions of fruits or vegetables. For extra nutrition, you may add one or more of the following products with any cleanse: Chlorophyll, Bee Pollen, Ginkgo formula, Blue-Green Algae and Malt-mineral formula.

Cleanse #2
Master Cleanser by Stanley Burroughs (a method of cleaning without enemas)

2 Tblsp. fresh lemon or lime juice
2 Tblsp. pure maple syrup
1/10 tsp. cayenne pepper
Pure water - combine in 10 oz. hot or cold water

Use 6 to 12 glasses daily
(You will not need anything else). If you become constipated, taking lower bowel cleanser in the morning and evening is helpful. Also, use lemon skin or pulp with the cleansing drink. Use Chlorophyll to minimize odors from the mouth.

Cleanse #3
Three-day Juice/Herbal Cleanse

For the first day, drink an eight-ounce glass or more of freshly-made carrot juice as often as desired.

For the second day, drink an eight-ounce glass or more of freshly-made apple juice as often as desired.

For the third day, drink an eight-ounce glass or more of freshly-made Concord grape juice as often as desired.

After the third day, incorporate the Transitional Cleanse into this program and continue on the Transitional Cleanse for seven days. Take the following supplements on a full stomach, at least fifteen minutes after meals.

- Take two Slippery Elm capsules three times a day and two Comfrey-Fenugreek Combination capsules also three times a day with juice. Twenty minutes before or after drinking the juice you may drink as much steam-distilled water as you desire.

- The second day of the Transitional Cleanse, add two Bone, Flesh and Cartilage Formula capsules (to rebuild flesh and cartilage) three times a day and one teaspoon of Red Clover Extract Formula (as a blood purifier and to support the liver) in juice or water three times a day.

- On the third day, add the following:

  - Two or more Lower Bowel Formula, capsules three times a day for regularity and to heal the colon.

- Two or more Nervine Formula capsules three times a day for nerves.

- Two or more Diabetes Formula capsules three times a day, to help the pancreas.

- Two or more Kidney Formula capsules three times a day, to support the kidneys as toxins are being flushed from the system.

- Two or more Calcium Herbal Formula capsules three times a day for a natural calcium supplement. (Acidophilus should also be added).

Spring and Fall Cleanses

Many people traditionally go on a "spring cleanse" to flush toxins from the liver and gallbladder. Drink the juices of fruits and vegetables which are in season. However, drink the fruit and vegetable juices separately, as they are assimilated better in the body that way. The diet should be comprised of moderate protein and complex carbohydrate foods such as whole grains.

The Chinese believe that fall is the time to strengthen the lungs and intestines because they are associated with the Metal element and autumn. A low-fat diet high in roughage from fresh fruits and vegetables; also plenty of greens and grains is recommended. Stay away from meats, dairy products, sweets and starches. The Master Cleanser program is a good choice to cleanse accumulated toxins from the system. Also, eating unsprayed Concord grapes and drinking their fresh juice for two days to a week will give you lots of energy. (If you are diabetic, check with a health professional before trying this regime). Take one tablespoon of compressed olive oil in the morning and evening with a cup of *Herbal Tea,* to keep the bowels moving. Be sure and keep the pores clean as this will assist the health of the lungs by not keeping congestion within the body. It is suggested that you use cold water to rinse at the end of a shower or bath to close the pores. This will help prevent heat loss in the body and will guard against susceptibility to becoming chilled by leaving the pores open to the cold.

The Successful Approach

In the book *Natural Healing With Herbs,* author and herbalist Hubert Santillo says: "One of the main reasons why therapies fail, whether herbal therapy or otherwise, is because the correct use of foods is not properly incorporated into the program. This difficulty is easily overcome if one understands the true meaning and use of a cleansing diet, proper food combining and a transition diet. A change from a traditional diet to a vegetarian or raw food diet is a progressive regime.

The Bloodstream should receive vitamins, minerals, amino acids, fatty acids, simple sugars and water from the intestines; not poisons. When proteins are digested properly, their end products, amino acids, pass from the intestines to the blood. If proteins are improperly combined with other types of food, putrefactive bacteria ferment them into skatole, intol, phenol, hydrogen sulfide and other poisons.

When starches and sugars are properly prepared for assimilation by good digestion, their final stage is simple sugars called monosaccharides which the body uses without difficulty. But when starches undergo putrification from staying in the intestines too long, or when mixed with incompatible substances, they are broken down into acetic acid, alcohol and carbon dioxide. These by-products of putrification are absorbed into the bloodstream and affect muscle tissues, joints, organs, glandular ducts and genetically weak areas, causing tumors, pains, arthritis, gout, etc.

The main objective of dietary therapy is to learn how to adapt to stressful situations and purify your body, particularly the intestinal tract, so larger amounts of nutrients can be absorbed. The cleaner you are internally, the more you absorb, the less you need to eat. The more congested you are the less you absorb, the more you must consume. In a pure body, more energy can manifest while eating small amounts of food."

Nutrition, Digestion and Assimilation

Famous nutritionist Dr. Bernard Jensen advises: "Our foods must be 60% raw. Raw fruits and vegetables and the juices made from them are the best sources of vitamins, minerals, enzymes, prostaglandins and fiber. Even low-heat, waterless cooking reduces the nutrient value a little, steaming takes away more and boiling almost any food causes great loss of nutrients. To provide the nutrients the body needs in as close to natural form as possible, we must have 50 percent of our foods raw.

Nature cures but she must have the opportunity. What does this law have to do with foods? We find that only foods build or replace tissue. Drugs, surgery or radiation may stop a disease, but only foods can correct the tissue damage caused by a disease...

...An imperfect digestion or underactive bowel may leave us malnourished even on a "perfect" diet. If we digest our foods well and they cannot be assimilated through the bowel wall because of toxic accumulations or putrid encrustations blocking the way, we remain malnourished. It is not always what we eat that counts, but what we digest and assimilate."

Healing Power of Fasting

Fasting is the quickest and easiest way to eliminate a toxic overload in the body. Toxins usually build up because of eating too much food, or eating non-food, or when enervating habits reduce the eliminative detoxifying capacities of the liver, kidneys, and skin and the excretory efficiency of the bowels, bladder and uterus. Fasting can be done both as a general health measure as well as a therapy for specific disorders. The following are benefits derived from fasting.

1. Fasting decomposes and burns those cells that are diseased, damaged, aged or dead. This includes tumors, abscesses, and fat deposits.

The essential tissues and vital organs, glands, nervous system and brain are not damaged or digested in fasting.

2. New and healthy cell growth is speeded up during fasting. When old or diseased cells are decomposed, the amino acids are not wasted but re-cycled and used again.

3. The concentration of toxins in the body can be 10 times as great as normal. The lungs, liver, kidneys and skin all help cleanse during the fast, and they do so efficiently because they don't have to worry about digesting food as well. All of their energy is used for cleansing.

4. Fasting provides a psychological rest to digestive, assimilative and protective organs.

5. During a fast, the nervous system is rejuvenated, the mental powers improved, the glandular chemistry and hormonal secretions are stimulated and increased, and the biochemical and mineral balance of the tissues is normalized.

During a fast, many people have felt a slight electric current or vibration of vitality that shakes and tingles throughout the body. Often, the soul has every reason to shout for joy and triumph. Some other physical and emotional benefits are the following:

- To lose unwanted weight the safest and quickest.
- To feel and look younger.
- To rest the digestive system.
- To boost mental and physical power.
- To improve better eating habits.
- To improve digestion.
- To normalize the colon.
- To achieve better sleep.
- To relieve tension.
- To lower cholesterol.
- To lower blood pressure.

How To Tell A Disease Crisis From A Healing Crisis

A healing crisis may develop when cleansing the body. Learn to listen to your body and rest when you are tired, drink plenty of liquids when thirsty, and eat only when you are hungry.

Fruits are cleansers and eliminate toxins and can sustain the body with its natural sugar, vitamins and minerals. If you are cleansing too fast on fruits, slow down by including steamed vegetables, vegetable juices or vegetable broths.

Vegetables are higher in carbohydrates and will slow down the cleansing process which may be needed when the body needs to be strengthened and built up in order to go through another cleanse.

Herbs, vitamin C complex and supplements help the body to dissolve mucus and toxins, by helping nature. Blood cleansers, colon cleansers, chlorophyll, or blue green algae are some agents that will help remove obstruction and congestion in the body. Enemas may be needed in case of stubborn cases of congestion.

Massage therapy will speed the cleansing process. Foot reflexology will help eliminate and break up toxins. Chiropractic treatments will help the body heal faster.

Some of the following symptoms may appear during a healing crisis.

- Food cravings
- Depression
- Diarrhea
- Fever
- Sore Throat
- Headaches
- Insomnia
- Skin rashes
- Sore muscles
- Nausea
- Discharge from nose, eyes, bowels or urinary tract
- Leg cramps
- Change in menstrual cycle

Healing will bring positive results such as a feeling of well being, less cravings for junk food, better circulation, clear skin, more energy, freedom from pain, improved digestion and disease elimination.

A Healing Crisis

1. This may happen when the body is naturally cleansed through fasting/or semi-fasting using wholesome and nourishing food.

2. A healing only happens when the body has enough vitality to withstand the cleansing symptoms.

3. It usually happens when the body feels its best.

4. A healing crisis usually develops about three months after a change of diet or fasting.

5. The healing crisis can last from two to seven days. If the vitality of the body is low, it could last longer than a week.

6. No crisis may appear if correct eating, colon and blood cleansing eliminate the waste a little at a time.

7. The body goes through three stages in order to completely clean the body. They are eliminative, transitional and building stages. The crisis will usually manifest during the transitional stage.

8. A chronic disease may cause aches and pains as the body is throwing off toxins. The chronic disease took years to develop. The pain during a healing crisis may be more severe than while the chronic disease was developing.

Some people may want to give up when they start experiencing the worst part of the healing crisis. They do not understand what is happening to their bodies when during a healing crisis. If they eat or take drugs, the disease is stopped, but it is pushed deeper into the system to manifest itself later in a more advanced disease symptom.

Eating during the eliminating process stops the cleansing because the body has to stop the cleansing to digest the food or to process the drugs.

Disease Crisis

A disease crisis happens when the body becomes congested, with built-up toxins and ceases to function properly. In cases of colds, flu and fevers, the body is trying to cleanse and restore health to a toxic body. These are acute diseases and should not be suppressed but need to be allowed to run their course.

1. A disease is produced when the body is overloaded with toxins and mucus.

2. When constipation develops.

3. When germs in the body have food to eat and are multiplying.

4. When the strength and vitality of the body is lowest.

5. Negative thoughts increase toxins and prolong their stay in the body.

6. Disease crisis happens in order to protect life. If the congestion would continue at the rate it was increasing, it would cause damage to the vital organs and could develop into chronic diseases such as cancer, heart disease, or asthma.

7. Disease can accumulate from negative thoughts, hate, fear or anger. Emotional stress cause a disease crisis.

Can Stress Cause Disease?

Stress can cause disease by dilating the capillaries. When the capillaries dilate, it causes the pores in the capillary walls to enlarge. The walls can become hard and brittle and give out.

When the pores of the capillary walls become enlarged, it allows the blood proteins to pass from the capillaries into the tissues between the cells. This causes an imbalance in mineral and symptoms of disease increase.

Stress causes the organs to tighten up and prevent the natural process of digestion, assimilation and elimination.

ATHLETE'S, ENDURANCE & HEALTH

Exercise is extremely important and an essential part of total body health. Studies continue to show however, that the majority of Americans live sedentary lives. Our society does not require intense physical activity for survival. We do not have to plant and harvest our own crops. We aren't required to walk where we want to go. In order to stay healthy, we need to make time for exercise, and it can be fulfilling as well as enjoyable.

The benefits from exercise are many. A fit body is more efficient. Studies show that physical inactivity can lead to serious health problems. Some believe that a lack of exercise is responsible for many of today's health problems. Coronary heart disease, high blood pressure, high blood cholesterol levels, hypertension, strokes, and even cancer are associated in part with a lack of exercise.

Another benefit in regular exercise is an increased sense of well-being. This has been found to occur due to an increased production of two chemicals in the brain. These seem to be produced more rapidly and frequently when an individual is physically fit. This increase in levels of certain chemicals may also be responsible for the reduction of stress that individuals who regularly exercise feel. They also are generally more able to cope with the stresses of life that everyone feels. A study done at the University of Southern California in the physiology lab suggests that a dose of exercise may be more helpful when dealing with anxiety than tranquilizers. This is certainly an interesting concept. Exercise is beneficial for many reasons.

Scientists speculate that exercise may enhance the immune system. Studies done recently seem to support this view. If this is possible, then exercise can help prevent many illnesses including cancer and other immune related disorder. Exercise may be more valuable to health than previously thought.

Exercise is also helpful when trying to lose weight. An overweight body is usually less healthy.

In studies conducted recently, individuals put on exercise programs were able to lose weight gradually, usually around two pounds a month, without dieting. Exercise helps to lose fat while increasing muscle mass. The benefits of exercise usually last throughout the day. The metabolism continues to run faster even after the exercise has ended.

Before beginning an exercise program, it is important to have a thorough medical examination if there is any doubt as to your health. Some may require in depth heart testing to determine problems that may exist. Exercise is important to health and most people can participate in a moderate exercise program without any problems.

Regular, moderate exercise is important to good health. Experts agree that exercise can increase circulation, increase the digestive process, strengthen the heart, reduce blood pressure, increase lung capacity and oxygen utilization, lower blood cholesterol levels, and promote an overall sense of well-being due in part to the release of endorphins. It also helps cleanse the body through perspiration, tone the nervous system, and strengthen the immune system to prevent disease.

Becoming more active is an important part of health. One important step is to use our bodies more. Take the stairs whenever possible instead of the elevator or escalator, park a few blocks away from an appointment and walk, put more energy into housework, walk or ride a bike to activities, and spend time working in the yard. These are a few suggestions.

A regular exercise program is needed to keep the body in optimum condition. Experts usually suggest a minimum of 20 to 30 minutes three to five times per week. It is a good idea however, to try and do some type of activity to increase the heart rate each day. It is important to start out slow and gradually increase activity. Doing too much in the beginning can cause pain and injury, which may discourage and end exercise routines.

Even a leisurely stroll is beneficial to health. Just do something to stay active!

Aerobic exercise is important to fitness. These are the activities that create a training effect. Aerobic activities provide more improvement in health than any other type of exercise. Aerobic means with oxygen, or activities which increase the breathing and heart rate for an extended period of time. They improve the ability of the heart and lungs through regular exercise. There are many different activities which are considered aerobic. Anaerobic means without oxygen. These activities are those that require quick action and bursts of energy and oxygen such as sprinting and are not continuous over a period of time.

It is important to monitor the heart rate when beginning an exercise program. There are different formulas to calculate maximum heart rate levels. This simple formula is recommended by the Institute of Aerobic Research. It is 220 minus your age to predict maximum heart rate. For men in great condition, it is 205 minus half your age. Aerobic exercise should work at 75 to 80 % of the maximum heart rate. The heart rate can be checked by placing the fingers on the artery of the neck.

Exercise should be enjoyable. Pick activities that are fun for you. Music can also help relax and make exercise enjoyable. Turn on the music when exercising at home, or wear headphones outside to run or walk.

ENDURANCE/STAMINA FOR THEMORE SERIOUS ATHLETE

Athletes strive consistently to increase their endurance and stamina. Exercise is important for everyone, but the more serious athlete seeks a strong body that will withstand stress, hardship, fatigue, and illness while pursuing his or her physical goals.

Endurance is the ability to keep going through pain and hardship. It is being able physically to continue when the stress is great and pain may occur. Stamina is related to endurance. It involves resistance to fatigue and illness. It involves strength, support, and solidity.

NUTRITION

Nutrition is an important part of life for the serious athlete. It is thought that nutrition can even help in preventing and healing injuries. Dr. Bernard Friedlander, a Santa Monica, California Chiropractor has this to say. "Many injury problems are food related. You'd be surprised, but by acquiring a bit of nutritional awareness and putting it into practice, there is no doubt you can maximize both prevention and healing of injuries. I've seen many athletes transform themselves from injury-prone to injury-free just by adding good nutrition to their training program." (*Let's Live*, Feb. 1987, p 10).

Dr. Friedlander has treated many athletes including world class competitors. He, as well as many sports nutritionalist agree that athletes need more complex carbohydrates and less protein and fat in their regular diets. This would mean using common sense. Junk food should be eliminated or greatly reduced in the diet. Add more whole grains, pasta, beans, and fresh fruits and vegetables to the diet.

Many experts used to believe that protein was the essential ingredient in building muscle. Now it is thought that exercise and complex carbohydrates work together to promote muscle strength and energy. Vitamins and minerals are needed more when the body is active. They can help promote the growth of muscle, bones, and cartilage. This can help in the prevention of injuries such as sprains and broken bones.

A high complex carbohydrate diet is beneficial. Complex carbohydrates give the body energy to sustain endurance. This energy helps to limit the fatigue which can lead to injury in and athlete.

Proteins such as eggs and meat sometimes require a full day before they are digested. They also require more energy to digest. Carbohydrates are stored in the muscles as glycogen and are readily available to be used in the form of energy. In the July 1985 issue of "Let's Live" on page 25 it says, "...only about half the calories of protein can be converted into energy, and in the process harmful by-products, such as ammonia, are produced. To dilute these toxins, the body uses seven times more water than it would need to burn carbohydrates. This, of course, makes the risk of dehydration that much greater."

Fresh fruits and vegetables are important for their mineral and vitamin content. They should be eaten regularly. Whole grains, pasta, and beans can fill the need for complex carbohydrates. These supply the athlete with energy that will be sustained and help relieve fatigue which often can lead to injury. Many nutritionists recommend that the athlete eat 65 percent of the diet in complex carbohydrates, 10 to 15 percent in the form of fat (mainly vegetable fat), and 10 percent in protein.

The February 1987 issue of "Let's Live" on page 10 quotes Dr. Bernard Friedlander suggesting a cause of fatigue in athletes. "One cause of fatigue can be too much animal protein and fat in the diet. They are difficult to break down. Loading up on milk and animal protein requires a tremendous amount of energy expenditure for digestion and assimilation. It can take up to several days to completely break down some protein and fatty foods, particularly for people who have weak enzyme systems due to overeating and poor eating choices. And there are many athletes in this category."

The August 1993 issue of "Better Nutrition for Today's Living" on page 26 lists some nutrients that athlete's need. "The first rule of supplementing for better athletic performance is to know your body and its needs and to take supplements as part of a balanced nutritional program. The following are some of the most important nutrients for top athletic performance.

Antioxidants

Vitamins C and E, glutathione and superoxide dismutase (SOD) are essential for peak athletic performance.

Calcium lactate

This salt of lactic acid can speed the clearance of lactic acid from the body. Lactic acid builds up in muscles during anaerobic activity, causing the fatigue, burning and aching that slow you down.

Phosphates

Phosphates, such as sodium phosphate, also help to reduce excess lactic acid and maximize oxygen uptake by muscle tissue.

Carnosine

This little known derivative of the amino acids alanine and histidine is responsible for about 40 percent of the buffering of skeletal muscles and is essential for reducing fatigue from lactic acid buildup. This compound also activates muscle enzymes, which helps them contract, and improves their energy metabolism.

B-complex

The B vitamins are essential for the effective use of energy for athletic endurance. The need for them escalates as our energy output increases; they are particularly important in the metabolism of carbohydrates. The B vitamins should always be taken in a balanced formula, rather than individually.

Minerals

Essential minerals are also keys to an athlete's optimal nutrition program, because they are cofactors in the forming of all our enzymes. Many of us, including athletes, may be deficient in calcium, magnesium, potassium, iron, zinc, chromium and boron."

DEHYDRATION

Dehydration can occur with strenuous exercise. Athletes must replace fluid lost as sweat during exercise. Pure water is important because it is easily assimilated by the body. Electrolyte loss may also occur. They regulate the activity of the nervous system and all the muscles including the heart. Sodium, potassium and chlorine are essential to the heart as well as the muscles. Exercise can deplete the body of essential minerals. A deficiency can lead to electrolyte imbalance which can cause respiratory failure, muscular weakness or even heart failure. When the body becomes dehydrated, the blood circulation and body temperature regulation is impaired. (*Better Nutrition,* Sept. 1992 p 17).

Many sports physiologists recommend that an athlete drink about two cups of water before any competition. Drinking eight ounces of fluid every 15 to 30 minutes during exercise is also advised.

Many drinks are available for athletes to help replace the essential elements lost during exercise. They can help by increasing the oxygen levels in the muscles and increasing energy and endurance. Endurance drinks should contain fructose, glucose polymers, electrolyte minerals (calcium, magnesium, sodium, potassium, and chloride), and amino acids. Magnesium is often deficient in athletes and very essential in endurance activities. There are some wonderful drink mixes available that contain these important elements.

LEG CRAMPS

Leg cramps while running or exercising can be a warning sign of a potassium, magnesium, calcium or zinc deficiency. The body needs these important minerals supplied daily. A calcium combination herbal formula supplement can help strengthen the bones, muscles, and cartilage while supplying important minerals to the body. It should contain the following: Alfalfa, Marshmallow, Plantain, Horsetail, Oatstraw, Wheat Grass, and Hops. An herbal potassium combination should include: Kelp, Dulse, Watercress, Wild Cabbage, Horseradish, and Horsetail. This may help regulate sodium levels and create a mineral balance. This combination contains important electrolytes and can help balance proper fluid levels.

IMPORTANT HERBS

Single Herbs which supply important minerals include: Alfalfa, Comfrey, Slippery Elm, Irish Moss, Kelp, and Spirulina. All herbs contain minerals.

Chromium Picolinate is an important supplement. It has been studied and found to improve and build muscle safely. Gary W. Evans, Ph.D, a professor of Chemistry at Bemidiji State University in Minnesota, has studied Chromium Picolinate extensively. He found that those taking this supplement had more endurance and energy than those who were not. Endurance and energy come from blood sugar and insulin, and chromium assures rapid intake of blood sugar and helps convert glycogen for use in the body. It may help lactic acid accumulation caused by the inability of the muscle tissue to burn glucose quickly enough to produce ATP, which stores and releases energy.

HERBS AND SUPPLEMENTS FOR THE ATHLETE

1. _____
ATHLETE TRAINING DRINK

Glycogen, Complex Carbohydrates, Chelated Minerals and Vitamins, Lipotropics, Amino Acids, Natural Flavors and Colors.

This formula is a high performance beverage containing glycogen. It is a high caloric, all natural, muscle and weight gain formula. The amino acids help promote rapid muscle growth. It is used for sports activities to aid in endurance and increased performance for the serious athlete involved in rigorous exercise. This formula is designed especially for the training process of an athlete.

2. _____
ATHLETE PERFORMANCE DRINK

Glycogen, Complex Carbohydrates, Fructose, Citric Acid, Sodium Citrate, Natural lemon and lime Flavors, Vitamins, Minerals, L-Carnitine and Natural Colors.

This formula is great as a fluid replacement beverage before, during and after sustained workouts. It is an excellent source of mineral, fluid and electrolyte replacement. It helps improve endurance by delaying fatigue. It can help reduce muscle cramping during prolonged exercise. This formula is for the athlete to use before, during and after a competition where peak performance is required.

3. _____
ENERGY BARS

Rice Syrup, Oat Bran, Rolled Oats, Peaches, Raisins, Almonds, Yogurt, Milk, and other natural ingredients.

This nutritious energy bar is a great meal replacement or snack. It provides a good tasting bar full of important nutrients which provide energy to the body naturally.

4. _____
MINERAL CAPS

Calcium, Magnesium, Manganese, Potassium, Silica, Iron, Zinc, and other minerals.

These mineral capsules are important for the body in replacing minerals lost from the body. Athletes require extra sources of minerals to replace those lost during training and competition. They help replenish the nervous system and strengthen the skeletal system. Minerals are very important in helping with the delicate balance of electrolytes in the body.

5. _____
ENERGY TONIC/HIGH FIBER DRINK

Fructose, Natural Flavors, Citric Acid, Sodium Bicarbonate, L-Carnitine, Potassium, Calcium, Vitamins, Glucose Polymers, Siberian Ginseng, Gotu Kola, Bee Pollen, and other ingredients.

This powder drink is specially formulated to build muscle tissue, increase energy, and create an over-all feeling of well being. It is useful for athletes in endurance sports and preventing muscle cramping. It is also known to increase energy in the body.

Aerobic Support: Alfalfa, Bee Pollen, Chlorella, Ginkgo, Ginseng, Suma, Blue-Green Algae.

Antioxidants: Ginkgo, Chlorella, Chaparral, Spirulina, Milk Thistle, Vitamins A,D,E, and C, Minerals Selenium and Zinc.

Athlete's Foot: Black Walnut, Echinacea, Chaparral, Tea Tree Oil.

Blisters: Comfrey Salve, Golden Salve, Aloe Vera, Slippery Elm.

Circulation: Ginger, Cayenne, Ginkgo, Prickly Ash Bark, Suma.

Cuts, Abrasions: Comfrey Salve, Golden Seal Salve, Black Walnut, Aloe Vera, Echinacea, Arnica, Witch Hazel.

Endurance: Ginseng, Ho Shou Wu, Schizandra, Ginkgo, Bee Pollen, Suma.

Fractures (to heal and prevent): Horsetail, Oatstraw, Comfrey, Slippery Elm, Alfalfa, Kelp, Dulse, Whole Grains, Buckwheat, Millet, Brown Rice, Whole Oats.

Muscle Spasms: Hops, Chamomile, Passion Flower, Scullcap, Valerian.

Sore Feet: Warm Ginger Bath, Rosemary Foot Bath, Tea Tree Oil, Aloe Vera.

Sore Muscles: Essential Oils with Wintergreen, Muscle Rub Down.

Stimulants: Ephedra, Ginseng, Bee Pollen.

CHILDREN & HEALTH

Parents want what is best for their children. They want to give their children a good start in life. They want to solve every problem immediately. They don't like to see their children suffer physically, mentally or emotionally, but sometimes what we think is best really isn't.

Nutrition for children begins before they are born. The absence of good nutrition and adequate vitamins and minerals can effect the health of the unborn child as well as their development. Neural tube defects in children have been linked to a deficiency of folic acid in the diet of the mother. Many doctors believe that a healthy diet may help prevent heart disease, strokes, diabetes and cancer.

PREVENTION

Prevention is the key to health. Preventive medicine is practiced in many different societies. The Asian cultures emphasize staying well and healthy more than treating the symptoms of an illness. This involves keeping the body in optimum health through nutrition, exercise, rest, and natural supplements. Even under the best of circumstances however, there will be problems. Illness will occur in our less than perfect environment. Accidents will happen no matter how hard we try to avoid them. Being prepared and knowledgeable can make things easier when problems do occur.

Children will become ill. It is important for them to experience common ailments in order to help develop and strengthen their immune systems. A cold or flu is nature's way of eliminating toxins from the body. No one is immune from the toxins that are in the environment. Most childhood diseases respond to the body's normal defense system.

Prevention actually begins while the fetus is developing inside the mother. The health of the baby rests to a great extent on what the mother ingests. The mother is responsible for nourishing the growing baby through the placenta. If the baby is given a good start nutritionally from conception, he will have a greater chance of being born with a strong immune system. A pregnant woman should probably take a nutrient supplement because of the needs and demands of the fetus. Dr. Lendon Smith suggests a pregnant woman take vitamin C, B-complex, calcium, magnesium, and zinc. (*"Let's Live,"* Sept. 1990, by Jack Joseph Challem, p 14). The pregnant woman should eat well, not trying to diet during her pregnancy to produce a healthy child with a strong immune system. Meals should be eaten regularly.

Breast feeding is a great choice when possible. Studies have shown that bottle fed babies are more prone to ear infections as well as other illnesses. Breast milk contains important substances that help prevent allergies in the baby. It also is a bonding time for mother and child. Breast feeding can help the baby develop a strong immune system. In addition, the breast milk contains everything that the baby needs for development during the first six months of life.

NUTRITION/BUILDING THE IMMUNE SYSTEM

The most important factor in strengthening the immune system is proper nutrition. Many individuals do not know exactly what this involves. Medical professionals usually have very little nutritional training during their educational experience. They look to drugs to treat the symptoms of illness.

Eating a variety of foods will help the body get the nutrients that it needs and also make meal time more enjoyable. There are a wide variety of fruits and vegetables available in the supermarket which are nutritious and delicious. Fresh fruits and vegetables are full of nutrients. Canned, dried, and frozen foods often lose some of their nutritional value through the processing procedure. Additives also can be undesirable. Remember to wash thoroughly or peel produce that has been treated with pesticides.

VEGETABLES AND FRUITS

Vegetables and fruits are important to a balanced and nutritional diet for all children. They are full of vitamins, minerals, enzymes, protein, complex carbohydrates, and fiber. There are many different varieties available.

If possible, it is important to buy produce that is free of pesticides, or grow as much produce as possible to ensure quality and safety. Local farmers can be used to be sure of the freshness of the produce.

Try and introduce new types of produce to children. If they refuse the new food, keep offering it to them. Some children need to adjust to new foods gradually before they will be willing to try them. There are many exotic and different varieties available at the local supermarket. Prepare them in different ways such as cutting them in clever shapes.

Raw as well as cooked vegetables should be included in the diet. Some should be cooked to make sure that the natural toxins are eliminated. These include broccoli, collards, kale, and brussels sprouts. Carrots, onions, garlic, salad greens, cucumbers, radishes, peppers, and tomatoes are great eaten raw. Again, variety is the key. Vegetables are essential to a healthy body.

Fruits should be sun ripened if possible. Unfortunately they are usually picked green and allowed to ripen on the way to the grocery store. This does not allow for the optimum amount of nutrients. Using the local farmer makes it possible to acquire sun ripened fruit.

WHOLE GRAINS

More and more research in combination with the medical community are pointing to the benefits of a diet rich in whole grain products. Processed foods are slowly losing their attractiveness in the eyes of many consumers. Whole wheat bread sales are on the rise, and there are a variety of delicious and nutritious grains available. It is now known that whole grains are important to ensure a nutritionally sound diet. It is important to remember that babies should not be given grains until they have enough teeth to chew thoroughly. This enables the digestive juices to do their part in the digestive process.

Grains are known to be low in fat and rich in complex carbohydrates. They have been used by many people in many cultures as a staple in the diet. They can be used to make all kinds of wonderful recipes, and they are a low cost source of nutrition, fiber, vitamins, and minerals.

They are best when grown organically to avoid contamination and pesticides. Grains can be cooked, sprouted, and ground into flour to make baked goods.

Whole wheat is probably the best known grain in our culture. It is full of nutritional value. It is often used for baking bread. Some use wheat in recipes as a meat substitute, and whole wheat can be used in soups and as a cereal. Most children are accustomed to white flour, which is the processed form of whole wheat. Unfortunately, the fiber and germ are eliminated in the processing. Whole grain wheat is a valuable nutrient.

Millet is a grain that has been used in many cultures. It is the only grain that is considered to be a complete protein. It can be added to cereals and breads and combined with other grains. It is a nutritious grain that can be introduced to babies. It can also be combined and cooked with brown rice.

Brown rice is a nutritious addition to the diet. Brown rice needs to cook longer than white rice, but the wait is worth the time. Most children are used to the white rice commonly used, but brown rice can be introduced and enjoyed by most everyone. A little butter and honey can sweeten the taste of the rice. It is full of nutritional value.

Buckwheat is a valuable grain. It is used as the main grain product in many northern European countries. The seeds of the buckwheat flower are ground into flour to make cereal and pancakes. Buckwheat is a hardy grain and it thrives in adverse conditions. It has few problems with insects and diseases and it seems to do well even in poor soil.

Barley is a wonderful and nutritious addition to soups and stews. It is a member of the same family as corn, oats, rice, and wheat. Barley flour is used in bread, cereal and as a thickening agent.

Corn is the only vegetable that is also considered a grain. Ground corn is great for muffins, tortillas, cereal and breads. It is also used as livestock feed and to make nonfood items such as drugs, paints, and paper goods. There are several thousand different types and varieties of corn.

Oats are a very important grain. The seeds of the plant are used in oatmeal, cookies, breads, and cereals. Oats have a high food value. The majority of the crop grown in the United States is fed to livestock. Oats however, are becoming more popular with the interest in the health benefits of whole grain oats and oat bran on the increase.

Rye is similar to wheat. Rye is used to make delicious breads. It is thought to have been cultivated from wild species found in Asia. Rye does not contain as much gluten as wheat and is preferred by some for this reason.

LEGUMES, NUTS, AND SEEDS

Legumes include peas, beans, and lentils. They are an inexpensive and nutritious addition to the diet. They contain complex carbohydrates, fiber, protein, vitamins, and minerals. They are low in fat and cholesterol.

Nuts and seeds are recommended only in small amounts because of their high content of fat. They are a good source of protein and fiber and contain some essential fatty acids, vitamins, and minerals.

EXERCISE

It is common knowledge that exercise is extremely important. It is an essential part of total body health, but studies continue to show that the majority of Americans live sedentary lives. They do not participate in regular exercise. Children today are less fit and weigh more than they did 30 years ago. They spend much of their free time in front of the television.

These statistics need to change and adults as well as children need to become more active.

It is the parent's responsibility to be an example where exercise is concerned. Participating with children can be enjoyable for the whole family. Take walks, hikes, and bike rides together. Make exercise a part of life.

HERBS AND SUPPLEMENTS

Staying healthy may include supplementing the diet. When children are old enough to make some of their own food choices, and when they venture to school and activities, they may eat foods that are not allowed or encouraged at home. It is important to given them some nutritional helps through herbs and supplements.

The usual diet may contain too much fat, sugar, and protein while too little of vitamins particularly B complex, E, and C and many of the trace minerals. Adding these to a child's diet can keep them healthy and build the immune system.

Herbal remedies can be very beneficial for children. Getting them to take them however, may not be easy. They are usually unable to swallow capsules and don't like the taste of herbal teas. The tea may be added to fruit juice. In addition, the herbal extracts often contain glycerine, which adds a slightly sweet taste to the product making it easier to swallow.

HERBS FOR CHILDREN

Chamomile
This can help settle an upset stomach as well as relax the body.

Catnip
This herb can help with colic, gas, indigestion, an upset stomach, and calm the nerves.

Scullcap
Scullcap works as a relaxant on the body. It can help induce sleep and reduce hyperactivity.

Peppermint

Peppermint is known to strengthen the body. It helps with stomach problems and digestion.

Ginger

This is great for nausea and motion sickness. It can soothe an upset stomach. It is also useful for colds and flu, aches and pains, and congestion.

Aloe vera

Aloe vera can be applied to scars, scalds, burns, and skin irritations. Taken internally, it can clean the stomach and colon.

Licorice

This herb has a pleasant taste. It can help with coughs, colds, flu, and lung congestion. It is also a mild laxative.

Lobelia

It is used for allergies, asthma, bronchitis, croup, and almost all childhood diseases. It aids with relaxation and is thought to help remove obstructions from the body.

Red Raspberry

This can help with colds, colic and fever in children.

Garlic

Although the odor may be unpleasant, garlic is a great natural antibiotic. It is found in some extract formulas. It is helpful for both viral and bacterial infections. It can be used for earaches, respiratory problems, colds, sore throat, fever, and injuries. It can be used as an enema, externally or taken in liquid or capsule form.

Tea Tree Oil

This is helpful in healing infections when applied externally. It can help promote healing and acts as a local anesthetic to relieve pain.

HERBAL COMBINATIONS

1. _____

Garlic, Gravel Root, Comfrey Root, Wormwood, Lobelia, Marshmallow, White Oak Bark, Black Walnut Hulls, Mullein Leaf, Scullcap, Uva Ursi, Apple Cider Vinegar, Glycerine, and Honey.

This herbal extract can help build the immune system and stimulate it to protect the body. It is helpful for childhood illnesses, common cold, flu, respiratory problems, coughs, and congestion.

2. _____

Peppermint, Elderberry, Sweet Orange Peel, Juniper Berry, Catnip, Marigold Flower, Angelica Root, White Pine Bark, Burdock, Peach Bark, Elecampane, Licorice, Honey, Glycerine, and Distilled Water.

This extract combination is helpful in relieving symptoms of colds and flu. It can help drain congested sinuses, relieve a sensitive stomach, and aid digestion problems.

3. _____

Chickweed, Licorice, Comfrey Root, Marshmallow, Mullein, Comfrey Leaf, Horehound, Lobelia, Cayenne, Distilled Water, and Glycerine.

This combination is great for coughs, sore throats, and hoarseness.

4. _____

Cloves Flowers, Bayberry Root Bark, Ginger Root, White Pine Bark, Capsicum Fruit.

This combination is great for the cold and flu season. It can help with cold symptoms and to stimulate the immune system.

IMMUNIZATIONS

The area of immunizations is certainly controversial. Parents who have decided not to have their children immunized, have felt the wrath of the public school system administrators. What are the controversies involved with immunizing?

There is a growing awareness in the public's eye of the dangers associated with immunizations. The trend began years ago with the production of mass immunizations in order to save our children from many of the natural childhood diseases. The evidence of the benefits of these immunizations however, are not clear.

It is thought by some that the better living conditions of our society today are responsible for the reductions in childhood diseases rather than the immunizations. The longterm effects of the immunizations are really not known. Dr. Robert S. Mendelsohn, M.D. suggests, "There is a growing suspicion that immunization against relatively harmless childhood diseases may be responsible for the dramatic increase in autoimmune diseases since mass inoculations were introduced. These are fearful diseases such as cancer, leukemia, rheumatoid arthritis, multiple sclerosis, Lou Gehrig's disease, Lupus erthematosus, and Guillain-Barre syndrome. An autoimmune disease can be explained simply as one in which the body's defense mechanism cannot distinguish between foreign invaders and ordinary body tissues, with the consequence that the body begins to destroy itself. Have we traded mumps and measles for cancer and leukemia?"(Mendelsohn, Robert S., *How to Raise A Healthy Child Inspite of Your Doctor*, Chicago: Contemporary Books, p 211).

Many health conscious individuals feel that these childhood diseases are nature's method of eliminating toxins from the body. They regard these diseases as a cleansing process. To not allow the body to use these diseases to cleanse may lead to a suppression of the toxins and to more deadly disease.

It has been proven that immunizations are not the only factor in determining who will get a particular disease. Nutrition, living conditions, and sanitation are also involved. If a child is healthy and has a strong immune system through proper diet, adequate sleep, and exercise, he will probably only suffer a mild case of a particular disease.

Dr. Lendon Smith recommends having children immunized. He feels that they are beneficial. "Sometimes infants will have a very bad reaction to DPT shots, and this is a sign of a poorly functioning immune system. To improve the baby's reaction, I recommends giving the baby a supplement of vitamin C the day before, one more the day of the shot, and another the day after." (Challem, Jack Joseph, *"Let's Live,"* Sept. 1990, p 20).

Whether to immunize or not is an individual decision. It is important to learn the facts before making that decision.

CHILDHOOD ALLERGIES

An allergy is the body's defense against a substance which is not normally harmful to the body. Pollens, cosmetics, dust, drugs, insect bites and stings, chemicals, foods, molds, and animal hair to name a few cannot really hurt the body. They are known as allergens. Just about any substance may cause an allergic reaction in someone somewhere. The immune system acts to safeguard the body against foreign bodies by using the white blood cells to fight them off. When the body wrongly identifies a substance as an invader, the white blood cells can cause symptoms and damage often causing more harm than the invader. The allergic reaction can become an illness.

There is no clear cut answer as to why some people develop allergies while others do not. Heredity certainly plays a part in the development of allergies. Children of parents with allergies more frequently have allergies. Babies who are not breast fed more often acquire allergies as well. This is why it is important if possible to breast feed the infant. There are many benefits transferred to the child. There also seems to be emotional and stress related allergy problems. Stress does cause some suppression of the immune system which may lead to the allergic response.

Stress may not always be emotional. It can come in other ways which attack the body's immune system and destroy its defenses. An onslaught of toxins is stressful, as in the case of sudden exposure to toxic chemicals. This causes an overload on the immune system.

All children come in contact with some form of foreign agents daily. They come in the form of germs, viruses, environmental chemicals, pollutants, pollen, etc. A child under stress is especially vulnerable whether it is physical, emotional, or environmental. This is why it is so important to keep the immune system in top shape.

When the immune system is working well, it can take care of the foreign invaders through the mucous membranes. The sinuses send the allergens down the throat where they travel to the digestive tract which neutralizes and destroys them. The tonsils, adenoids, and lymphatic system each play an important role in the process of eliminating these harmful substances.

Allergies seem to have increased as industrial technology increased. Chemicals, pollutants, food additives, herbicides, pesticides, synthetic drugs and processed foods may have added to this rise.

There are many problems that some doctors have linked to childhood allergies. Some include:

BEDWETTING

Nocturnal Enuresis commonly called bedwetting which persists beyond the age of three may be linked to allergies. Some believe the major allergens affecting this problem are 1. milk and milk products; 2. wheat; 3. eggs; 4. corn; 5. chocolate; and 6. pork. Inhalants such as pollens, house dust, molds, and animal hair may also cause bedwetting. The problems seems to be in the decreased bladder capacities due to allergies. Fluid builds up in the layers of the bladder and cause it to swell. When the allergen is removed, the bladder will most likely return to normal size.

HYPERACTIVITY

Allergies may also be linked to hyperkinetic activity in children. The most common offenders include milk, wheat, eggs, chocolate, sugar and food dyes. Some children can't sit still, concentrate, control emotions, and sleep. This may be due to allergies which cause them to feel out of control and unable to sit for any amount of time.

RESPIRATORY

The respiratory system is often linked to allergies. Many think of sniffles, itchy eyes and a cough when they think of allergies. This type of allergic response is often caused by milk and wheat products as well as pollens and pollutants in the air. Some allergy symptoms include asthma, coughs, colds, hay fever, sinusitis, nose bleeds, wheezing, shortness of breath, and tightness in the chest.

CEREBRAL

It has just been in recent years that cerebral or brain allergies have been recognized. These may show up in the form of schizophrenia, depression, hallucinations, delusions, catatonia, etc. These symptoms are caused by a swelling of the lining of the brain. Many patients have been helped with these problems through controlling allergies. Many different substances, among them auto exhaust, corn, plastic, environmental toxins, etc. may trigger symptoms in sensitive individuals. Some other forms of cerebral allergies include anxiety, dizzy spells, nervousness, insomnia, learning disorders, restlessness, and fatigue.

GASTROINTESTINAL

Gastrointestinal allergies often accompany respiratory allergies in a majority of cases. These allergies have the same symptoms as ailments such as ulcers, colitis, appendicitis, heartburn, indigestion, nausea, diarrhea, constipation, and intestinal gas.

CARDIOVASCULAR

Allergies can affect the cardiovascular system. When an allergen is introduced into the body allergic symptoms may include hypertension, rapid pulse, high or low blood pressure, and irregular heartbeat.

SKIN

Skin problems have been linked to allergic responses. Some types of allergies may be caused by a toxic colon or contact with detergents or other topical substances that a person is sensitive to. Some symptoms include acne, blisters, blotches, flushing, dark circles under the eyes, eczema, hives, itching, and psoriasis.

NERVOUS SYSTEM

Allergic responses by the nervous system can be caused by many different factors including poisonous substances, foods, chemicals or preservatives. These are often linked with cerebral allergies and symptoms include migraines, drowsiness, depression, anger, anxiety, irritability, restlessness, and lack of concentration. Some health professionals feel that Attention Deficit Syndrome (ADD) and other problems dealing with concentration may be linked to allergies.

EAR

These manifestations of allergies are often linked to respiratory allergies. Children who often suffer from ear infections may have allergy problems. Most common allergens are wheat, sugar, milk, chocolate, pollens and other inhaled allergens. Some symptoms are frequent ear infections, itching in ears, dizziness, imbalance, sensitivity to noise, and earaches.

WEIGHT LOSS

Living in a nation where people are obsessed with dieting has lead to many different quick weight loss diets and programs. Some people are in constant battle with their bodies. Overweight people are often shunned or looked on with disapproval. They turn from one diet to another in order to develop the perfect size and shape which will lead to happiness for them. This obsession has lead to many of the eating disorders which plague our society. Anorexia nervosa and bulimia are common. The female population in particular think that their bodies must be perfect in order to be happy with themselves.

The problem with quick diet fixes is, that they are not permanent. Studies have shown that weight lost quickly will almost always return. Unfortunately, fad diets not only don't work and the weight is usually regained, but the body is more likely to gain back extra body fat with each diet tried. The only sure way to lose weight for the long term is a slow and gradual approach incorporating improved diet and exercise.

There is no miracle cure to the fat problem. Obesity can be controlled but not by taking a simple pill or supplement, and pounds will not be shed while eating a high fat diet. Quick fixes may sound great, but it takes long term goal commitments and permanent life style changes to ensure a healthy body.

Rapid weight loss usually consists of water loss. Some claim, "Lose ten pounds in one week." Yes, this is indeed possible but it won't be fat that is lost. Most of the weight will probably be water, and this will most definitely reappear. High protein diets cause the kidneys to work extra hard to remove the urea out of the body. This leads to the water loss. Returning to a normal diet will lead to return of the water and weight. This type of diet is hard on the body especially the kidneys.

The most efficient and healthy way to lose weight is by concentrating on health and fitness. By changing the diet to a low fat, high complex carbohydrate diet with some protein, the weight will drop gradually. The changes need to be lifelong, and a commitment must be made. Add to this an aerobic exercise program and heath and fitness can be attained.

AUTOINTOXICATION

Autointoxication may add to the problem of obesity. If the body does not eliminate each day all of its waste material, it can build up and lead to obesity. This is a result of constipation and can lead to a condition where the body poisons itself through reabsorbing into the bloodstream harmful bacteria. This can weaken the immune system and the entire body. Purifying the blood and cleansing will help with this problem. Studies done at the Mount Sinai Medical Center in New York City have found that too much body fat can cause liver malfunction. Fat deposits in the liver can increase the production of enzymes needed to help the liver function properly and eliminate toxins. The excess fat puts added pressure on the liver, and it has to work harder. Obese people are at higher risk for liver disease.

MODIFYING THE DIET

Changes can be made gradually to a healthier lifestyle and eating habits. Trying to change the family's diet in a day is probably unrealistic. They will most likely rebel. Introduce a few new items per week, and try not to make it a big deal. Concentrate on one step at a time. Learn to look for the fat content of foods and limit the fat intake. Add more whole grain products to the diet. Incorporate a variety of fruits and vegetables.

Recipes can be modified to fit with an effective diet. Choose recipes low in fat. Concentrate on using 10 to 20% of the calories in the form of fat. This would be approximately 13 to 30 grams of fat per day. Add whole grains to the recipe. Eat protein, sugar and salt in moderation.

Chew food slowly. This helps with the digestion

process. The food can be better assimilated by the body.

Complex carbohydrates are important to add to the diet. Stick to whole grains, beans, lentils, baked potatoes, sesame seeds, brown rice, pasta, and other nutritious foods.

Fruits and vegetables make great snacks. Have a variety on hand ready to eat.

FOODS TO HELP WITH OBESITY

Food intake should correlate with foods associated with good health and nutrition. Fats eaten in abundance slow digestion. They also limit the hydrochloric acid in the stomach causing digestion and assimilation problems. Refined foods also upset digestion and metabolism. They lack vitamins, minerals, and enzymes that are essential to glandular regulation and digestion.

Fruits and vegetables should be eaten in abundance. Fresh and steamed vegetables provide vitamins and minerals. Fruit is considered a cleanser for the body and vegetables help build the body. High fiber foods are essential. Carrots, celery, beets and apple juice are thought to help stimulate and feed the glands. Lettuce, broccoli , celery, asparagus, scallions, cucumbers, kale, carrots, cabbage, parsley, watercress, and cauliflower are all good vegetables to add to the diet to encourage weight loss.

Lemon juice in a glass of water first thing in the morning is considered helpful for cleaning the liver and eliminating toxins from the body.

Whole grains are good to provide fiber and enzymes to the body.

FIBER AND WEIGHT LOSS

In cultures where fruits, vegetables, and whole grains are eaten in abundance, there is less incidence of obesity, colitis, cancer and polyps of the colon, and appendicitis. The diets of our so called civilized society contains mainly refined and processed foods which eliminate the fiber and roughage along with many of the nutrients. The fiber adds bulk and also the elimination time is increased speeding up the process. It seems that the quicker that the food is eliminated through the system, the greater the benefits. This may make the body less susceptible to storing the fat which is a natural tendency. Fiber can keep toxins from building up in the colon by keeping the bowels moving. High protein and fat diets are absorbed mainly in the intestines. This may lead to constipation problems. Also cholesterol and fats are excreted from the body at a faster pace as well as toxins. The theory is that the less time toxins and carcinogenic substances remain in the bowels, the less chance of them causing problems. Diets low in dietary fiber allow the food to remain longer in the intestines causing toxins to build up and disease to begin. The fiber will not cure all physical problems, but it may help in preventing some illnesses in susceptible individuals. With a high fiber diet, the bowel wall may remain strong and clean.

There are many benefits to a high fiber diet. The foods high in fiber usually are lower in calories and fat than other foods. Fiber often fills up the stomach because it swells with moisture and leaves a feeling of being full. Fiber foods pass through the intestinal tract at a faster pace reducing the calorie absorption and possible toxins to enter the body.

The best method of increasing fiber is to include whole grains, brown rice, oats, pasta, and ample amounts of fruits and vegetables to the diet. Be aware of what you are eating. Fast foods are not only high in fat, but very low in fiber. Fiber should be gradually introduced into the diet as to avoid intestinal problems such as diarrhea, bloating, and flatulence.

There are fiber supplements available which can increase the amount of fiber in the diet. Some of them are listed below.

1. _____

Psyllium Husk, Fructose, Maltodextrin, Fructooligo Saccharide, Citrus Pectin, Natural Orange Flavor, Hibiscus Flower, Natural Banana Flavor, Guar Gum, Caa

Inhem Extract, Peppermint Leaf Powder, Cinnamon Bark Powder, Papaya Fruit Powder, Garlic Powder, Rhubarb Root Powder, Alfalfa Powder, Fenugreek Seed Powder, Slippery Elm Bark Powder, Ginger Root Powder, Cape Aloe, Burdock Root Powder, Black Walnut Hulls Powder, Red Raspberry Leaf Powder, Pumpkin Seed Powder, Yucca Root Powder, Marshmallow Root (Althea), Uva Ursi Powder, Buchu Leaf Powder, Capsicum Fruit Powder, Clove Seed Powder, Chickweed Powder, Cornsilk Powder, Dandelion Root Powder, Echinacea Root Powder (Augustifolia), and False Unicorn.

There has been much research done as to the benefits of a high fiber diet. This product can help put fiber in the diet that is missing from the food that we eat. It contains two kinds of fiber both insoluble and soluble. The insoluble fiber passes through the system without dissolving in water. Its bulk helps make digestion cleaner and faster. Soluble fiber dissolves in water and may, with the help of a low fat diet, lower blood cholesterol levels.

PSYLLIUM (Plantago ovata)

Psyllium: considered a *colon* and *intestine* cleanser. It lubricates as well as heals the intestines and colon. It does not irritate the mucous membranes of the intestines but strengthens the tissues and restores tone. It absorbs acids and toxins in the intestinal tract. It is reported to be good for *auto-intoxication,* which can cause many diseases, by cleansing the intestines and removing toxins. It creates bulk and *fiber* which is lacking in the typical American diet. It is considered a food and may be used daily for healthy bowels.

SINGLE HERBS TO HELP WITH WEIGHT LOSS

Some herbs thought to help with obesity and losing weight include cascara sagrada, dandelion, ephedra, fennel, kelp, papaya, parsley, and yarrow.

CASCARA SAGRADA:

Cascara Sagrada is an herb known to help with chronic constipation. Keeping bowel function healthy is important to health and weight control.

DANDELION:

Dandelion is a great blood purifier and strengthener. It can help individuals suffering from anemia and supply the body with essential nutrients for a healthy body. It contains all the nutritive salts that the body uses to purify the blood. It can help balance gastric acids to promote digestion and assimilation. Dandelion is useful as a diuretic which can help with weight loss. It is also a mild laxative.

EPHEDRA:

Ephedra has been studied and found to promote weight loss. It seems to have an appetite suppressing effect. Many people are finding success in controlling and losing weight from taking a combination containing ephedra. Some studies relate the weight loss to an increase in the metabolic rate of adipose tissue. It may actually help reduce the rate of fat tissue reduction. It also is known to increase the basal metabolic rate which causes the body to burn calories faster.

Some studies have shown ephedrine to have some side effects. The studies done used the component ephedrine alone and not the entire herb. The whole herb is considered safer by most herbalists. Some of those side effects include increased blood pressure, increased heart rate, insomnia and anxiety. Ephedra is generally used in combination with other herbs such as white willow and kelp to avoid possible problems. It is recommended to lessen the amount taken if some side effects do occur and modify the dosage for individual use.

FENNEL:

Fennel is very good for the digestive system. Good digestion and food assimilation are essential for weight loss. The essential oils in the fennel seed are probably responsible for its soothing effects.

KELP:

Kelp contains many essential minerals. It contains iodine which is important for the function of the thyroid. This natural iodine is absorbed slowly and safely by the body. Decreased thyroid function can be a cause of obesity. The thyroid gland is responsible for metabolism, energy and proper growth. It can help increase the body's metabolism.

PAPAYA:

Papaya is well know for its ability to aid in digestion. It contains papain which is an enzyme that breaks down protein into a more digestible state.

PARSLEY:

Parsley is a natural diuretic. This can help when water retention is a problem. It is better for the body than diuretic drugs because it will not deplete the body of potassium. It also helps with digestion.

YUCCA:

Yucca is thought to strengthen the intestinal flora. It is used as an aid in digestion by keeping the wrong type of bacteria out of the digestive tract. It helps to break down accumulations of undigested waste that can collect in the colon.

HERBAL FORMULAS

2. _____
WEIGHT LOSS COMBINATION

Ma Huang (Ephedra), Salix Alba (White Willow), and Fucus Vesiculosis (Kelp)

This combination contains a blend of herbs that contribute to weight control. It is a well balanced blend of nutritional supplements. It can help increase energy, suppress the appetite, and increase the metabolism. This formula can help the body maintain a proper balance and function well. Ma Huang is thought to help reduce the size of the fat cells through thermogenesis. This process can help burn the stored fat that accumulates in the body.

3. _____
WEIGHT SUPPORT

Glycine and L-Methionine

This formula containing amino acids is helpful with the weight loss process. It is thought to suppress the appetite. It is helpful in preventing excess accumulation of fat in the liver. It also aids in the control of fat levels in the blood and in the prevention of cholesterol buildup.

4. _____
WEIGHT LOSS TEA

Senna, Buckthorn, Peppermint, Caa Inhem, Uva Ursi, Orange Peel, Rose Hips, Althea, Honeysuckle, and Chamomile.

This blend of herbs is used as a natural laxative. It is helpful when used as a digestive aid. It is also a natural diuretic and as an appetite suppressant. It is useful for people interested in achieving an optimum body weight.

5. _____
HIGH FIBER/ENERGY DRINK

Fructose, Natural Flavors, Citric Acid, Sodium Bicarbonate, L-Carnitine, Potassium, Calcium, Vitamins, Glucose Polymers, Siberian Ginseng, Gotu Kola, Bee Pollen, T64X (special herbs in a lactose base) and other ingredients.

This is a powder formula which is added to water or juice to help increase energy and control weight. It is high in fiber and contains valuable minerals which can help with fluid balance in the body. It can aid with sports and endurance activities.

6. _____
NUTRITIONAL WEIGHT SUPPORT

L-Carnitine, Zinc, Amino Acid Chelate.

This combination is thought to help build muscle while reducing excess fat accumulations. It also helps increase energy, prevent cholesterol build up, and strengthen the heart.

7. _____
METABOLISM FORMULA

Manganese, Iodine (kelp), Amino Acids (glutamic acid, proline, histidine).

This formula is designed to increase the metabolism in the body to promote weight control. These ingredients are combined to help stimulate the body's metabolism to work more efficiently.

8. _____
ENERGY/APPETITE SUPPRESSION

Vitamin B6, Lecithin, Apple Cider Vinegar, Kelp, Choline, Inositol, Calcium, Magnesium, Juniper Berry, Uva Ursi, and Essential Fatty Acids.

This combination is designed to provide the body with essential vitamins and minerals to ensure proper nutritional support. It is known to increase energy in the body and help suppress the appetite.

9. _____
ENERGY/DIGESTION

Parthenium, Chickweed, Licorice Root, Saffron, Gotu Kola, Guar Gum, Cascara Sagrada, Red Clover, Echinacea, Fennel, Black Walnut, Kelp, Dandelion Root, Hawthorn Berries, and Papaya.

This formula is useful with weight loss. It contains ingredients essential to nutrition and the assimilation of food. It also helps with increasing energy and digestion.

10. _____
THERMOGENIC FORMULA

Ephedra Sinica, Ilex Paraguairenis, Arruda Brave, White Willow, Licorice, Dandelion, Kelp, and GTF Chromium.

The ingredients in this combination are designed to increase energy and the metabolism in the body. It is known to increase the body's thermogenic (fat burning) ability. It can help reduce hunger and promote weight loss.

11. _____
IMMUNE BUILDER

Ginseng, Echinacea, Psyllium, and other ingredients.

This combination can help enhance the function of the immune system. The immune system is the first line of defense in the body against disease. It can aid digestion and assimilation of food while promoting energy and strengthening the body. It also contains ingredients which have a laxative effect.

12. _____
CHROMIUM SUPPLEMENT

Gymnena Sylvestre, Papaya, and Chromium Picolinate.

This formula is useful for weight control. It also helps with digestion and food assimilation. It is thought to promote body toning. It is used by some for diabetes and related problems of blood sugar and the pancreas.

13. _____
COMPLETE DRINK

Fructose, Whey Protein Concentrate, Soy Protein Isolate, Malto-Dextrin, Gum Arabic, High Oleic Sunflower Oil, Natural Flavors,, Jerusalem Artichoke Flour, Dipotassium Phosphate, Tricalcium Phosphate, Xanthan Gum, Potassium Chloride, Carrageenin, Magnesium Oxide, L-Methionine, Vitamin A, L-Carnitine, Potassium Gluconate, Ferric Orthophosphate, Citrus Pectin, Vitamin C, Vitamin E, Niacin, Copper Gluconate, Zinc Oxide, Manganese Sulfate, Pantothenic Acid, Biotin, Pyridoxine Hydrochloride, Calcium Chelate, Garcinia Cambogia, T64X Special Herb Blend in Lactose, Gotu Kola, Siberian Ginseng, Bee Pollen, Folic Acid, Thiamine Mononitrate, Vitamin D3, Riboflavin, Potassium Iodide, and Lactobacillus Bifidus.

This combination of ingredients is full of nutrition. It contains an ingredient which can help combat lactose intolerance by helping improve the digestability of milk products. It contains an enzyme which aids the digestive process. It restores beneficial bacteria to the body. It is a great source of fiber and can help relieve constipation. The complete formula also helps increase energy and increases the metabolism in the body. It also contains ingredients which are known to aid in lowering blood cholesterol levels. It also helps suppress the appetite.

14. _____
BREATH SPRAY/APPETITE SUPPRESSION

Alcohol, Water, Glycerin, Anacardum 8x, Ignatia 8x, Graphites 8x, Antimonium 8x, Cruden 8x, Argentum Mitricum 8x, Pulsatila Ngicans 8x, Sepa 8x, Hypothalamus 10x, Caa Inhem, Essential Orange Oils.

This is a homeopathic remedy which can help reduce cravings for sweets and snacks. This can help when trying to lose or maintain weight. It is also used as a breath freshener.

15. _____
ENERGY/NUTRITION

Chinese Ephedra Sinica, Ilex Paraguairensis Leaf, Kelp, Dandelion Root, Arruda Brava Leaf, Capsicum, and Chromium AAC (GTF Chromium amino acid and niacin complex).

Losing weight is on the minds of many individuals. This blend of nutritious ingredients are designed to help the weight loss process. It helps by increasing the metabolism in the body and also serves as a nutritional support.

16. _____
ENERGY AID

Garcinia Cambogia Fruit, Bissy Nut, Bdellium Gum, Uva Ursi Leaves, Pippali Fruit, Arruda Brava Leaves, Kelp, White Willow Bark, L-Carnitine, and Chromium (AAC).

This product works with Energy/Nutrition to aid with weight management.

17. _____
ESSENTIAL FATTY ACIDS

The essential fatty acids are important to the body. They help the central nervous system and must be replenished daily. They can help reduce cravings for fatty foods and eliminate hunger feelings. The body needs the good fat to function. It also helps stimulate the use of the bad fats for energy.

VITAMINS, MINERALS, AND SUPPLEMENTS TO AID WITH WEIGHT LOSS

VITAMINS AND MINERALS

B-COMPLEX:

The B-complex vitamins are thought to help with appetite control and with the production of hydrochloric acid. This is known to aid in the digestion process. B6 works with magnesium to break down proteins, fats, and carbohydrates. B12 aids the body in utilizing B6, folic acid, and vitamin C.

VITAMIN C:

Vitamin C is important in glandular function. It is an essential element of a strong immune system. It may also help cholesterol from depositing to the arterial walls and lower serum cholesterol levels.

VITAMIN E:

Vitamin E helps with metabolism. It also is thought to increase the HDL Cholesterol levels which is protective against heart disease. It is also an immune system enhancer. It is important for fat metabolism in the body.

IODINE:

This is essential for proper functioning of the thyroid gland. The thyroid is important to regulate the metabolism of the body.

LECITHIN:

Lecithin is known to be a fat emulsifier. It breaks down fat in the body.

CHROMIUM:

Chromium is being marketed in formulas as a weight loss aid. It indeed plays a vital role in a healthy body. It is a trace mineral needed daily by the body. In its active form, it is referred to as Glucose Tolerance Factor or GTF. It aids in the metabolism and regulation of blood glucose levels. It is also involved in muscle development and energy production. Chromium also helps synthesize cholesterol, fats, and protein. It helps stabilize blood sugar levels through insulin utilization. Because of the poor diets of the average American, it is thought to be deficient in most diets. It is estimated that 80% of chromium is lost in processed food. Refined foods and high sugar diets required more chromium because of the loss in the urine.

But how does chromium aid weight loss? Chromium or GTF helps maintain insulin activity and also aids in the utilization of glucose which leads to appetite suppression. It seems to help with the hunger center in the brain. It may actually reduce the false feelings of hunger or cravings for junk food.

"It is thought that the regulation of the appetite for food occurs in the hypothalamus region of the brain. There is evidence of lateral "feeding center" in the bed nucleus of the medial "satiety center" in the ventromedial nucleus. The activity of the "satiety center" is believed to be governed by the level of blood sugar utilization of the cells within the center. These cells are often referred to as "glucostats," when their glucose utilization does vary with the amount of insulin in circulation." (Ganung, W.F. 1973. Rev. Med. Phys., Los Altos: Lange Med. Publ., p. 161.) quoted by (Passwater, Richard A., Ph.D.1982. GFT Chromium, New Cannen, Conn., p. 21.)

Another positive effect of chromium for dieters is the prevention of fluctuation in blood sugar levels. Eating less sometimes causes mood swings because of low blood sugar levels. The stored glycogen can be retrieved for use with the help of chromium. It aids in the production and storage of glycogen.

Chromium is probably more widely known for recent studies linking chromium to a reduced risk of heart disease. It may help prevent plaque buildup in the arteries. Low levels of chromium are thought to be a risk factor for developing heart disease. It also may help increase the beneficial HDL cholesterol and aid in lowering LDL cholesterol.

Chromium is also being studied with regard to diabetes. Diabetes results from a deficiency of insulin. Proper amounts of chromium may help decrease the requirements of insulin.

This important trace mineral may be a factor in reaching and maintaining optimum body weight. It is also important for many body functions.

ESSENTIAL FATTY ACIDS

It is important to remember that we do need some fats in our diet. They are essential in that they carry the fat-soluble vitamins A, D, E, and K. The right kind of fat is important for good health.

The essential fatty acids (EFA's) are important for a healthy diet and required by everyone. Some of the common EFA's include omega-3, alpha-linoleic, and omega-6 linoleic acid. These cannot be made in the body and must be consumed. Every single cell in the body requires daily doses of EFA's. Cold-water fish, dark green leafy vegetables, walnuts, soybeans flaxseed oil, linseed oil, evening primrose, and gooseberry oil are some sources that contain EFA's. The EFA's help improve the function of the glands which can help in weight loss. Some individuals on low or no fat diets experience symptoms of fatigue and periods of no weight loss. This could be due in part to the absence of EFA's in the diet. A small amount of the EFA's in the diet can actually help in the weight loss process. Some research has found that the

right kinds of fat can help balance the body to achieve weight loss.

ARTIFICIAL SWEETENERS AND WEIGHT LOSS

There is a lot of controversy regarding the use of artificial sweeteners. Many support the belief that these sweeteners have many advantages over natural forms of sugar. Dieters are often seen consuming diet drinks because they think they will help them lose weight.

NutraSweet® and Equal® are the trade names for aspartame. Advocates claim that aspartame is natural made from two building blocks of protein similar to those found in fruits, vegetables, grains, and dairy products. But others claim that this product is far from natural. It is composed of two amino acids which are phenylalanine and aspartic acid and found in nature. The problems seems to be that they are isolated from the other amino acids that they usually are found in combination with. The two amino acids that aspartame does contain are delivered in the body in a highly concentrated form, which the body does not ordinarily have to deal with.

Artificial sweeteners are hundreds of times sweeter than sugar. Some researchers believe that the body is tricked into thinking it is getting a large amount of sugar. This causes the metabolic process to speed up leaving the individual hungry and tired. This in return may cause more food to be eaten. Some studies have shown that dieters who use artificial sweeteners may actually gain more weight than those eating regular sugar products.

In *Health and Fitness Excellence*, page 340, and written by Robert K. Cooper Ph.D, states, "Don't rely on artificially sweetened foods and beverages to help you lose weight or prevent fat gain. According to an ongoing study by the American Cancer Society involving more than 78,000 women aged fifty to sixty-nine, long-term users of artificial sweeteners are more likely to gain weight than non-users over the course of one year. In addition, fake sweeteners usually don't satisfy hunger. A recent study on aspartame conducted at Leeds University in England reported that not only was this sweetener generally ineffective in suppressing appetite, but in some people it actually increased feelings of hunger. In contrast, sugar (glucose) was found to reduce hunger and produce a feeling of fullness."

Some information has brought to light some new facts about NutraSweet®. It contains the amino acid phenylalanine. It is known to cause problems with some of the brain neuro-transmitters. It seems to affect some of the brain levels of amino acids and affects the production and release of some neurotransmissions. This could affect many different brain functions such as blood pressure, appetite, and mood changes.

There are also some who have claimed other side affects associated with the use of aspartame. These include dizziness, nausea, diarrhea, headaches, seizures, and mood changes. Reports have been sent to the National Center for Disease Control concerning this issue. The company responsible has also been sent many complaints.

Cyclamates, which were banned some years ago, are now being reconsidered. Saccharin is know to cause cancer and is still present as an artificial sweetener.

Most natural health advocates recommend using natural sugar in small amounts and staying away from artificial sweeteners. There is really no evidence to support the use of artificial sweeteners as beneficial. Studies done seem to show that more weight is gained by individuals who choose to use artificial sweeteners.

EXERCISE AND WEIGHT LOSS

Exercise is extremely important and an essential part of total body health. It can help with weight loss by increasing the metabolism of the body and by burning more calories even after the exercise as ended. Exercise often decreases the appetite. Cardiovascular and respiratory function increase with regular exercise It also makes individuals look as well as feel better.

The benefits from exercise are many. A fit body is more efficient. Studies show that physical inactivity can lead to serious health problems. Some believe that a lack of exercise is responsible for many of today's health problems. Coronary heart disease, obesity, high blood pressure, high blood cholesterol levels, hypertension, strokes, and even cancer are associated in part with a lack of exercise.

BODY SYSTEMS & DISEASES

THE CIRCULATORY SYSTEM AND LYMPHATIC SYSTEM

DISEASES OF THE CIRCULATORY SYSTEM

Anemia	Hemorrhoids
Angina Pectoris	Hypertension
Arteriosclerosis	Nosebleeds
Bruising	Myocardial Infarction
Cholesterol	Raynaud's Disease
Circulation, Poor	Rheumatic Fever
Gangrene	Stroke
Heart Palpitations	Thrombosis & Phlebitis
Hemorrhage	Varicose Veins

The circulatory system consists of the blood, heart, arteries, veins and capillaries. Every cell of the body must receive nourishment and it is the job of the circulatory system to see that rich, nourishing blood reaches all cells and organs of the body for health and vitality.

The American Heart Association has estimated that every 30 seconds there is a death in the United Stated caused from cardiovascular diseases. Heart disease is the number one killer in the United States. It is becoming a natural way to die. They call it death from "natural causes." It is not only a disease of the elderly but is killing people in their prime of life, suddenly and without warning. The very young are showing signs of hardening of the arteries. It is estimated that over half of Americans are accumulating plaque and toxins in their veins. One doctor stated in 1941, when heart attacks started increasing in the United States "atherosclerosis is a disease and not the inevitable consequence of age, since it appears in the young."

John Harvey Kellogg, M.D. in 1916 stated the following: "Diseases of the heart and blood vessels are a common consequence of an acute accumulation of feces in the colon, probably the result of the excessive absorption of toxins to which such accumulation give rise." Fatty deposits in the blood vessels are mainly caused by a toxic colon. An unhealthy colon causes damage to the blood vessels, as well as the small capillaries.

Before World War II, doctors used to treat circulatory diseases as intestinal toxemia or autointoxication. A common statement used was "every physician should realize that the intestinal toxemia are the most important primary and contributing causes of many disorders and diseases of the human body."

Chinese statistics show that "constipation is one of the most common symptoms in ischemic stroke," so Chinese healers often treat stroke by looking for-and treating-constipation. This is what the U.S. doctors used to do before drugs and surgery became the standard way of treatment. As for the cause of stroke, the Chinese include "fatigue and worry," "excessive eating," "dissatisfaction," and "climatic changes," as well as purely Chinese factors like "blood stasis" and "stagnation of liver-qi."

Chinese studies of stroke patients show recovery rates as high as 88%, suggesting that "Chinese medicine is of significance not only in preventing the occurrence of [stroke] but also in treating it." (Keji and S Jun, "Progress of research on ischemic stroke treated with Chinese medicine," *Journal of Traditional Chinese Medicine* 12 (1992): pp 204-10.)

Symptoms of circulatory problems could be the following:

• Chest pain, fatigue on climbing, anxiety, water accumulation in the lower legs, restlessness, dizziness,

• Clogging of the arteries takes place without pain. Fat accumulates around the heart before the veins become clogged.

- Stress has a profound effect on heart attacks when the body has accumulated toxins in the veins and around the heart.

- Nicotine, caffeine, and all drugs, sugar and white flour products add to the fatty buildup on the artery walls causing decreased blood flow and a high risk of heart disease.

- Blood vessels become brittle and break easily, increasing the danger of hemorrhage, blood clots and strokes.

- Uric acid found in meat can clog the small capillaries.

- A congested liver and kidneys causes a back pressure of blood in the veins and weakens the heart as well as the entire circulatory system.

- Proper bowel function prevents accumulation of toxic waste in the liver and blood stream. Most people eat a low fiber diet and do not completely eliminate after each meal. This leaves a residue to accumulate on the large colon walls.

- The "peak hour" for heart attack starts in the early morning hours. The blood thickens with a heavy meal, caffeine, alcohol, smoking, rich desserts, and is heightened with stress.

- Temperature extremes affect some susceptible people's blood viscosity and in hot summers and in cold weather, heart attacks are increased.

THE LYMPHATIC SYSTEM

The lymphatic system is a part of our immune system and is a part of our detoxifaction center. It has the job of carrying nutrients throughout the body as well as removing waste material from all the tissues. The lymph's fluid has the ability to go deep into the tissues where blood cannot penetrate and pick up toxic material in the form of acids and catarrh that has to eliminated for our protection. These toxins are then passed through the eliminative channels of the lymph glands. These lymph glands or nodes collect the waste material and dump them in the blood stream. They are then transported to the colon, kidneys, lungs or skin to be eliminated.

The lymph is a clear fluid which bathes all tissues of the body. The vessels that carry this lymph also carry lymphocytes. They act like complex miniature computers, being able to recognize foreign matter, and producing antibodies to combat them. When the body is supplied with proper nutrition, these antibodies destroy poisons before they can cause serious damage and health problems.

The tonsils and appendix are two of the organs that protect the lymph system from becoming overloaded. The tonsils help in the throat area. The toxic material that is eliminated through the tonsils is usually swallowed and with the help of the lymph fluid is reabsorbed into the system and then carried through the bowels. If the tonsils have been removed, this protection is gone and any infection that enters the mouth goes directly into the lymphatic system, which can cause an overload for the lymph glands to eliminate.

Exercise is very important for the lymphatic system. It needs a pumping action to fulfill its job. The up and down movement on a mini-trampoline causes the lymph vessels to expand and compress, to stretch and relax. This is an action that the lymph fluids need to do their vital job, and eliminate wastes and toxins.

DRUGS THAT CAN CAUSE CORONARY ARTERY DISEASE

The following drugs can cause the symptoms of circulatory diseases and with long use can cause a deterioration in the veins and capillaries. In most cases, the drugs prescribed for a certain ailment usually create the same symptoms.

INDERAL (Propranolol) is used to treat several serious cardiovascular disorders: 1.) Angina. 2.) Heart rhythm disturbance. 3.) High blood pressure. 4.) Myocardial infarction. 5.) It is also prescribed to reduce the frequency and severity of migraine headaches.

The commonly used drugs for circulatory problems such as Propranolol (Inderal), may actually increase "hardening of the arteries," according to a study of the Norwegian Oslo Heart Study Project reported in July 1980. (Weitz, Martin, *Health Shock*, p 156.)

EPINEPHRINE is used for acute attacks of bronchial asthma and allergy sensitivities such as sting reactions. It can cause heart palpitation, and rise in blood pressure and possible stroke in predisposed individuals. It can gradually wear and tear on the artery walls, causing a build-up of plaque and toxins.

BROMOCRIPTINE is used to treat manifestations of Parkinson's disease. This drug can affect heart function adversely and induce or intensify angina in susceptible persons. This drug will eventually weaken the arteries. One side effect of this drug is constipation. If there is impaired liver function, this drug can increase liver damage because of a backed-up colon.

INDOMETHACIN is used to relieve mild or moderately severe pain associated with musculoskeletal acute and chronic gout, rheumatoid arthritis and osteoarthritis, dental, obstetrical and orthopedic surgery, menstrual cramps and migraine like headaches. This drug is not recommended for older adults according to the USP, Drug Information for the health Care Provider. 6th edition. This drug may also make epilepsy or Parkinson's disease worse, cause more stomach and intestinal bleeding than aspirin, and hide the signs of any infection in the body.

DRUGS PRESCRIBED FOR THE CIRCULATORY SYSTEM

NADOLOL prescribed for angina pectoris can cause impotence, mental depression, nausea, vomiting, may mimic Raynaud's phenomenon, may activate bronchial asthma and abrupt withdrawal can cause severe angina (what it is supposed to prevent).

ATENOLOL prescribed in angina pectoris could cause congestive heart failure in advanced heart disease, could worsen angina in coronary heart disease with abrupt withdrawal.

DIURIL and other thiazide diuretics to treat high blood pressure can cause potassium and other mineral deficiencies, leading to cardiac arrhythmia. Potassium and other minerals are essential for the heart.

THE DIGESTIVE SYSTEM

DISEASES OF THE DIGESTIVE SYSTEM

Acidosis	Gingivitis
Alklosis	Heartburn
Anorexia Nervosa	Hepatitis
Appendicitis	Hiatus Hernia
Bad Breath	Indigestion
Celiac Disease	Motion Sickness
Dyspepsia	Pyorrhea
Cirrhosis	Tooth Decay
Gall Stones	Thrush
Gastritis	Ulcers

The digestive system is our first line of defense against disease. It is the digestion and assimilation of the food we eat that determines how efficiently our entire body works. Digestion is the breakdown of food by the digestive system for proper assimilation by the blood and lymph vessels so it can be distributed to all the body cells and be oxidized for healing and rebuilding the body.

Digestive diseases are becoming a national health problem. Over 20 million Americans suffer from digestive problems. Half of all cancers are found in the digestive system. T.V. commercials are a good indication of how many people suffer from digestive problems. The typical American diet contributes to the diseases of the digestive tract.

A Russian scientist named Kouchafoff, found that after cooked food is eaten, white blood cells increase in the intestines. The white blood cells are part of the immune system, and always increase in number when there is a need to eliminate hostile invaders. This would indicate with their concentration on cooked food that it is the beginning of an inflammation or disease. Cooked food places an added burden on the immune system as well as contributes to digestive disturbances. It is no wonder we have so many auto-immune diseases plaguing us today. Eating of raw food does not increase in white cell numbers. Eating of raw vegetables before cooked food prevents the appearance of the extra white cells. This was discovered by a famous Swiss nutritionist, Dr. Bircher-Benner. A salad with endive or watercress included is very beneficial for digestion and will heal and repair the stomach.

Proper digestion depends on a healthy appetite. A healthy appetite depends on live, nourishing food and the images it creates in our minds. The smell and taste of food helps create a proper image in our minds for proper digestion. Digestion begins when hunger enters the scene and starts the saliva gland working. Saliva is important for digesting carbohydrates. Improper digestion of carbohydrates can cause auto-intoxication and gas in the large intestines.

The small intestine is vital in the digestion and absorption of the food we eat. The small intestine changes the food we take in our bodies into useable material like glucose, fatty acids, and amino acids. The type of food we eat determines the nutrients we will receive in our blood stream. Digestion is completed by enzymes secreted in the intestinal juices in the small intestine. Any disruption of the small intestine or disease or digestive problems interferes with the small intestine's main job of absorption, which leads to malabsorption. If the small intestine is healthy, the nutrients move at a normal rate, and are absorbed and assimilated and the waste material is carried on to the large intestine. If there is a large coating of mucus on the intestinal lining, or if the intestines are irritated and moves nutrients too fast, the body will receive very little nourishment. If proteins are not properly digested, they ferment into poisons such as phenol, indol and skatol. These poisons are then absorbed into the bloodstream and cause a breakdown in the system.

Emotional stress plays a major role in stomach digestive disorders. The stomach is a very sensitive organ and nervous problems can slow down or speed up digestion. Under acute stress, the stomach has a tendency to shut off acid production. Chronic stress causes an excessive excretion of hydro-chloric acid, which can cause acid indigestion. This irritation of the mucous membrane lining of the stomach is what causes ulcers and hiatal hernia. It is a big mistake to eat while under emotional stress.

ACID AND ALKALINE BALANCE

Before food can be used in the body for energy it must be digested. Food, after it is digested is called ash, which is either an "acid ash" or an "alkaline ash." For the body to sustain life, the blood needs to be alkaline. If it drifts toward the acid side, death results. Eating an "acid ash" food diet forces the buffering organs of the body to go into a state of hyperactivity. This is done as a "buffer" in the blood, in order to keep it in an alkaline state (a buffer will change acid to alkaline). If the body is exposed too frequently to a hyper-activity state, it causes the organs like the liver, gallbladder and kidneys to wear out. The result is toxicity and illness.

The high protein diet Americans eat is a major cause of the buffering system breaking down. Protein is an acid ash and causes the body to move into a state of hyper-activity to buffer the acid.

An overacid condition of the body is called acidosis. It occurs when the liver, colon, and glands have been overburdened with too much cooked food, a high meat diet, drugs, alcohol, tobacco, sugar and white flour products. Stomach ulcers, diabetes, arthritis, and many health problems are associated with acidosis. Anger can also cause a weakness in the digestive process. Anger, hate, frustration, and depression weaken the nervous system and stomach secretion.

The cause of acidosis is eating too much acid forming foods and not enough alkaline forming foods which causes a toxic colon and affects the liver, and kidneys. Acid is absorbed into the blood stream, causing many diseases in the body.

When the body becomes too alkaline, it is called alkalosis. Alkalosis is caused when foods are not properly digested. In the colon an alkaline medium encourages the growth of strep bacteria and kills the beneficial bacilli in the mucus of the colon walls. Many toxins accumulate and pass through its walls directly into the bloodstream. These toxins can cause fatigue and tissue poisoning. One strong alkaline poison is guanidine, which is one of the strongest alkaline poisons known. This doesn't happen too often. It is easier to become more acidic than alkaline. Overalkaline in the blood can result from extended vomiting or hyperventilating. It can be caused by excessive use of antacids, lack of hydrochloric acid in the stomach, and a deficiency of certain minerals. Certain drugs can cause an alkaline condition, along with high cholesterol, glandular imbalance, poor diet, diarrhea and diseases such as diabetes.

Symptoms of Digestive Problems could be the following:
- Aching muscles
- Headaches
- Indigestion
- Belching, often
- Excessive gas
- Heartburn
- Abdominal Pain
- Bloated Feeling
- Nausea
- Burning in the Stomach
- Wrong Food Combining can create indigestion and acid stomach. Protein and starch are a poor combination. Sugars and starches eaten together can cause and alcoholic stomach. Sugars and proteins are a poor combination. Fruits should be eaten alone.

DRUGS THAT CAN CAUSE DIGESTIVE PROBLEMS

ANTACIDS: They reduce HCL in the stomach and prevent protein from being digested. They will neutralize acids that are causing fermentation but they also reduce the natural HCL production. More natural HCL is needed to treat the cause rather than the symptoms.

ANTIBIOTICS: They destroy the friendly bacterial flora in the colon. This causes deficiencies of the B-complex vitamins and vitamin K and other minerals and lead to dysentery. Most drugs cause disruption in the digestive system.

XANAX: Along with similar tranquilizers, this can disrupt the digestive system. Xanax has over 60 side effects. It is used to treat short-term symptoms of anxiety or panic attacks. Side effects are abdominal discomfort, constipation, diarrhea, dry mouth, increased or decreased appetite, increased or decreased salivation, vomiting and nausea.

COMPAZINE used to control severe nausea and vomiting can cause nausea and vomiting, which severely disrupts the digestive system.

ACTIGALL: It is prescribed to help dissolve certain kinds of gallstones. It can cause abdominal pain, appetite loss, constipation, gas, indigestion, metallic taste, diarrhea, nausea, severe pain in the right side of the abdomen, and vomiting.

ALDACTAZIDE and other high blood pressure drugs are used to eliminate excess water from the body, and can cause disruption in the digestive system and cause abdominal cramps, change in potassium levels, diarrhea, inflammation of the pancreas, loss of appetite, nausea, stomach bleeding, stomach inflammation, stomach ulcers, and vomiting.

ENDOCRINE SYSTEM
(Glandular)

DISEASES OF THE GLANDULAR SYSTEM

Addison's Disease   Hypoglycemia
Cushings Disease   Hypothyroidism
Cystic Fibrosis   Mononucleosis
Diabetes   Pancreatitis
Goiter   Parathyroid Disease
Hyperthyroidism

The glandular system has many important functions necessary for health and well being. The endocrine glands secrete hormones for activities of the body directly into the blood stream. The glands get their orders directly from the brain and spinal cord and have life and death control of the entire body. It is essential that we keep these glands healthy with the finest nutrition possible. It is important and vital that the blood stream be pure and that the veins and arteries be clear and free of fatty deposits. The blood must be flowing freely and the heart functioning normally to get pure blood to all the glandular areas at all times if we expect excellent mental and physical health.

Scientists used to believe that the brain was insulated from the rest of the body by the blood/brain barrier, and that diet did not have much to do with a healthy endocrine system. A major breakthrough occurred when Dr. Richard J. Wurtman and his colleagues at the Massachusetts Institute of Technology demonstrated that diet does contain precursors of brain neurotransmiters which modulate aspects of mood, mind, memory and behavior.

Dr. Wurtman has demonstrated in his research that carbohydrates in a meal stimulate the production of insulin which, in turn, facilitates the uptake of the amino acid tryptophan which is then used by specific regions of the brain for the synthesis and secretion of the neurotransmitter serotonin, which has a calming effect upon mood.

We know that an iodine deficiency has an impact on the thyroid and can produce goiter. Recent studies have demonstrated that zinc insufficiency may have an adverse impact upon thymus secretion of the hormone thymosin which, in turn, has a T-lymphocyte regulatory effect.

Nutrition also has an impact upon the behavior mechanisms of the hypothalamus and pituitary. Animal studies over the past several years have shown that marginal deprivation of certain nutrients and calories can result in suppression of normal appetite mechanisms in the hypothalamus, resulting in eating disorders. This may shed a new light on eating disorders as anorexia nervosa, bulimia and compulsive eating, and the effect of lack of nutrients has on the endocrine and nervous systems.

Proper nutrition does have an impact on a healthy endocrine system. Each gland plays an important role to overall health of the whole body. When one gland isn't working properly, it can affect other glands. It is important that we understand the gland, and the nutrients that will clean, build and strengthen them.

GLANDULAR SYSTEM AND RAW FOOD

Raw foods are necessary for the glandular system. Cooked food kills the enzymes and causes the endocrine glands to become overworked which leads to body intoxication and diseases such as hypoglycemia, diabetes and obesity. Cooked foods over stimulate the glands and cause the body to retain excess weight. The enzymes from live food helps the body to maintain proper metabolism.

The problem arises when the glands do not receive the nutrients necessary to satisfy the body's needs. When this happens, the glands over-stimulate the digestive organs and demand more food (because the body is not nutritionally satisfied) This produces an over secretion of hormones, and an unhealthy appetite, which finally results in exhaustion of the hormone producing glands.

GLANDULAR FUNCTION

The glandular system consists of the pituitary gland, thyroid gland, parathyroid gland, thymus gland, pineal, male sex glands, the testes, female sex glands, the ovaries, pancreas, hypothalamus and adrenal glands.

The glands work together in producing and excreting chemical substances known as hormones. The hormones are responsible for coordinating and controlling various organs and tissues so the body works smoothly and efficiently. The hormones are released into the bloodstream. The hypothalamus, located at the base of the brain, regulates the network of glands along with the nervous system and the pituitary gland. When disorders of the endocrine system develop, they usually consist of either underactivity or overactivity of one or more glands. An imbalance is usually created by the lack of nutrients to the glands.

THE ADRENALS

The adrenals protect us from stress. Aching joints are one sign that the adrenals are exhausted, too exhausted to produce the hormones that prevent pain and inflammation.

Healthy adrenals improves digestion, burn fat more efficiently and give the body strength throughout the day. Herbs which help in a crisis situation for the adrenals are lobelia and cayenne. The Adrenals benefit from Vitamin A, C, B-Complex and Pantothenic Acid. The herbs for the adrenals are licorice, hawthorn, camomile, skullcap, rose hips to nourish and build, capsicum and ginseng to nourish and strengthen the adrenals.

THE THYMUS GLAND

The Thymus gland is considered the youth gland. It helps the removal of negative charges from the body. It helps create an attitude of good thoughts and feeling. It needs beta-carotene, B-complex and zinc. It especially needs calcium and phosphorus. For circulation, cayenne and ginger are good. Also prickly ash, ginkgo, suma and gotu kola. The nervine herbs are beneficial like lobelia, hops, passion flower, scullcap and St. Johns wort. Cleansing herbs are lobelia, mullein, bayberry and echinacea.

THE PINEAL GLAND

The pineal gland puts us at peace with ourselves. It needs stimulation from electro-magnetic impulses from the optic nerves. Sunlight entering the eyes triggers retinal nerve impulses which travel to the pineal gland. The nerve impulses from the pineal gland are fed to the hypothalamus and pituitary which affect many of the vital functions of the body.

THE PITUITARY GLAND

The pituitary is the "Master Gland" acting as a synergist to most all of the glandular extracts. The pituitary, when healthy, protects us from fatigue due to excessive mental stress.

Those who cannot tolerate stress and cannot work under pressure, need the pituitary strengthened.

Vitamins B-6, Vitamin E, and B-Complex are needed as well as manganese, selenium, trace minerals, and amino acids ornithine, tryptophan and taurine. Herbs that help the pituitary are kelp (helps all the glands), gotu kola, and ginseng.

THE PANCREAS

The pancreas is important in the digestion of food, the secretion of insulin for the maintenance of proper blood sugar levels and for activating enzyme processes in the body.

Nutrients for the pituitary are B-complex, minerals, chromium, selenium, manganese and sodium. Amino Acids are Isoleucine, and leucine. Herbs that help are alfalfa, juniper berries, uva ursi, saw palmetto, golden seal, and ho shou-wu.

THE THYROID

The thyroid gland secretes a hormone called thyroxin which regulates the rate of metabolism of human cells. Hyperthyroidism occurs when there is an excess of thyroid hormone and this creates a feeling of heat and the body tends to lose weight because more fuel is being burned, even with a big appetite. Bulging eyes, nervousness and mental fatigue are common.

Hypothyroidism exists when there is insufficient thyroid hormone. The body tends to feel cold and the individual becomes puffy faced, obese, sluggish, and dull-witted.

Nutrients necessary are vitamin B-6, all the B-complex. All minerals are vital but especially, iodine, potassium, sodium, and the amino acid tyrosine. Herbs which help are kelp, dulse, black walnut, white oak bark and gentian.

DRUGS THAT CAN CAUSE DIABETES AND THYROID PROBLEMS

The following drugs can cause latent diabetes in susceptible persons. All drugs cause damage to the inner organs, especially to the delicate glandular system.

CORTICOSTEROIDS used for anemia, eczema, dermatitis, hives and nasal polyps, to name a few can cause problems with the pancreas.

TRICYCLIC ANTIDEPRESSANTS such as Tofranil, Pamelor and serotonin blockers such as Prozac. Used for persons who have feelings of despair and hopelessness, Prozac is a strong drug with many side affects.

INDOMETHACIN such as Indocid is used to reduce inflammation and pain. It can irritate the stomach and intestinal tract, cause gastric ulceration and blood disorders, liver damage and toxic hepatitis.

DRUGS USED TO TREAT DIABETES

ORASONE the generic name is Tolbutamide. It is used to treat Type 11 diabetes (non-insulin-dependent). Orinase-type drugs may possibly lead to more heart problems than diet treatment alone. (The P.D.R. Family Guide). A study done between 1961 and 1969 using tolbutamide showed that diabetics who took drugs to reduce the sugar levels in their bloodstream suffered from more fatal heart attacks. Some doctors felt morally obliged in 1969 to stop giving patients tolbutamide. Yet this drug is still listed drug guides.

CHLORPROPAMIDE It is used in regulating blood sugar in noninsulin-dependent diabetes. Side effects include hypoglycemia, severe and prolonged liver damage, and rare blood cell and bone marrow disorders.

The *New England Journal of Medicine* printed an article commenting on useless diabetic drugs. "There is no reason to use a drug that does not work...even the safest drug is of no value if it has no efficacy...diabetes can probably be controlled in many patients with diet alone." (S.W. Shen, New England Journal Of Medicine,1977, no. 14, page 296.)

IMMUNE SYSTEM

SOME DISEASES OF THE IMMUNE SYSTEM

AIDS	Epstein-Barr Virus
Allergies	Gastritis
Ankylosing Spondylitis	Legionnaires' Disease
Bacteremia	Erythematosus Lupus
Cancer	Reye's Syndrome
Candida	Toxic Shock Syndrome
Chylamydial Disease	

NEW DISEASES

There are several new viruses in the news lately. One that has caused great concern is called "Flesh Eating Virus". There have been several fatal infections reported from England. This infection spreads as fast as one inch per hour and is put in the same category as Hantavirus and Legionnaires' disease. It progresses rapidly to a fatal stage. Although these strains of viruses remain rare, the U.S. centers for disease control report 500 to 1000 of these unusual diseases every year in the United States.

LASSA FEVER

Lassa fever is one of a dozen viruses that scientists call hot agents—viruses that spread easily, kill quickly and have no cures or vaccines. It is found in the blood and urine of infected patients. Those handling these fatal viruses must wear suits hooked to outside air supplies and enter a lab through airtight hatches that seal behind them. All equipment is sterilized or burned to prevent any contamination. This virus is found in West Africa.

One species of rat carries the virus and can contaminate food and household items. This disease becomes fatal when the patient bleeds. One man bled from his nose and mouth. It burst out of his capillaries beneath his skin and eyes.

EBOLA FEVER

This virus was first documented in 1976 when it struck Sudan, a small village in Africa. The victims began to bleed and ran a fever. Ebola killed half the people it infected. The same year it struck in Zaire and 50 other villages killing 90% of its victims.

The immune system is our body's major defense against all viral diseases. Every strain of virus has on its surface uniquely shaped molecular configurations called antigens. These antigens are spotted by the helper T cells in the white blood cells and are able to mobilize the body's defenses. A healthy immune system will have the helper T cells patrolling the bloodstream to recognize a specific antigen and destroy it.

Viruses and germs are all around us. They have been around since the beginning of time. They will not harm a clean body. They are scavengers, waiting for the opportunity to invade the filth in the system. Viruses cannot produce on their own. They need a host to survive.

A germ is a bacterium. It is easily seen with an ordinary microscope. It multiplies and spreads by itself, given the proper conditions. The body can recognize a germ and alerts the macrophages or "germ eaters" of the immune system that the foreign organism has invaded the body's territory. The macrophage then "eats" the germ and gets rid of it. When the macrophage (which is a white blood cell) eats enough germs, it has done its duty and then dies. When there is an accumulation of these dead macrophages, it creates the substance known as pus.

Viruses are a different story. They are very sneaky. The word "virus" comes from the Latin word for 'slimy liquid' or 'poison'. Viruses are very selective about choosing their hosts. Some viruses, like those which cause the flu or rabies, can infect either man or animal, but most favor certain cells or species. "If it's AIDS, it commonly goes to the T cells," states Dr. Bernard Fiels, chairman of the department of microbiology and molecular genetics at Harvard University. "If it's polio, it goes to certain subsets of nerve cells in the spinal cord. If it's hepatitis, it goes to the liver."

Viruses are very tiny in comparison to germs. The difference has been likened in size to a pin head beside a basketball. Viruses are ten to one hundred times as tiny as the average bacterium. They can only be detected by an electron microscope.

How do viruses know which cells they can invade? The answer lies in the protein shell which encases the virus. The protein shell has markers on its exterior which mesh exactly with the receptors found on the surface of certain cells. The virus attaches itself to specific areas on the cells exterior, is then covered by part of the cells membrane and taken inside, like a guest. Some viruses use other means to enter the host cells. Once the virus is inside the cell, it sheds its protein coat and integrates its DNA with the host cells genetic code. The cell does nothing to extricate the virus, believing it is part of itself. Once the genetic reprogramming is set in motion, the cell's genetic apparatus reproduces viruses over and over again. This reaction ultimately leads to the host cell's demise, because eventually the viruses multiply to the extent that it bursts the cell and destroys it. The body, invades more cells and promotes additional destruction of the body's defenses. The key to avoiding the harmful microbes is embracing positive health habits.

INVADING VIRUSES

Leprosy is increasing rapidly in South America. There are an estimated million people in Brazil that have leprosy. It is very common in the Amazon rain forest and growing fast. The treatment they are using is a drug that killed and crippled many babies in the late 50's and early 60's, called Thalidomide. They are finding deformed children from ages 13 to 3. This is a cruel trick to play on the innocent and unsuspecting victims. Thalidomide is being tested in the United States to use on Tuberculosis patients. We need to come to the realization that drugs do not cure. They only suppress the disease further in the body. In fact the wide use of drugs, vaccinations and life style has helped to weaken and break down the immune system. This helps the viruses increase more rapidly.

AIDS is the most devastating virus to the immune system. It completely breaks down the body's defense system. The AIDS victim usually dies from another disease because of no protection from the immune response.

According to Dr William Campbell Douglass, M.D., in which he states in his book, *AIDS The End of Civilization,* "A careful study of World Health Organization (WHO) literature reveals the careful planning that went into the seeding of AIDS in various nations. They used smallpox vaccine for their vehicle and the geographical sites chosen in 1972 were Uganda and other African states, Haiti and Brazil. The recent past of AIDS epidemiology coincided with these geographical areas." Dr. Douglass calls, "AIDS, the greatest Biological disaster in the history of mankind." I am inclined to believe these doctors. We are seeing too many people with immune related diseases. It is estimated that by the year 2000 over 100 million people worldwide will have been infected with HIV. The immune related diseases will increase at about the same rate. We need to protect our immune systems, which is our only protection.

A lecture I attended listening to Eva Snead, M.D., also confirms what Dr. Douglass states. She said, "All viral vaccines are made from Green monkey kidney." We make polio, measles, mumps and rubella with the monkey virus vaccines.

ENVIRONMENTAL POLLUTANTS

Environmental poisoning may be the cause of such diseases as Alzheimer's disease, lupus, multiple sclerosis and Lou Gehrig's disease. The leading causes of death in the United States are coronal heart disease, cancer, and diabetes, which were either nonexistent or were extremely rare before the Industrial Revolution.

These diseases and many more are caused by the slow, chronic poisoning from our polluted environment. The pesticides in our food, the heavy metals in our air, the inorganic minerals, toxins, and chlorine in our water and in white flour products contribute to this poisoning.

These environmental poisons are less then 200 years old, and new ones are constantly being produced. The liver does not have the ability to deal with all these poisons especially when the colon is congested, which blocks the ability of the liver to detoxify. Also, the colon and liver can convert toxic chemicals into poisons and free radicals. Since the body is not used to detoxifying these pollutants, it stores them in the tissues, which will cause diseases of all kinds.

There is also an increase in viral diseases. These are diseases that didn't exist 50 years ago. It is believed that most of our infectious diseases declined because of poisons accompanying the Industrial Revolution. But now these viruses have adapted to the poisons in our environment and are more deadly then ever.

We are made to believe that as a nation we are living longer and have healthier lives than ever before. This has been based on the idea that the average life expectancy has increased. The fact is, our average life expectancy is higher, but that's because we had a very high infant mortality rate 100 years ago. Many individuals who might have died in infancy years ago now live to old age. But they are not healthier. It is life expectancy that has increased, and not the number of years we live.

Eating grains, beans, fruit and vegetables will protect us from the pesticides especially if they are organically grown. Toxins are less of a problem in fruits and vegetables even when they are sprayed with chemicals, than those in animal foods. The animals eat grasses and grains full of pesticides and fungicides and are given hormones and antibiotics. The toxins collect in their fat or tissues. Meat products can have 20 times more poisons than our grains, fruit and vegetables.

DIOXIN DANGER

Dioxin is one of the most potent synthetic chemical toxins that man has ever produced. Dioxin is developed by a chlorine bleaching process. Wood pulp fiber is bleached with dioxin. There are many products made from this wood pulp fiber that we use every day, such as toilet paper, sanitary napkins, tampons, paper towels, tissues, milk cartons, juice cartons, coffee filters, tea bags, paper plates and cups, the packaging of TV dinners as well as other foods. The list could go on and on.

Dioxin is also found in our environment in the air and the water. It is suspected that immune suppression, liver disorders, cancer and birth defects are caused by dioxin. Toxic shock syndrome is an example of how dioxin may be related to this problem. Tampons, for the most part, are treated with dioxin. The bleaching process sensitizes the vagina, making it more vulnerable to infection. If the immune system is low, toxic shock syndrome could develop.

Fluoride in the drinking water damages the body's repair and rejuvenation capabilities. It causes a breakdown of collagen, the protein which binds the body together. Dr. John Yiamouyiannis, author of *Fluoride—The Aging Factor*, says that "Our immune system is the body's defense mechanism against bacteria, infections, viruses, and foreign proteins that get into our bloodstream. It attacks and destroys them. Fluoride interferes with the body's ability to reach and destroy the target. It reduces by 70 percent the ability of these white blood cells to reach the target."

IMMUNE PROTECTION

An excellent formula for protecting the immune system contains: Milk Thistle, which is a potent antioxidant and helps prevent harm from free radicals, bioflavonoids and vitamin C which work together, synergistically enhancing absorption, which have anti-inflammatory, anti-allergy and auto-viral properties, grapefruit pectin, which is a fiber that helps carry toxins from the body, acerola fruit, which is extremely high in natural vitamin C, and indoles, an extraction from cruciferous vegetables, which have been scientifically shown to balance hormone levels, detoxify the intestines and liver and strengthen the body's immune system. Building the immune system is the only sure defense we have against diseases.

DRUGS THAT CAN CAUSE IMMUNE RELATED DISEASES

All drugs will eventually weaken the immune system. Vaccinations and antibiotics are widely used and are considered one of the main causes of these disorders. Autoimmune diseases have increased since mass inoculations were introduced.

In the book, *The Essential Guide To Prescription Drugs*, 1992, by James W. Long, M.D., the following is stated, "It is estimated that 15,000 to 20,000 cases of drug-related lupus occur annually in the United States. More than 50 medications have been thought to be responsible for inducing lupus. The following drugs have a definite association.

CHLORPROMAZINE Brand names are Largactil, Thorazine, Stelazine. These are major tranquilizers and neuroleptics. They are prescribed for serious mental illness, particularly schizophrenia. Possible side effects are loss of white blood cells, liver damage and damage to the central nervous system causing trembling and rigidity (Parkinsonism). Hormone problems are common, breast enlargement, absence of menstrual periods, and impotence. It can also cause depression, agitation, insomnia, a fall in blood pressure and weakness.

HYDRALAZINE Some brand names are Alazine, Apresazide and Apresoline. These are used for moderate to severe hypertension. This has been known to induce Lupus Erythematosus-like Syndrome. It can also cause rare blood disorders and liver damage.

ISONIAZID Some brand names are Isotamine, Laniazid, and Rifamate. This drug is used to prevent and treat active Tuberculosis. This disease is increasing in the United States and around the world. It can induce Lupus, liver damage, nervous system disorders, bone marrow depression and mental disturbances.

DRUGS USED TO TREAT IMMUNE RELATED DISEASES

AZT was used as an experimental drug on AIDS. The drug companies have been trying to find a chemical that will kill the virus and rebuild the Immune System. To date, none of the AIDS drugs have proven to cure the disease. There has been talk of a vaccination for the AIDS plague and yet this disease was brought upon mankind through smallpox and other vaccinations.

INTESTINAL SYSTEM

The Large Intestine or Colon

SOME DISEASES OF THE INTESTINAL SYSTEM

Appendicitis	Crohn's Disease
Colitis	Diarrhea
Constipation	Diverticulitis

It is estimated that 90% of all ailments plaguing mankind begin in a toxic and constipated colon. Poisons from the colon can weaken and stress the heart, can lodge in the joints and cause stiffness and pain, can invade the muscles and cause fatigue and weakness, can enter the brain and cause senility and brain fatigue, and can cause the skin to eliminate in the form of blemishes, psoriasis, liver spots, wrinkles and bumps, and can irritate the lungs and cause asthma, bronchitis and bad breath.

The following are poisons from a toxic colon which can cause diseases and discomfort to mankind.

Phenol—Agamatine—Indol—Cresol—Butyric Acid—Botulin—Histidine—Ammonia—Indican—Idoethylamine—Ptomarropine—Neurin—Sepsin—Uric Acid—

Dr. Henry A. Cotton, in 1932 wrote a paper about the pathology of intestinal toxemia. He had studied the colons removed from insane patients for years and on examination revealed one or more of the following characteristic changes in the bowel.

1. Destruction of the epithelium and mucosa; the mucous membrane may be denuded and eroded over large areas, there may be edematous thickening of the muscular wall and congestion of the peritoneal coat.

2. Areas of hemorrhage, pigmentation and ulceration.

3. Extreme atony and atrophy of the muscular coats with the bowel wall thinned in places to a parchment-like consistency, resulting in dilated, pouchy areas referred to by Cotton as "segmental blowouts".

4. Marked thickening of the bowel wall due to chronic fibrous tissue growth.

5. Adenitis of the mesenteric glands. This is invariably present. Cultures made by Cotton from enlarged lymph nodes in the mesentery of the colon and small intestine, after colectomy or a postmortem in every instance showed various types of streptococci and virulent colon bacilli.

6. Diverticulosis.

It is significant to know that the colon is in even worse shape in the majority of people today than it was at the turn of the century. Diets are low in fiber, the body needs 30 to 40 grams of fiber a day. Waste material accumulates because of the glue-like food we ingest daily. The body needs pure water. Inorganic minerals, toxic metals, worms and parasites help create constipation and accumulate in the body and produce toxic waste material. When eating under stress, it causes free radicals, indigestion and constipation. Lack of nutrients in the food increases constipation.

Eating regular wholesome food, proper sleeping habits, and regular exercise will help proper elimination. Food combining, finding a regular time to eliminate every day, and finding peace within oneself helps the body regulate itself.

SOME DRUGS THAT CAN CAUSE CONSTIPATION

Aluminum is very constipating. It is found in food processing, (pickles and relishes), aluminum cookware and foils, (Do not use foil to cook baked potatoes), antacids, baking powder, beer, bleached flour, buffered aspirin, deodorants, FD&C color additives, municipal water sources, salt, soda and tobacco smoke.

PEPTO-BISMOL This is used for ulcers to coat the stomach. It contains bismuth subsalicylate and can cause constipation. It also can cause confusion, drowsiness, headaches, hearing difficulty, anxiety and other side effects.

PEPCID AND TAGAMET This drug is used for ulcers. It can cause constipation, insomnia, dizziness, mental confusion and other side effects.

ASPIRIN It is in common use today. It is used for relief of mild to moderate pain and inflammation and to reduce fever and prevent blood clots. It can cause constipation as well as irritate the stomach, heartburn, skin rashes, hives, nasal polyps and nasal discharge.

ATROPINE It is prescribed to prevent motion sickness. It has an antispasmodic action. Side effects are constipation, blurring of near vision, dry mouth and throat, and hesitancy in urination.

DICYCLOMINE It is prescribed to relieve gastrointestinal spasms. It can cause constipation, urinary retention, headaches, weakness, dizziness, nausea, and vomiting to name a few side effects.

ANTIDEPRESSANT DRUGS The following can cause constipation ELAVIL—SINEQUAN—TOFRANIL—They can also cause impaired urination, dry mouth, blurred vision and many other side effects.

DRUGS USED FOR CONSTIPATION

LAXATIVES These are used in abundance in the United States. The advertisements in magazines and on T.V. would indicate that it is very common. Regular use causes an inactive and lazy bowel. They are habit forming. They do not rebuild the colon but can cause depletion of minerals such as potassium. Loss of potassium can lead to a heart attack.

INTEGUMENTARY SYSTEM
(Skin, Sweat Glands, Hair, Nails)

SOME DISEASES OF THE INTEGUMENTARY SYSTEM

Acne	Cysts
Abscess	Dandruff
Frostbite	Nail Problems
Athlete's Foot	Psoriasis
Baldness	Warts
Bug Bites	Wounds
Burns	Wrinkles
Corns and Callouses	

The health of the hair, nails and skin is an indication of the over-all health of the entire body. When the skin has eruptions, rashes, and allergic reactions, it means the inner skin or mucous membranes also have eruptions. The skin is the largest elimination organ. The skin underneath the hair also eliminates constantly.

Lack of essential minerals is also a cause of hair loss and unhealthy skin. Any disease that impairs the vitality of the body has an effect upon the hair and skin. Hair loss and problems with the scalp and skin are symptoms of an imbalance within the body.

The hair and skin need to be treated internally and externally. The proper shampoo, without chemicals, and harsh detergents which contains nutrients is the first line of defense. Loss or discoloration of the hair is generally due to the lack of hair building elements in the blood or to sluggish circulation in the head and skin. Many experts advise shampooing daily to remove dirt and impurities from the environment. Also toxins are eliminated constantly through the skin and the scalp. Massaging the scalp before washing will help to loosen up dead skin and increase circulation.

The skin needs natural ingredients in its cleansers and moisturizers to insure that the pores are clean and free from dirt and other toxins for healthy looking skin. Diet has a profound effect on the health of the skin and hair. The blood needs nourishment through vitamins, minerals, live food, and herbs, which are beneficial to healthy hair and skin. The hair and nails need protein and minerals.

Acne is the leading skin disease. Teenagers and young adults account for the largest number of skin patients. Other skin disorders are skin cancer, warts, fungal infections and psoriasis.

The nails can also mirror the health of the body. White spots can indicate a lack of minerals, or poor assimilation of nutrients. Ridges going lengthwise can indicate anemia or having had anemia in the past. It could also be a lack of B-vitamins and adequate protein. Iron supplements containing yellow dock and dandelion would help in the assimilation of iron. Bulging or too flat nails means a diet change is needed. Pink nails indicate good circulation.

Brittle nails that break in layers may indicate a deficiency of B-vitamins or iron, or of silica found in horsetail or oatstraw. Splitting nails may be due to lack of hydrochloride acid. Horizonal ridges may reflect a deficiency of protein, calcium, silica or sulphur. It could also stem from illness or severe stress, which could cause a deficiency of B-complex vitamins.

SOME DRUGS THAT CAN CAUSE HAIR LOSS

MACRODONTIN An antibiotic to treat urinary tract infections. It can cause hair loss, liver damage and nervous disorders.

CYTOXAN It is used to treat cancer of the breast, leukemia, Hodgkins, skin, adrenal gland, retina and cancer plasma cells. It can cause hair loss, bladder damage and a secondary cancer may occur up to several years after the drug is given. It may cause nausea, vomiting, stop menstruation, initiate prolonged impairment of fertility or temporary sterility in men. Many more side effects may occur.

COUMADIN It is a blood thinner. It can cause severe bleeding, pain in chest, joints, abdominal pain as well as hair loss, and many more side effects.

TEGRETOL Used to treat seizures. It may cause heart, liver or kidney damage, hair loss, dizziness, drowsiness, nausea, vomiting along with dozens of other side effects.

HALDOL Used to treat schizophrenia. It can cause permanent liver damage, hair loss, muscle spasms, and twitches in face and body.

RIDAURA A gold preparation to treat rheumatoid arthritis. It has to be taken for 3 to 6 months to get beneficial results. It may suppress joint swelling but does not cure rheumatoid arthritis. It may cause hair loss, diarrhea, indigestion, stomach pain, gas,

vomiting nausea, and many other problems.

NALFON An anti-inflammatory to treat arthritis. It can cause constipation, nausea, diarrhea, hearing loss, nervousness, ringing in ears, tremors, upper respiratory infections and hair loss as well as many more.

Other drugs that can cause hair loss are asthma drugs, Atrovent, Choleclyl, beta blockers such as Corgard and Inderal, blood pressure drugs such as Catapres, and Lopid, depression drugs such as Elavil Sinequan and Prozac, gout drugs such as Zyloprim, and Colfbenemid, thyroid drugs such as Synthroid, and Methimazole, ulcer drugs such as Tagamet, Pepcid, Zantac and Cutptec.

DRUGS USED TO TREAT SKIN DISORDERS

One treatment is a synthetic vitamin A derivative called Tegison (why not use the natural vitamin A?). It is considered an effective treatment for severe, resistant psoriasis. Major drug-induced effects include: birth defects, hepatitis, adverse effects on eyes and vision, musculoskeletal structures, and blood cholesterol and triglycerides. Also coal tar preparations, steroid creams, methotrexate (an anti-cancer drug), and anthralin have many side effects.

A DRUG DEVELOPED FOR HAIR GROWTH

Rogaine, a highly advertised hair growth treatment, is found only moderately effective in treating male, pattern baldness in 39% of users. It is also advertised to treat thinning hair in women. There are over 40 side effects of Rogaine, some of these are excessive body hair growth in 80% of users, (what woman would want more hair on her face back, arms and legs),retention of salt and water, excessively rapid heart beat, scalp irritation, aches and pains, anxiety, back pain, blood disorders, bone fractures, bronchitis, depression, eczema, exhaustion, facial swelling, faintness, genital infections, headaches, vomiting and weight gain.

THE NERVOUS SYSTEM
(Nerves, Brain)

SOME DISEASES OF THE NERVOUS SYSTEM

Alzheimer's Disease	Memory Loss
Anorexia	Meniere's Syndrome
Autism	Meningitis
Bruxism	Multiple Sclerosis
Bulimia	Muscular Dystrophy
Depression	Neuritis
Down's Syndrome	Parkinson's Disease
Dyskinesia	Schizophrenia
Dyslexia	Senility
Epilepsy	Shingles
Fatigue	Spina Bifida
Headaches	Vertigo
Hyperactivity	Tic Douloureux
Insomnia	
Manic-Depressive Disorder	

The central nervous system consists of the spinal cord and brain. The peripheral nervous system comprises the nerves that extend out from the spinal cord and the base of the brain to other parts of the body. The autonomic nervous system regulates the internal organs.

The nervous system is a very delicate and vital part of the body and needs to be treated and fed properly. The central nervous system and the immune system are closely connected. When one system fails, the other is affected. The brain has the job of transmitting information back and forth from the immune system.

The brain is our most sensitive organ and reacts to poor nutrition, prescription drugs, air pollution, poor food and water. When a brain neuron dies, it can never be replaced. The brain is vulnerable to lack of oxygen or glucose. It can be destroyed by drugs, alcohol and drugs together, concussion, stroke, toxic metals such as mercury and aluminum, and inflammation. Malnutrition during gestation and in early childhood causes irreparable damage to the structure of the brain.

Brain starved infants lose their ability to develop properly. Alzheimer's disease creates a loss of memory, and autopsies on these individuals have disclosed extremely low brain levels of biochemical raw materials essential for synthesizing neurotransmitters, which helps make remembering and thinking possible. The lack of nutrients to the brain can cause serious problems with memory.

Brain and nervous system disturbances can start early in life and gradually increase. Researchers have found that dyslexia, learning problems, writing difficulties and other problems of the nervous system are connected with cerebral diseases such as Alzheimer's. It may take years to manifest itself in a serious dementia disease as it is a gradual process. Just because we all age doesn't mean we have to have memory and brain dysfunction.

In researching nervous disorders, I came across literature written by medical doctors at the turn of the century that proved there was an actual connection between the health of the colon and brain and nervous disorders. Many women I have interviewed with nervous disorders had excellent success when they cleaned their colon with herbs and changed their diets.

SOME DRUGS THAT CAN CAUSE NERVOUS SYSTEM DISORDERS

Benzodiazepines are psychotropic. Ativan is a brand name and Lorazepam in a generic name. These drugs can contribute to violent behavior, such as murder and suicide. The have also been associated with an increased risk of babies form with a cleft lip. It is believed they can also effect children with behavioral problems when mothers have taken them in mid term. (Melville, Arabella and Johnson, Colin, *Cured To Death*).

ATIVAN is prescribed to treat anxiety and nervous tension. Some side effects are: unsteadiness, lethargy, drowsiness, hangover effects, fainting, indigestion, disorientation, depression, agitation, amnesia and insomnia.

BITOLTEROL with the brand name Tornalate is prescribed for prevention and relief of asthma. Side effects are nervousness, irregular heart rhythm, dizziness, insomnia and fine tremor of hands.

BROMOCRIPTINE the brand name is Parlodel and it is prescribed for Parkinson's disease, prevention of lactation following childbirth and correction of infertility. Side effects are abnormal involuntary movements and altered behavior, Raynaud's phenomenon, dizziness, nervousness, and nightmares. Serious side effects are confusion, hallucinations, incoordination, visual disturbances, depression and seizures.

CYCLOBENZAPRINE the brand name is Flexural. It is prescribed as a muscle relaxant. Side effect are confusion, depression, skin rash, hives, swelling of face and tongue, fatigue, weakness, numbness, and unsteadiness.

SOME DRUGS USED TO TREAT DEPRESSION

NARDIL usually prescribed only after anti-depressant treatment has failed. It is used for anxiety or phobias mixed with depression. Common side effects are constipation, dizziness, drowsiness, fatigue, headache, muscle spasms, sexual difficulties, tremors and weakness. There are a whole list of foods and beverages to avoid when taking Nardil, and some of them are caffeine and chocolate to excess, cheese, except cottage cheese and cream cheese, dry sausage, flava bean pods, pickled foods, wine, yeast extract and yogurt.

AVENTYL is prescribed for depression. There are over fifty side effects listed including agitation, anxiety, constipation, diarrhea, dizziness, fatigue, hair loss, hallucination, heart attack, insomnia, nausea, nightmares, numbness, panic, tremors and weight gain.

HERBS FOR NERVOUS DISORDERS

Nervous disorder diseases are becoming more common. Almost all nervous disorders are affected by auto-intoxication. This is self poisoning by chronic constipation. Stress, heavy metal poisoning, air pollution and diet can affect the nervous system.

The following herbal combinations will help build up the nervous system: Blood purifier, calcium combination, combination for digestion, glands, and nerves, relaxants, lower bowels, potassium and stress.

Nervine and antispasmodic herbs strengthen the functional activity of the nervous system. They strengthen the mind and promote good mental health and clarity as well as aiding imbalances and mental diseases. Most nervine herbs are also antispasmodics; herbs that relieve spasms of muscles to help stop tremors, convulsions and cramps. They also serve as broncho-dilators, relieving spasms in the bronchial tubes. Others help to relieve menstrual cramping and headaches. Many of these herbs nourish the mind and nerves and restore the flow of energy in the body and mind.

Emotions, like anxiety and fear, weaken the kidneys and adrenals. They damage the nerves and cause insomnia, mental instability, numbness, cramping and nerve pain, which may lead to damage of nerve tissue.

Negative emotions cause an imbalance in the brain. These are emotions like anger, envy, and hatred. They can cause hypertension, insomnia, irritability and other mental and nervous imbalances.

HERBAL HELP TO STRENGTHEN THE NERVES AND PROMOTE NATURAL, PEACEFUL SLEEP

Daily relaxation techniques need to be practiced. Massage therapy is relaxing for the nerves. Daily intake of B-complex, vitamin C and herbal calcium are essential for the nerves.

Confusion - Gotu kola, red clover and scullcap.

Depression - Blue vervain, cayenne, damiana, gotu kola, kelp, rosemary and scullcap.

Exhaustion - Gotu kola, dong quai, ginger, lady's slipper, licorice, passion flower and valerian.

Grief - Black cohosh, damiana, dong quai, hops, lady's slipper, sage, scullcap, valerian.

Hysteria - Catnip, chamomile, crampbark, hops, lady's slipper, licorice, lobelia, mistletoe, passion flower, scullcap and valerian.

Insomnia - Catnip, chamomile, hops, lady's slipper, passion flower, pappermint, scullcap and valerian.

Muscle Twitching - Blue vervain, hops, lady's slipper, passion flower, scullcap, and valerian.

Nerve Tonic - Dong quai, hops, lady's slipper, passion flower, and scullcap.

Nerves, Soothing - Black cohosh, catnip, chamomile, hawthorn berries, hops, passion flower, peppermint, scullcap and valerian.

Nervousness - Catnip, blue vervain, hawthorn, and valerian.

Nevous Exhaustion - Blue vervain, gotu kola, hawthorn, hops and scullcap.

Nervous Excitement - Black cohosh, chamomile, gotu kola, hawthorn and scullcap.

Nervous Headaches - Blue vervain, chamomile, feverfew, gotu kola, passion flower, scullcap, valerian and wood betony.

Nervous Indigestion - Catnip, chamomile, gentian, ginger, hops, papaya, and peppermint.

Nervous Irritability - Catnip, chamomile, gotu kola, hawthorn, lady's slipper, and wood betony.

Nightmares - Chamomile, hops, passion flower, scullcap, and valerian.

Sleeplessness from Jangled Nerves - Black cohosh, passion flower, scullcap, and valerian.

Soothing for Female Problems - Black cohosh, chamomile, dong quai, lobelia, passion flower, safflower, and valerian.

Stress - Hawthorn, kelp, licorice, wild yam.

Tension - Chamomile, lady's slipper, passion flower, scullcap, valerian and wood betony.

Wakefullness - Passion flower and scullcap.

Weakness of Nerves - Blue vervain and valerian.

THE RESPIRATORY SYSTEM

SOME DISEASES OF THE RESPIRATOY SYSTEM
(Nose, Throat, Trachea, Bronchi)

Allergies	Hay Fever
Asthma	Laryngitis
Bronchitis	Pharnygitis
Coughs	Pleurisy
Cold	Pneumonia
Croup	Sinusitis
Emphysema	Tuberculosis
Flu	

The respiratory system depends on clean oxygen and it may well be the most essential nutrient for health and well-being. Almost all the body's vital functions depend on oxygen especially energy production in the muscles. Lack of oxygen depletes the body of energy.

The lungs are one of the channels of

elimination in the body. The lungs and the kidneys expel the greatest percentage of worn-out phosphorus, and all waste material is removed from the cells through proper breathing. The problem arises with respiratory diseases when the kidneys and colon are congested. The lungs are not meant to eliminate toxic material for the kidneys and colon, but when they are backed up, the lungs eliminate. The delicate lungs become irritated and cause discomfort and infections. Breathing properly with fresh, clean air is essential to cleanse the body and utilize nutrients. Exercise in fresh air helps the lungs increase their ability to pump oxygen. The vessels and circulatory system are kept healthy by the blood vessels. The bone marrow stimulates to produce more red cells, and carbon dioxide and waste material are removed from the cells. Metabolism in all body organs is stimulated with intake of oxygen.

The most frequent cause of illness in the United States is acute respiratory infections. Air pollution, bad diet, tobacco, and constipation are the main causes of lung problems. Air pollution causes serious health problems. Respiratory infections include asthma, emphysema, chronic bronchitis, coughing and chest pain and are caused and aggravated by toxic air pollution. Burning eyes, an irritated throat, breathing difficulties and impaired immune function can also result from excessive toxic air pollution.

There are six known pollutants that are causing serious damage to the lungs and they are lead, ozone, carbon monoxide, nitrogen oxides, sulfur oxides and fine particulates (PM10). PM10 suppresses the body's immune system and may even cause cancer.

Carbon monoxide binds with hemoglobin in the blood and decreases the ability of the blood to transport oxygen and can result in dizziness, headaches, and slowed reflexes. Recent research indicates that prolonged exposure to carbon monoxide may cause arterial or heart disease.

Ozone is a very serious pollutant that can cause permanent lung scarring and decreases pulmonary function at levels found in our air. At lower levels ozone also causes eye irritation, wheezing and burning in the nose and throat.

Lead is a very dangerous pollutant. Lead can effect blood forming tissues, reproductive and nervous system and kidneys disorders. Lead also damages neurological tissues and diminishes learning potential, especially in children.

SOME DRUGS THAT CAN CAUSE RESPIRATORY DISORDERS

PINDOLOL is an antihypertensive and beta adrenergic blocker used to treat high blood pressure. It can cause bronchial asthma (in asthmatic persons), depression, anxiety, insomnia, abnormal dreams, nausea, constipation, diarrhea, fluid retention and joint and muscle discomfort.

HYDRALAZINE is used to treat hypertension and severe congestive heart failure. It can cause nasal congestion, constipation, delayed urination, headaches, dizziness, tremors, nervousness, confusion, depression and bleeding into lung tissue.

KETROPROFEN is used to relieve pain and inflammation. Side effects are drowsiness, ringing in ears, and fluid retention. It can also cause depression, confusion, impaired memory, changes in kidney function, asthma, kidney failure, vomiting blood and many more. Aspirin, oral contraceptives, penicillin, and resperine can also cause the symptoms of asthma.

DRUGS USED TO TREAT ASTHMA

THEOPHYLLINE is used to treat acute bronchial asthma. Side effects are nervousness, insomnia, rapid heart rate, headache, dizziness, irritability, tremor, fatigue and weakness. It can also cause loss of appetite, nausea, vomiting, abdominal pain and diarrhea.

PROVENTIL is used as an inhaler or in tablet form. It is prescribed for the relief of bronchospasm. Side effects include, nervousness, palpitation, headache, dizziness, restlessness, insomnia, hand tremor, nausea, heartburn and vomiting.

BECLOMETHASONE A cortisone-like drug used to treat the relief of allergic rhinitis and control severe chronic asthma. Side effects are thrush, skin rash, sore throat, bronchospasm, and asthmatic wheezing.

THE STRUCTURAL SYSTEM

(Bones, Muscles, Cartilage)

SOME DISEASES OF THE STRUCTURAL SYSTEM

Arthritis	Muscular Dystrophy
Carpal Tunnel Syndrome	Osteomalacia
Bursitis	Osteoporosis
Fractures	Rheumatism
Gout	Scoliosis
Lumbago	Sprains
Muscle Cramps	Swellings
	TMJ

The bones provide the foundation for the muscles. Symptoms of osteoporosis are chronic neck, shoulder muscle, and back pain at the end of the day, and pain and stiffness when sitting up. Fibrositis is another common disease with which women suffer. The muscles, nerves and bones are affected. Muscle tightness, spasms and chronic back pain are common in fibrositis.

When we have aches and pains of the bones, muscles and ligaments, the body is trying to warn us that something is wrong.

We need to respond and find the cause of the aches and pains. The sooner we deal with the causes, the sooner the aches and pains will go away.

One of the main causes of bone loss, and muscle aches and pains is lack of nutrients or the ability to assimilate them. The diet we eat may be causing bone loss. Calcium is abundant in many foods, and if we eat a natural diet, we should get plenty of calcium. What we eat may be leaching calcium and essential minerals from the bones. Caffeine, soda drinks, high meat diet, sugar products, and white flour will all leach calcium and essential minerals from the system. Many of the lifestyle variables and nutritional habits that contribute to the loss of bones mass are the same ones that increase the risk of many other degenerative diseases. When we nourish the body to prevent bone loss, we may be avoiding many other diseases.

Bruising, inflammation, and injured ligaments are common. When the bones, and muscles are nourished properly, there is less chance of sustaining injuries. The best way to deal with bones, muscle and nervous aches and pains is nutrition and chiropractic approaches.

Bones and muscles can be strengthened with vitamins, minerals and herbs. The right diet will also give strength to the structural system. A lot of fresh and steamed vegetables, fruit, whole grains, nuts, seeds, sprouts, supplements such as essential fatty acids, chromium and an herbal bone combination, containing oatstraw and horsetail are essential.

Science has proven Silica's crucial role in calcium metabolism, bone formation, normal growth and healing properties for many ailments. Horsetail and oatstraw, with its rich content of silica have been found to play a crucial role, both preventively and therapeutically, in the following: Arteriosclerosis, Atherosclerosis, Osteoporosis, Arterial and connective tissue related diseases; for the synthesis of elastin and collagen fibers in the ligaments, discs, skin, tendons, nails and hair. Silica helps arthritis, assists normal growth in children and adults, pregnant and lactating women, Pagets disease, and practically all bone degenerative situations.

In Louis C. Kervran's book, *Biological*

170

Transmutations, his findings revealed that significant amount of bone-breaks and fractures could be avoided altogether if sufficient silica were included in the daily dietary intake. He also found that the number one food to use during bone healing is whole grains (which are generally high in magnesium and low in calcium). He found that a high meat or flesh food intake, on a regular basis, can have a demineralizing effect upon the total body, as it is both acidifying to the system as well as relatively poor in minerals. The grain, buckwheat affords an excellent source of minerals including manganese as well as magnesium, and brown rice rates high in magnesium and also is valuable for its silica content. Millet is high in calcium and magnesium and is easy to digest and assimilate.

DRUGS THAT CAN CAUSE STRUCTURAL PROBLEMS

METHOTREXATE

An anticancer drug used to treat severe psoriasis, childhood cancers, and prevention of rejection of bone marrow transplant. Side effects are sores in mouth and throat, vomiting, cramping, diarrhea, bloody urine, weakness, fatigue and bone marrow depression.

CORTISONELIKE STEROIDS

These are used for many diseases such as asthma, arthritis, skin problems and side effects include bone thinning sterates, and can also cause Cushings Syndrome where bone fragility is manifested.

ZIDOVUDINE

An antiviral drug used in AIDS infected individuals to reduce the risk of infections. Side effects are serious bone marrow depression, brain toxicity, skin rash, hives, headaches, weakness, insomnia and nervousness along with many more.

DRUGS USED TO PREVENT BONE LOSS AND MUSCLE ACHES AND PAINS

PREMARIN It is used for menopause and to prevent osteoporosis. Side effects are increased risk of endometrial carcinoma and cancer of the lining of the womb.

CODEINE It is used for pain, and is found in empracet, phenaphen and tylenol. Side effects are addiction, nausea, constipation and drowsiness.

IBUPROFEN It is prescribed for sprained muscles, inflamed joints and tennis elbow. Side effects are digestive tract irritation, heartburn, indigestion, ulcers and can cause damage to the kidneys.

THE URINARY SYSTEM
(Kidneys, Bladder)

SOME DISEASES OF THE URINARY SYSTEM

Bedwetting
Bladder and Kidney Infections
Bright's Disease
Cystitis
Kidney Stones

The kidneys are working constantly. A constant drip, occurs day in and day out, all day and all night, three to four times more by day than by night, from the kidneys into the bladder. The kidneys are the chief organs for cleansing the body's internal fluid. They are our filtering system, and they absorb and excrete toxins. If the filters are plugged up, it may cause infections, and when the kidneys lose their ability to filter toxins and filter the blood, they can become diseased and cause the loss of protein in the blood which is lost in the urine. Poor kidneys will also lose essential nutrients such as potassium, calcium, magnesium and zinc. Kidney disease causes toxins to remain in the blood and poison the tissues. Kidney failure can cause high blood pressure, stroke, heart attack or glaucoma.

The kidney's job is to maintain a constant and healthy internal environment in the body. They adjust the body's electrolyte balance. They manufacture hormones that regulate blood pressure, calcium metabolism and red blood cell production. The kidneys are very smart. They eliminate whatever is bad for the body and brain and any excess of the good. If you go on a candy spree, sugar rises in the blood, reaches a concentration too high for safety, and the kidneys have the job of throwing out the excess.

The kidneys try to maintain the health of the body, but when distress hits, pain, pallor, swelling, high blood pressure, blood in the urine, burning and stinging—you know your kidneys are in trouble. Its not their fault! They would take care of you if you would let them.

Toxins can accumulate in the blood and cause kidney damage. Alcohol, drugs and smoking can cause damage to the kidneys as well as exposure to heavy metals such as cadmium, lead and mercury. These can accumulate and cause damage to the kidneys. Drinking water contains metals as well as air pollution. Smokers have higher incidences of kidney failure than nonsmokers.

About 12 million Americans experience urinary incontinence, and it affects all ages, not just the elderly. There are many diseases that can cause this as well as pregnancy, infections, surgery, and obesity.

Kidney stones are common and about 90 percent are caused by calcium deposits. The concentration of calcium can be eliminated without surgery. Distilled water, herbal calcium formula, and kidney formulas to heal, and dissolve toxins and strengthen the kidneys are helpful.

DRUGS THAT CAN CAUSE KIDNEY DAMAGE

There are many pain killers that can cause kidney damage.

TOLMETIN It is prescribed for the relief of pain in acute and chronic rheumatoid arthritis, osteoarthritis and juvenile rheumatoid arthritis. Side effects are liver and kidney damage with painful urination and bloody urine, pain in intestinal tract, ulceration, headache, dizziness, blurred vision, ringing in the ears, and abnormal bleeding or bruising.

SULFISOXAZOLE These are used against susceptible bacteria and protozoa. Side effects are skin rashes, rare blood disorders, anemia, drug induced kidney and liver damage, headaches, dizziness, unsteadiness, ringing in the ears, nausea, vomiting, abdominal pain and diarrhea.

RIFAMPIN A strong antibiotic used in treating tuberculosis in combination with other drugs. It is used in prevention of meningitis. Side effects are: skin rash, hives, drug fever, headaches, drowsiness, dizziness, numbness and tingling, drug induced liver and kidney damage with impaired urine production, and bloody or cloudy urine.

DRUGS USED TO TREAT URINARY INFECTIONS

PENICILLIN It is used to treat infections due to susceptible microorganisms. Side effects are yeast infections, drug induced colitis, skin rashes, black tongue, nausea, vomiting, mild diarrhea and dizziness.

CLINDAMYCIN An antibiotic used for serious infections in the respiratory tract, abdominal cavity, genital tract in women and blood stream. Side effects are multiple joint pains, skin rash, toxic liver reaction with jaundice, severe colitis, persistent diarrhea, and rare reduction of white blood cell and platelet counts.

CHANNELS OF ELIMINATION

THE LIVER

There are seven channels of elimination that need to be considered when it comes to health and vitality. They are the Liver, Kidneys, Lungs, Bowels, Skin, Blood and Lymph System. The Liver is the key channel of elimination. It is the most important and the last to be considered when it comes to health. Good health is impossible without proper function of the liver. The typical American diet contributes to a damaged liver, and you can go for years and not be aware of it. The high meat, high fat, sugar, white flour products contribute to a dysfunctional liver. Dr. A. Vogel, an herbalist for over sixty years says, "Everything that enters the liver through the portal-vein must be detoxified and transformed. This is the reason proper liver function is so enormously important for the health of the whole body-more important than is generally presumed."

Dr. Andrew Weil, M.D., author of *Natural Health, Natural Medicine,* says, "High-Protein diets impose a considerable work load on the digestive system and may contribute to feelings of fatigue and lack of energy. A frequent complaint of patients who consult me is lack of energy. If I can convince them to cut down on the amount of protein they eat, increase their intake of starch and vegetables, and do more aerobic exercise, most of them find that they feel better and have more energy.

Another problem with protein as a fuel is that it does not burn clean. Because of its nitrogen content, protein leaves "ashes" when it burns, toxic nitrogen wastes that must be eliminated from the system. After a high-protein meal, amino acids flood into the bloodstream. The liver has to work hard to metabolize them to a simple compound, urea, which is poisonous and must be removed by the kidneys. For this to happen, large amounts of water have to be excreted to flush the urea from the blood. In addition to the general workload on the entire digestive system, protein metabolism especially taxes the liver and kidneys."

Dr. Vogel says, "There are several well-known cancer researchers who, on the basis of their experience, affirm that cancer cannot develop in the body, nor can other cell degenerations occur if the liver is functioning in an efficient, healthy way. Usually, a reduction of the liver activity is at the basis of the formation of tumors, when the purification and regeneration of this vital organ is not working satisfactorily."

Everything we breath, eat and absorb through our skin is purified and refined in the liver. The heavy metals we breathe, and drugs we take are the most destructive elements that the liver has to deal with to detoxify. Pain killers and sleeping pills are a heavy burden on the liver. The side effects from drugs have a profound reaction on all the other organs of the viscera as well as the liver itself. When the liver is overburdened in trying to expel poisons, this puts an overload on the kidneys, where the toxins are ultimately expelled. The strain is then placed on the kidneys, and it is no wonder the elderly have kidney problems and are ill all the time.

Liver injury can cause vague symptoms such as digestive problems, constipation, low energy output, allergies and hayfever which is caused by the inability of the liver to detoxify harmful substances. Liver dysfunction can cause mental disturbances, because the liver is unable to detoxify excess hormones, these enter the blood and travel to the brain. A healthy liver inactivates hormones when they are no longer needed. Toxic accumulation in the liver and the inability of their normal removal from the brain cells can result in numerous mental disturbances. Many ailments can benefit from liver detoxification, such as arthritis, allergies, anemia, diabetes, hypertension, obesity, alcoholism, and infertility.

Many studies done on subjects who had no apparent liver damage showed that each person had degeneration of liver cells, much scar tissue, a high infiltration of fat or enlarged liver. When the liver is damaged, a lower amount of bile is produced. This causes chronic indigestion, and many people are plagued with digestive problems. Just watch the ads on television, they alone indicate that digestive problems are widespread.

Lack of exercise has an indirect effect on the liver. It damages the liver with an overload of toxins that should have been eliminated through the lungs, which need to do their share of cleansing. The excess toxins are then passed along to an overburdened liver. Overeating, especially overcooked food, puts a strain on the liver as these do not supply the enzymes and amino acids essential for proper digestion.

According to the American Liver Foundation, liver diseases are the fourth leading cause of death up to the age of 65. It is not commonly known that there is a wide incidence of liver disease in America. There are indications that liver problems are on the increase. In the past, liver damage was thought to be a problem of chronic alcoholics, but now it is seen among social drinkers, overweight persons, people over exposed to drugs or chemicals and those whose nutrition is not adequate to protect them. Children are not exempt, we are seeing tens of thousands of American children with liver diseases and many hundreds of them die.

Proper Diet for the Liver

The diet needs to be high in fresh raw fruits and vegetables, lots of lightly steamed vegetables, especially greens, salads and lots of sprouts. Foods which are high in natural sodium have been used for relief of liver congestion. They include kelp, dulse, ripe olives, Swiss chard, beet greens, celery, watercress, parsley, turnips, mustard greens, sesame seeds and sunflower seeds.

Lemon juice in warm water, first thing in the morning will help cleanse the liver. Lemon juice with cold pressed olive oil, in the morning before breakfast, is an excellent tonic and a gentle natural laxative. Olive oil in its natural state is a good source of healthy fats and cholesterol and is easily digestible. Fruit juices stimulate, cleanse and relieve congestion, especially citrus fruit, such as grapefruit, lemons, limes and oranges. Carrot juice upon waking is a tonic to the liver and helps liquify bile. Spinach, onions and string beans also can be eaten raw or juiced but are much harder to digest when cooked.

An herbal combination, which was developed for those who have severe liver problems as well as for those who need to keep their liver healthy and functioning properly is Barberry Bark, Dandelion Root, Golden Seal Root, Red Beet Root, Oregon Grape Root, Yellow Dock and Pan Pien Lien.

Single herbs that help heal and restore liver function are: Burdock (restores function of the liver and gallbladder), Cascara Sagrada (heals the liver and strengthens the bowels), Dandelion (clears obstruction of the liver and detoxifies), Gentian (strong biter, helps digestion and liver function), Golden Seal (helps regulate liver function, heals), Licorice (combines well with bitters to balance formulas), Milk Thistle (heals damaged liver), Pau D'Arco (protects the liver from further damage, strengthens the entire body), Parsley and Watercress (help Wild Yam (remove toxic buildup of bile), Wormwood (stimulates the liver, eliminates worms), and Yellow Dock (protects the liver, rich in iron for a healthy liver).

THE KIDNEYS

The kidneys, located below the waist on either side of the spine, are bean-shaped organs, measuring approximately four inches by two inches by one inch. These small organs have a big and important job to perform constantly for the body. When we have a nagging backache and it persists, we should realize that the kidneys are located close to the spinal column. The kidneys also suffer when high blood pressure isn't corrected. Each kidney contains about one million individual filtering units. These filtering units, called nephrons, consist of receptacles called glomerule that are attached to tubules. Glomerulus is the name of the combination of a tuft of capillaries and the cupped end of the tube. Tubule is the name of the tube that leads off from the glomerulus. If the tubules of both kidneys are spliced they would make a tubule fifty miles long. The kidney's job is to maintain a constant and healthy internal environment in the body. They adjust the body's electrolyte balance. They manufacture hormones that regulate blood pressure, calcium metabolism, and red blood cell production. The kidneys are very smart. They eliminate whatever is bad for the body and brain and any excess of good. If you go on a candy spree, sugar rises in the blood, reaches a concentration too high for safety, and the kidneys have the job of throwing out the excess. But it is not true that they need no thought or consideration. It is wise to remember that prevention is better than a cure when it comes to your kidneys.

The kidneys work constantly! The kidneys constantly drain, but they also retain. They try to maintain the correct amounts of glucose, nitrogen, water, acid, alkali, and all of what the body needs.

The kidneys try to maintain the health of the body but when distress hits—pain, pallor, swelling, high blood pressure, blood in the urine, burning and stinging—you know your kidneys are in trouble. If they are given the proper nutrients to stay healthy, they will protect the body.

Pure water is essential for healthy kidneys. Few people drink enough water, instead they consume large amounts of coffee, tea, soft drinks and alcohol. Even too much fruit juice is hard on the kidneys. There are certain nutrients that are essential for healthy kidneys. They are vitamins A, C and E. The B vitamins are also very important nutrients for healthy kidneys. They are usually lacking in the average american diet. The reason common table salt and baking soda is not good for the body is 99 percent of baking soda is reabsorbed and more than 95 percent of common salt.

Natural sodium is good for the body. Dr. Bernard Jensen stresses the value of whey as an ideal source of nutritional sodium so effective in keeping the joints limber. Whey also contains vitamin B13, used as a carrier to guide other nutrients past the blood brain barrier, especially in the treatment of multiple sclerosis and other neuromuscular conditions.

Kidney stones develop when mineral salts in the urine form crystals that clump together and continue to grow. Usually, under normal conditions these crystals are eliminated from the body through the urine, but sometimes they adhere to the lining of the kidney or settle in an area where they cannot be carried out through the urine. These crystals may grow into a stone ranging from the size of a grain of sand to a golf ball.

Herbs are very beneficial for the urinary system. Since the kidneys are vital to life, it is not surprising that nature has provided an abundance of herbs to aid their function.

A potassium formula is needed as well as sodium to help regulate the water balance within the body. It helps to normalize the heartbeat and nourish the muscular system. It also stimulates nerve impulse for muscle contraction, as well as the kidneys to eliminate poisonous body toxins. Potassium assists in the conversion of glucose to glycogen, the form in which glucose can be stored in the liver.

Two excellent formulas for the kidneys help clear mucus in the bladder and kidneys, increase the flow of urine, provide antiseptic properties, strengthen and tone the urinary tract, neutralize uric acid, soothe the nerves, clean the blood and increase circulation:

#1. Juniper Berries, Parsley, Uva Ursi, Golden Seal Root, Marshmallow, Watermelon Seeds, Pan Pien Lien, and Ginger.

#2. Juniper Berries, Uva Ursi, Shavegrass, Cornsilk, Parsley, Queen of the Meadow, Buchu Leaves, Goldenrod, Cubeb Berris, Cranberries, and Watermelon Seed.

Single herbs to help the kidneys are: Cornsilk (strengthens and heals), Garlic (Natural antibiotic), Hydrangea (natural diuretic to clean the clogged up filter of the kidneys), Juniper Berries (natural diuretic, healing), Parsley (diuretic), and Uva Ursi (strengthens and tones the urinary system).

The following herbs are also very beneficial for the kidneys: Alfalfa, Burdock, Dandelion, Golden Seal (cleans and heals the urinary tract), Kelp, Marshmallow (soothing and healing), Pau D'Arco (cleans the blood), Red Raspberry, Rose Hips (rich in vitamin C for healing), and Yarrow.

THE COLON

The colon, or large intestine, is usually considered a storage place for the semisolid remains of our diet, to be eliminated through the bowels. However, it functions to absorb fluids and electrolytes (sodium, potassium, chloride, etc.) from the undigestible food residues that form its content. The colon also takes up short-chain fatty acids which are produced by intestinal bacteria during the fermentation of fiber. These in turn can be used by the body for energy.

The colon has the essential function of sustaining intestinal microbes. There are over three pounds of them. Mainly benign, they form thirty to fifty percent of the dry weight of the stool, creating its texture and also its odor. They have the job of breaking down any remaining proteins, fats and fiber from the chyme of the small intestine.

The beneficial intestinal flora can keep disease producing microorganisms under control. Our diet determines which bacteria we grow. A diet rich in meat and/or fatty foods has been linked with colon cancer, or tumor formation in different parts of the body. A high fat, high meat, low fiber diet promotes longer storage time of fecal matter in the bowel and greater potential of unfriendly bacterial and cancer growth.

A 1982 article published in the *Saturday Evening Post,* "Constipation and Breast Cancer,"
made the following statement, "We found that 70 percent of the women we tested had [foreign] chemicals in the breast fluid. . .the breast cells are in contact with the bloodstream, which will contain certain foreign substances absorbed into the circulation system from the skin, lungs, and the gastrointestinal tract."

Many physicians today as well as in the past have found that the bacterial poisons absorbed from the intestine can affect almost every chronic disease. Dr. Bernard Jensen states, "In fifty years of sanitarium practice, I have had the opportunity to work with over 350,000 patients. Of all these people, not one of them was free from some form of bowel mismanagement. All sick people have bowel trouble. All sick people are tired, worn out and toxin laden. In working with patients, I spend the major part of the time in an effort to get the bowels back into proper functioning condition. Without this prerequisite, all other therapies, treatments, vitamins or other aids fall far short of their potential good. Proper bowel function is an essential precondition for staying healthy, and if ill, to overcome sickness and disease. The "sewer system" must work properly or the body remains soaking in its own putrid waste, encouraging disease process and forever eluding health-building and vitality-producing forces." (taken from *Iridology, The Science and Practice in the Healing Arts,* Volume II, page 407).

Dr. Arbuthnot Lane, who was surgeon for the King of England, spent many years specializing in bowel problems. He was an expert at removing sections of the bowel and stitching it back together. After doing surgery on his patients and during recovery, some of his patients experienced remarkable cures of diseases that had no apparent connection with his surgery. He tells of a young boy, who had arthritis for many years, and was in a wheelchair when he did the surgery. Six months later, this boy was entirely free from arthritis. One woman had a goiter, and when a specific section of the bowel was removed in surgery, there was a remission of the goiter within six months.

These experiences by Dr. Lane had impressed him in discovering a relationship between the toxic bowel and various organs in the body. He spent the last 25 years of his life teaching people how to care for the bowel through nutrition and not surgery. He made the following statement: "All maladies are due to the lack of certain food principles, such as mineral salts or vitamins, or to the absence of th normal defenses of the body, such as the natural protective flora. When this occurs, toxic bacteria invade the lower alimentary canal, and the poisons thus generated pollute the bloodstream and gradually deteriorate and destroy every tissue, gland and organ of the body."

Some of the many types of poisons which can be found in a toxic colon are: Phenol, Cadaverian, Agamatine, Indole, Sulphurrettd Hydrogen, Butyric Acid, Botulin, Putrescin, Urrobilin, Cresole, Histidine, Ammonia, Muscarine, Indican, Neurin and Sepsin.

These poisons can weaken and stress the heart, go to the skin and cause blemishes, paleness, psoriasis, liver spots, wrinkles and other facial conditions, can irritate the lungs and cause foul breath, go to the brain and disturb mental function and cause senility, go to the joints and cause pain and stiffness. They can affect the muscles and cause weakness and terrible fatigue and can rob you of your youth and vitality and cause you to become old long before your time.

Colon health depends on the maintenance of beneficial intestinal bacteria and one of the most important supplements to maintain this friendly bacteria is Acidophilus. The benefits of using Acidophilus are:

- Produce their own vitamins which are absorbed into the blood.
- Synthesize many of the B vitamins, including biotin, folic acid, and B12.
- Increase the absorption of calcium, phosphorus, and magnesium.
- Help normalize cholesterol levels of the blood.
- Help keep the intestinal tract free of unwanted bacteria.
- Produce digestive enzymes.
- Generate large amounts of lactase and may assist persons with lactose intolerance.

- Help maintain bowel regularity.

A formula to help strengthen the bowls contains: Cascara Sagrada, Barberry, Raspberry Leaves, Pan Pien Lien, Ginger, Rhubarb, Golden Seal Root, Fennel, and Cayenne.

THE LUNGS

Breathing is something we don't think about until we are confronted with some disease that affects our lungs. Asthma, bronchitis, croup, pneumonia or emphysema are diseases of the respiratory system that interfere with our breathing. When any of these diseases strike and breathing becomes difficult, then we consider the health of our lungs. We should not take breathing for granted. Proper breathing plays a vital function to our internal organs. Oxygen is the most essential nutrient for life and almost all the body's vital functions depend on oxygen, especially energy production in the muscle cells. Insufficient oxygen results in malnutrition, low energy, softening of bones, emaciation wasting, abnormal functions and premature demise.

Proper lung exercise is essential to increase the lungs ability to pump oxygen and keep the blood pumping through the vessels. The bone marrow is stimulated, which produces more red blood cells. The lungs and kidneys expel the greatest percentage of worn-out phosphorus and all waste material is removed from the cells through proper breathing. Metabolism in all the organs of the body is stimulated. Exercise is the proper way to build healthy lungs and produce a wonderful sense of physical and emotional well-being. Exercise also helps to regulate the appetite center in the brain and produces true sensations of hunger rather than eating out of boredom or confusion.

Breathing is the most important function that we need to consider for a healthy body. With increased air pollution; bodily gases and waste being sent constantly into our lungs to be discharged into the air, we need to increase our lung health.

All breathing should originate from the region of the diaphragm with a full, slow, steady breath. We should breathe as much as possible through the nose. The nose filters the pollutants and air reaches the lungs in a cleaner and purer form than it would be when inhaled through the mouth. Breathing through the nose also warms the air before it reaches the lungs; cold air irritates sensitive airways.

Another requirement for proper breathing is to breathe from and into the stomach. Suck the air deep into the abdomen to the point where this organ expands. This along with breathing deeply and nasally reduces the respiration rate.

Excess weight can also interfere with proper breathing. Even one inch of excess fat around the diaphragm is going to make it harder to breathe. For individuals with asthma or emphysema, being overweight is like wearing tight clothes constantly.

The benefits of proper breathing are:
1. Builds healthy lungs, preventing asthma, bronchitis and colds.

2. Improves brain function.

3. Thinking responses are quicker.

4. Relaxing for the nerves, improves nerve function.

5. Increases proper digestion and elimination.

6. Increases flexibility in the neck, spine, muscles, ligaments and creates a feeling of youthfulness.

7. Health of abdominal organs are increased; liver and kidneys.

8. Improves heart function.

9. Increases proper waste elimination through the skin. Skin brushing is also encouraged.

10. Improves eyesight and hearing.

11. Energy is increased, prevents fatigue.

12. Increases kidney health to prevent high blood pressure.

Mucous Membranes

The lungs are protected by the mucous membranes of the body. The inside of the nose is equipped with a lining called mucous membranes with its special ability to secret mucus. Nasal mucus performs a very necessary function of eliminating dust and debris and carries it out of the nose. It protects against particles entering the body such as bacteria, viruses, fungi and all kinds of air pollution.

Mucus has been defined as a secretion as well as an excretion. The secretion has a constructive purpose while an excretion is destructive, when the body tries to rid itself of toxins. Mucus becomes an excretion when the lungs, the skin, the bowels, kidney and menses are unable to rid the body of wastes that have accumulated, and mucus production increases to take over for the elimination channels.

If the mucus becomes too thick, then it dries out and sticks to the cilia and mucous membranes and this causes crusts to build up providing an environment for microbes to invade. This is usually the beginning of a cold. When the mucus is too liquid and runny it drips down around the cilia and a water nasal drip develops. This brings on inflammation and is usually a component of hayfever.

Diet determines the composition of mucus. Too much starchy food and milk products are well known for developing a thicker and more viscous mucus.

Liver and Kidneys

The liver and kidneys play an important role in healthy lungs. The liver and the kidneys are vital and important channels of elimination. The liver performs its job through the natural elimination channel which are the bowels. The kidneys cleanse through the bladder and urethra.

The problem arises when the liver becomes congested and is unable to perform its normal eliminative function. The toxins build up and are thrown into the blood stream. When the kidneys are congested, the toxins are also thrown into the blood. When toxic blood becomes congested and has no where to eliminate, it has to find a substitute avenue of elimination or the person would literally die. The lungs are the next channel of elimination to rid the body of toxins. The lungs have to take over eliminating the waste that should have gone through the kidneys. When the liver is congested and cannot eliminate properly, then the largest elimination organ takes over which is the skin.

The lungs should not have to do the eliminating for the kidneys, for this causes undue stress and strain of the respiratory system which weakens the lungs and causes asthma, bronchitis, colds, pneumonia or tuberculosis. The lungs are the most delicate organ in the body and should be taken care of properly.

DISEASES OF THE RESPIRATORY SYSTEM

The respiratory system is constructed with a series of specialized structures designed to efficiently exchange gases in the system to sustain life and body functions. This will promote good health throughout the entire body.

Nutrients are necessary to maintain elasticity in the lung membranes, which are by nature very thin, in order to expand and contract. They function as a two-way filter and when they do not function properly, emphysema may develop. A poor diet, with incomplete digestion along with free radicals, rancid fats and toxic air pollution can result in particles of matter which gradually close the "pores" of alveola and the lungs lose their elasticity.

With changes in the weather, the lungs are particularly vulnerable to the colder winter air and the quick changes from warm to cool. A diet low in mucus-forming foods are considered a must for those prone to respiratory diseases. The stomach and kidneys can handle just so much mucus forming foods and when the kidneys are backed up, the lungs try to take over their cleansing job. This becomes very irritating to the lungs and causes respiratory diseases.

Herbs are used very successfully to treat the respiratory system. They are designed to feed and nourish the lungs. Anti-catarrhal herbs will decrease mucus production. Expectorant herbs help to expel mucus. Demulcents herbs help to soothe inflammations. Antispasmodic herbs help to stop coughs. Antibacterial herbs help to stop infections. Nervine herbs help to calm the nerves and strengthen the body against stress.

Asthma

There can be many causes of asthma. An attack of asthma occurs when the tubes through which air is carried in and out of the lungs become narrowed. This leads to shortness of breath, cough and wheezing. Anxiety and panic tend to make the attack worse.

Sometimes asthma will respond well to the use of nervine herbs. Fear is one of the most potent triggers of an asthma attack. It could even be caused by fear of an asthma attack itself. The nervine herbs are black cohosh, hops, lady slipper, lobelia, scullcap and valerian.

Those with asthma should never use salt (sodium chloride) because it stimulates the adrenal glands. It is considered a high corrosive drug which cannot be utilized by the body. Organic salt found in herbs and vegetables is useful and necessary to the body.

Herbs for asthma are capsicum, cascara sagrada (colon), comfrey, ephedra, fenugreek, garlic, marshmallow, mullein, oatstraw, and slippery elm.

Acute attacks have been treated to open the air passages by using lobelia extract directly under the tongue. A dropper full every 15 to 30 minutes.

Maurice Messegue, a french herbalist,

recommends for lung conditions: five grams of garlic, five grams of lemon, one pinch of mint, one pinch of sage added to a liter of water (five grams is slightly less than a fifth of an ounce, while a liter is slightly more than a quart.)

Two cups a day will help soothe asthma. When using garlic, eat a handful of fresh parsley, it will help the bad breath.

Bronchitis

This is an infection in the upper respiratory tract with a dry violent, hacking cough. This is an inflammation of the mucous membranes of the bronchial tubes. Bronchitis is a warning that a state of imbalance is present in the body. A short fast for two or three days would help the body create a balance.

A cough may persist from two to four weeks. The cough is nature's attempt to expel the hard encrusted toxic mucus. After the lungs have eliminated and healed, then there is an improved state of health until the toxins become concentrated and accumulate again.

The herbs best used for bronchitis are pectorals (agents which aids in pulmonary disease), that combine with expectorant action to clear the mucus, and emulcent herbs to soothe the inflamed tissues. The anti-bacterial herbs are usually needed to fight infections.

The best herbs for bronchitis are boneset (helps aches), capsicum, cascara sagrada, comfrey, echinacea (fights infections), golden seal eucalyptus, garlic (antiseptic), ginger, licorice, lobelia (chest constricter), ma huang, marshmallow, mullein, pau d'arco, and slippery elm. Red clover is also very good to build up the immune system.

Coughs

A cough is the body's way of clearing phlegm and accumulated mucus from the lungs. The cough could start from mucus caught in the throat, from infections, congestion because of phlegm or foreign matter in the lungs. Herbs are beneficial for coughs. They nourish and soothe the irritated areas. For cough and hoarseness with mucus, use comfrey, fenugreek, licorice and slippery elm. For a dry cough, open a capsule of slippery elm and mix with aloe very juice, add a capsule of licorice root, eat it slowly and let the mixture coat the throat. Lobelia extract under the tongue can help control a cough. Let it slowly go down the throat.

Herbs for cough are: blue vervain, bugleweed, chamomile, cherry bark, comfrey, horehound, hops, horseradish, iceland moss, kelp, licorice, lobelia, mullein, passion flower, peppermint, red clover, saffron, and scullcap.

Croup

Croup usually results from viral infection. It is a childhood disease that affects boys more than girls. It usually occurs during the winter months. It is a very frightening disease giving a feeling of suffocation and difficulty in breathing. It develops in spasm of the larynx with a harsh, brassy, and gasping cough. There are different kinds of croup and each form of croup has additional characteristics. One is a form of bronchitis, one is laryngitis, which results from vocal edema and is usually mild, and there is one called acute spasmodic laryngitis which usually affects those with allergies and a family history of croup.

A humidifier with warm or cool moist air is very helpful. A few drops of a tincture of lobelia in comfrey and fenugreek teas is very useful. Lobelia extract on the tongue will help stop the spasms. Lobelia rubbed on the chest and back is very relaxing for the croup.

Herbs for croup: comfrey, chamomile, hops, licorice, lobelia, mullein, peppermint, slippery elm, and scullcap.

Emphysema

Asthma and emphysema are closely related. Read all the material written on asthma. The asthmatic suffers from sensitivity, while the person with emphysema suffers from a real physical change in the lungs. In emphysema the walls of the alveola start to break down, altering the structure of lung tissue. One physician said that emphysema stricken lungs resemble moth-eaten wool.

The relationship of cadmium to emphysema does exist. Autopsies have show high amounts of cadmium in the lung tissue of former emphysema patients. Those who suffered more severely from the disease contained the largest amounts of cadmium. The livers of people dying from emphysema and bronchitis contained three times as much cadmium as those dying of other diseases. Cadmium is found in the atmosphere. Refining metals in industry, burning modern products such as plastic, and rubber tires contain cadmium. Cigarette smoking exposes one to cadmium. Each cigarette contains a microgram of cadmium and inhaling the smoke of tens of thousands of cigarettes over the years can eventually takes its toll through emphysema.

Nutrients and herbs listed under lung protection and asthma should be utilized. Blood purifying herbs and herbs to cleanse the liver should be used.

Pleurisy

Pleurisy is an inflammation of the membrane sacs that surround the lungs. The pain in pleurisy is caused by the inflammation or irritation of the sensory nerve endings in the parietal pleuria.

It is essential to treat the infection with herbs. An herbal combination to fight infections is Golden seal, black walnut, althea, echinacea, plantain and bugleweed.

Single herbs to help are boneset, cascara sagrada, comfrey, garlic, pleurisy root, mullein, and slippery elm. A poultice made with flaxseed and put on the chest can be very beneficial.

Pneumonia

This is a acute infection of the lungs where the air is trapped in the lungs and there is trouble with gas exchange. The tiny air sacs in the lungs become inflamed with mucus and pus.

Some of the causes of pneumonia are severe colds, alcoholism, malnutrition and foreign material in the respiratory passages. The primary causes are bacteria, viruses, chemical irritants, allergies and can be a result of surgery in many cases; frequently causing death as a complication of major surgery.

The disease usually sets in with a severe and prolonged chill after which the temperature of the body rapidly rises to a high point. This rise is accompanied by the customary symptoms of fever. Pain is commonly felt about the chest region and is sharp, stabbing and aggravated by breathing. It is characterized by extremely frequent, shallow breathing.

Although germs are present in the body at all times, it is when the body becomes weakened that it becomes vulnerable to the attack of these germs. Use the same methods suggested for bronchitis. Enemas are very important to clean and rid the body of toxins and helping clear up the infection. Juices and vitamin A and C are very important to help the body fight the infection. Comfrey, chickweed, marshmallow, mullein and lobelia are very important herbs for pneumonia.

THE SKIN

Our skin is a complex organ and vital to overall health. The mucous membranes are the internal coverings, and the skin is the outside covering. The skin protects the internal organs, regulates temperature, and helps rid the body of toxins in the form of gas, vapor and perspiration.

The skin is the largest organ of the body and the largest elimination channel. The skin's health depends on the health of the inner organs. If the glands in the walls of the stomach do not secrete sufficient hydrochloric acid, the skin can lose its surface acidity and this increases the chance of infections.

Digestion, assimilation and elimination are vital to beautiful, healthy skin. If the skin is abused with frequent washing with harsh soaps, that are highly alkaline, it removes all the protective oil as well as the acidity. A soap that is pH balanced won't dry the skin. It is better to use soaps containing natural ingredients such as lanolin, cocoa butter or glycerine. Avoid soaps with coloring, perfumes, harmful dyes and chemicals. Avoid face creams containing mineral oil which will destroy vitamin A necessary for healthy skin.

Proper cleansing is essential for a radiant, clear complexion. Dead cells, rancid oil, perspiration, toxins and bacteria need to be removed daily or black heads, pimples or whiteheads will form and clog the pores. A film of dirt and pollution accumulates daily on the surface of the skin. A combination of fat and protein are the most common cause of fatty pimples, acne and boils.

When the body is overloaded with mucus, fat and protein, the kidneys, liver and digestive organs cannot process and eliminate fast enough, and therefore the body expels through the skin. In fact, the skin helps the kidneys. The skin has been called the third kidney because of its eliminative functions in cleansing acids in the blood, toxins and mineral wastes. Waste material accumulates in the intestine when meat ferments and produces indole, skatole, methane, and other toxic gases. These toxic gases dissolve in the water and enter the bloodstream through the intestinal wall. The kidneys are mainly responsible for cleansing the blood of these waste products, working constantly day in and day out without stopping.

The Skin and The Kidneys

The body becomes excessively acid when too much meat is eaten. The kidneys become overloaded, and the toxins not cleaned by them have to get out of the body. The stability of the cells or homeostasis must be achieved and the back up for the kidneys is the skin. The skin is considered the third kidney. The kidneys can only do so much elimination, and they are overloaded, it is up to the skin to help keep the blood clean. When the blood is clean and pure, diseases cannot invade the body. Skin diseases are very numerous,

but the cause is always the same. The kidneys are not able to handle all the waste produced by the type of food we eat. Bacteria or fungi along with the rich food combinations account for many varieties of skin problems.

The foods responsible for an over acid condition of the blood are: sugar, milk, cheese, ice cream, fatty meats, peanut butter, pastries and processed salty nuts. Excess fat, protein and malfunction of protein metabolism can also discharge in the form of callouses, moles, tumors and warts. It is also felt that too much sugar in the diet surfaces to the outer skin in the form of brown spots and freckles brought out by the heat of the sun.

The skin has three layers: The epidermis, dermis and a subcutaneous fat layer. Beneath these layers are muscle, cartilage and bone. The top layer is the sensitive, elastic covering that is abused and exposed to disease and injury more than any other organ of the body. This layer protects us from external drying and toxic materials such as chemicals, dust, poisons and radiation to name just a few of the pollutants that affect us.

The second layer is the dermis which shields and repairs injured tissues. It contains the nerves, blood vessels, ceraceous glands and sweat glands. The deepest layer of the skin is the subcutaneous, which produces lipids, fat globbules for subcutaneous tissue, and cushions muscles, bones and internal organs against shock. It also acts as an insulator and stores energy for release when needed.

Henry G. Bieler, M.D., who was a nutritional health doctor states in his book, *Food is Your Best Medicine,* "When the liver is congested and cannot eliminate, waste matter (toxins) is thrown into the blood stream. And when the kidneys are inflamed, toxins are also dammed up in the blood. Toxic blood must discharge its toxins or the person dies, so nature uses vicarious venues of elimination or substitutes. The lungs will take over the task of eliminating some of the wastes that should have gone through the kidneys, or the skin will take over for the liver.

From the irritation caused by the elimination

of poison through these 'vicarious' channels, we can get bronchitis, pneumonia or tuberculosis. As is determined by the particular chemistry of the poison being eliminated. If the bile poisons in the blood come out through the skin we get the various irritations of the skin, resulting in the many skin diseases, or through the mucous membranes (inside skin) as the various catarrh eliminate or through the skin as boils, carbuncles, acne, etc.

The skin's function is to exhale gases, sweat, and certain toxic salty substances. The vicarious elimination, which results from forcefully exuding gases, acid sweat or toxic oils and greases through the outer skin, has given name to enough diseases to fill a large dermatology textbook, chronic eczema, ichthyosis, psoriasis, are common examples. Skin diseases which are really signs of toxic irritation, respond well to a treatment dietary, directed toward neutralization and elimination of the poisons. This brings the hyperthyroidism under control."

The Skins Function in Acute Disease

The skin has a very vital function in eliminating toxins, gases, pollution and vapor from the system. Two quarts of toxins, in the form of sweat, gases and vapor ar released everyday if the pores are clean and free from built-up dead cells. If the skin is closed off because of dead cell build-up, these toxins are thrown back into the body for the other organs of elimination to take over its job.

Many people have a fear of being exposed to cold and wet weather. They think they will catch cold, bronchitis or pneumonia. It does not necessarily mean that you will get sick if you are exposed to drafts unless the organs of elimination are in poor working order. If the system is not filled with an accumulation of toxic matter, and if the kidneys and colon are in fairly good working order, these organs will assist the temporarily inactive skin function to take care of the extra amount of waste and toxic materials and eliminate them without serious side effects.

When the body has enough energy and vitality and the blood is clean, then channels of

elimination will take care of the toxins of vapor, gases and water which were not eliminated from the skin. But if the body is overloaded with waste and toxic material; and if the bowels and kidneys are already weakened through continued overwork and over-stimulation, along with toxic blood and low vitality, this is when you can come down with an acute disease. This is when the body says, "we have to get rid of the waste in the body somehow."

When the body is loaded with toxins and is exposed to drafts, cold, and wet weather, the toxic matter is thrown into the circulation by the chilling of the skin. By exposing the skin, with these toxic conditions in the body, it closes the skin off from doing its job. If the other normal channels of elimination are also shut down, then the toxins are thrown into the mucous linings of the nasal passages, the throat, bronchi, stomach, lungs, or the genito-urinary organs.

When the skin is chilled, the pores of the skin close and cause the blood to recede into the internal organs. As a result, the elimination of poisonous gases, vapors and toxins is suppressed. The waste material and toxins being eliminated through the internal membranes cause irritation and congestion and produces the symptoms of inflammation, infections and catarrhal elimination, sneezing, coughs, runny nose, diarrhea, leucorrhea, etc.

The elimination process does not occur through the ears, nose, throat, stomach, or lungs, until it becomes necessary for the body to eliminate excessive accumulation of toxins in order to protect the body from shutting down altogether from ultimate death. All acute diseases are a way of protecting the body; the way nature saves our lives.

We can understand that the chilling of the surface of the skin is only the spark that ignites the combustibles trapped within th body. When cold, flu, fevers and all acute diseases appear, the membranes of the internal organs are doing the work of the inactive sluggish and atrophied skin, kidneys and intestines.

The more accumulation of toxic material in the system, the lower the vitality and energy of the body. The more toxic the composition of the blood and lymph glands, the greater the chances of catching a "cold" or any other acute disease.

The skin must be kept clean, the blood pure, and the bowels, and kidneys in proper working order. For correct skin health, use herbs, daily dry brushing, frequent fasting, fresh air and sunshine along with proper food.

Skin Brushing

Regular bathing and washing will not remove the layers of dead skin. It takes a gentle and light abrasion on the skin when it is dry to rid the body of the dead unwanted skin. The dead layers need to be peeled away so the skin will be able to breath and live properly. This is what is referred to as dry skin brushing. Acne, pimples, excessive dryness or oiliness can all be greatly helped by this activity. It increases rapid cell production beneath the surface of the skin. It is considered the same body stimulation as compared to twenty minutes of jogging or fast walking. Rubbing the skin with a turkish towel will make sure the lymphatic system and bloodstream are exercised. Use a skin brush made from natural bristles with a long but detachable handle so that you can reach the back. It is a wonderful feeling, and so stimulating to brush just before your shower. It leaves a tingling and refreshing feeling.

Skin brushing is an effective way for cleansing the lymphatic system through physical stimulation. It also stimulates the bloodstream, is excellent for poor circulation and is a must on a colon cleansing program. It helps to dislodge mucus in the area that is needed. Start by brushing the soles of the feet and work up each leg; up the bottom and up to the middle of the back (avoid the genitals). Work towards the heart and bring all toxins toward the colon. Then start at the fingertips and brush up the arms, across the shoulders, down the chest and the top of the back; again avoiding sensitive parts like the nipples. Don't forget the arm pits, for this is where glandular inflammation collects in the lymphs. Then brush down towards the colon. On the area

below the navel, brush in movements starting on the right hand side, going up, across and down, following the shape of the colon. Women should brush the breasts, it cleans and protects against lumps.

The face should always be cleaned with a wash cloth or a natural soft brush.

Another type of skin brushing or a brisk scrub is done with stone ground corn meal while the skin is wet, followed by a tepid or cold rinse. This thoroughly cleanses the skin while stimulating circulation. The natural oil in the corn meal prevents irritation and leaves the skin baby soft.

THE BLOOD

One of the important jobs of the blood is to supply oxygen to each of some sixty trillion cells. The blood transports nutrients, eliminates toxic waste material and sends messages via the hormones it carries from the endocrine glands. So if the blood is contaminated, you can be pretty sure the whole body will be effected. In fact the blood stream is considered the "River of Life." Dr. Christopher taught that all disease stems from the blood stream. He said, "While I was in the Army I had many soldiers come to me with bad cases of furunculosis (boils). So I would lance, top and drain the boil, as was routine, and I could have said, 'Well, I've drained the boils, so you will have no more trouble.' But had I said this, the soldier would know I was not telling the truth, because the outbreak of boils often, or usually, recurred!"

Boils along with tumors, cysts, dermatitis, cancer and many other diseases come from impurities and poisonous waste accumulations in the blood. Cleansing the blood stream would be working on the cause of the disease. A boil is a symptom of toxic blood.

Blood Purification

Blood purification therapy is the ultimate of all herbal therapies. When the blood is purified and toxins and acids neutralized, all disease will disappear. This is especially useful for treating infections. The blood and lymph carry a multitude of toxins that have accumulated from chemicals, drugs, toxic metals, overeating, etc. Most of the toxins come from meat, starch, and white sugar products. This therapy is usually used along with other needed therapies.

Blood purification will effect the whole body. The principle of cleansing the blood stream is to use alterative herbs. Dr. Nowell gave us guide lines to follow for cleansing the blood.

"Alternatives, or, as they are sometimes called Antiscorbutics, are remedies which gradually alter and correct impure conditions of the blood. It is because of this that many of these agents are commonly called "blood purifiers" or "blood sweeteners." They alter the character of the blood stream because of being possessed of certain properties which the Vital Force can use in stimulating or strengthening the organs of nutrition and secretion, building up so that waste materials may be carried and a supply of helpful pabulum may be provided for the organism.

Removing impurities from the blood stream is only part of the work of the rational physician. All such conditions arise because of the improper functioning of one or more organs...most frequently the secretory organs...which fail to carry out the impurities of the blood. It is; however, possible that impurities may arise from improper food or impure air. Whatever the cause, the only means of cleansing the blood stream that would attend also to removing the cause while seeking to purify the blood."

The true alterative is an herb which slowly but surely cleans and purifies the blood stream and, at the same time, steadily tones up the organ or organs which may not be able to secrete impurities from the blood.

The liver, kidneys ad skin are the chief organs of elimination. They are responsible for carrying off impurities and waste matter from the system. If the liver is congested and bile retained in the system, this will have a negative effect on digestion. If the kidneys fail to secrete as they should, the blood stream is polluted. The skin may

be retaining impurities, or the lungs may be unable to oxygenate the blood due to impure air being breathed.

Alterative is intended to mean that certain herbs gradually alter and correct a bad condition of the blood, without necessarily producing evacuations of the bowels beyond normal evacuation. Alterative herbs help restore the toxic organs of the system to healthy action. They promote absorption of inflammatory deposits chiefly by stimulating the lymphatic glands, although this is not all they do. Better digestion results when the entire blood stream is purified.

Alterative herbs are: Burdock, Cascara Sagrada, Dandelion, Echinacea, Oregon Grape, Pau D'Arco, Red Clover, Sarsaparilla. Other alterative herbs are Alfalfa, Aloe Vera, Angelica, Comfrey, Golden Seal, Gotu Kola, Marshmallow, Dong Quai, Ginseng, Ho Shou Wu, and Uva Ursi.

An excellent herbal combination for cleansing the blood is: Red Clover Blossoms, Sheep Sorrel, Peach Bark, Barberry Root, Echinacea, Licorice Root, Oregon Grape Root, Stillingia Root, Cascara Sagrada Root, Sarsaparilla Root, Prickly Ash Bark, Burdock Root, Kelp and Rosemary Leaf.

THE LYMPHATICS

The lymphatic system is a part of our major "garbage-disposal" as well as our immune system. This wonderful protective network has the job of carrying nutrients throughout the body as well as removing waste material from all the tissues. The lymph glands do the job of collecting rubbish from our cells and bloodstream. The lymph's fluid has the ability to go deep into the tissues where blood cannot penetrate and pick up toxic material in the form of acids and catarrh that has to be eliminated for our protection. These toxins are passed through the eliminative channels of the lymph glands. These lymph glands or nodes collect the waste material and dump them in the bloodstream. Waste products are then transported to the colon, kidneys, lungs or skin to be eliminated from the system.

The lymph is clear fluid which bathes all

tissues of the body. The vessels that carry this lymph fluid also carry lymphocytes (a type of white blood cell and other substances essential for the body's natural defense system.) This is part of the immune process. Lymphocytes are vital for our overall health. They act like complex miniature computers; having the ability to recognize foreign matter (anything that does not belong in the body) and then having the ability to provide a blueprint so that the essential antibodies can be manufactured. If the body is supplied with proper nutrition, these antibodies challenge and destroy dangerous material before it causes serious damage and health problems.

The lymphatic system needs a pumping action to fulfill its job, and it cannot accomplish this alone. Exercise is the simple answer. The up and down movement on a mini-trampoline causes the lymph vessels to expand and compress, to stretch and relax. This is an action that the lymph fluids need to do their vital job. This type of exercise will provide the pumping system to stimulate the fluids helping in eliminating wastes and toxins.

The lymphatic system is the most important and vital one of the body and also the most neglected. This essential network helps nourish the body by transporting various nutrients to all parts of the body. This nutrition goes directly to the cells from the lymphatic fluids. When the lymph glands are full of toxins, the body will be filled with acids and catarrh. This needs to be corrected because it can cause the beginning of many diseases. It can promote fluid retention, loss of energy, constipation, congested sinuses, low back pain, aches and pains and a general sluggish feeling. The diseases it can cause are: allergies, arthritis, sinusitis, cancer, colitis, erythematosis, lupus, obesity and skin disorders.

The tonsils and appendix are two of the organs that protect the lymph system from becoming overloaded. The tonsils help in the throat area. The toxic material that is eliminated through the tonsils is usually swallowed and with the help of the lymph fluid is reabsorbed into the system and then carried through the bowels. If the tonsils have been removed, this protection is gone and any

infection that enters the mouth goes directly into the lymphatic system, which can cause an overload for the lymph glands to eliminate.

Lymphatic Nutritional Formula

The lymphatic system is usually neglected or ignored until the nodes become so enlarged that they become sore and painful. The nodes become enlarged when the body's accumulation of toxins is greater than the lymphatics can process and eliminate. Changing the diet from heavy protein to a cleansing one is beneficial for the lymphatics. Adding digestive enzymes such as hydrochloric acid and pancreatic enzymes, while cleansing and resting the lymphatic system, will speed the healing process.

This formula contains vitamin A, B6, C, and D. It contains magnesium, lecithin, coenzyme Q10, and sodium copper chlorophyllin. The following herbs enrich this formula: bayberry, alfalfa, chamomile, echinacea, parthenium, Siberian ginseng, yarrow and garlic.

Lymphatic Rosary

Lymphatic Rosary is the name given by Iridologists to the iris of the eye as the way of determining whether the lymphatic system is congested. LaDean Griffin, in her book *The Essentials of Iridology*, describes the lymphatic rosary, "The lymphatic rosary on the iris appears like globs or nodules of white, yellow, or brown beads strung around the sixth zone. Sometimes they connect all the way around, other times they are disconnected and show only sparsely around the circumference on the sixth zone. Anytime these globs show on the iris anywhere on this zone, it is an indication of an accumulation of mucus waste in the lymph of the body. If the color is extremely white, almost blue, and appears to be super-imposed on the top of the fibers of the iris, it is considered as an index of arsenic retention in the lymph system. When the lymphatic rosary appears white, yellow or brown and has a thickening of the fibers themselves, this indicates congestion. Often there is arsenic retention as well as a mucus congestion of the lymph, making it difficult to distinguish. The arsenic retained in the lymph is related to neuritis conditions and will become neuritis later as it becomes more chronic. It can also be related to arthritis.

There are seven zones from pupil to peripheral line. The sixth zone, where lymphatic rosary is found, has to do with circulation. When circulation is poor, the lymph nodes and the body begin to retain waste. As waste is retained in the lymph, the thyroid works overtime to send iodine into the body to kill germs living in accumulating mucus. When thyroid activity is increased, pituitary activity is decreased, as if it were on a balance scale; overactivity of the thyroid increases oxidation to assist the body in expelling waste, much the same way we breathe faster when we have a cold or fever. When the thyroid gland is overactive, the pituitary decreases its activity causing a slow-down of all other glandular activity. All glands are subservient to the pituitary. An all-out effort is directed through the thyroid to fight against bacteria in lymphatic waste which is accumulating, as indicated by the presence of a lymphatic rosary. The spleen is also noted in conjunction with a lymphatic rosary. The spleen is the organ of the body related to the production of red blood cells, but another activity of the spleen is to retain waste from the lymphatic system. It is much like a holding tank. When the lymphatic waste becomes alarmingly full, the spleen acts like a vacuum, drawing as much waste as possible to itself until such time as the body can overcome the waste. At that time the spleen will the eliminate retained waste. The appendix does a similar thing with the colon when an impaction in the ascending colon threatens to cause a back-up of waste into the small intestines.

The appendix protects the body as an overflow valve, because when waste backs up into the small intestines where absorption of nutrients takes place, it could poison the whole body. When the spleen and lymphatic system become full the body immune system is lowered. When the spleen area and the lymphatic system become full the body immune system is lowered. When the spleen area and the lymphatic rosary on the iris appears full all the way around an overlay of hite is superficially imposed on the top of the color of the iris, this is indicative of Hodgkin's disease.

A problem in the lymph system can develop into Hodgkin's disease if the rosary remains white for too long. To clean the entire lymphatic system a milk food diet and cleansing herbs, particularly laxatives are used. Flush the body's lymph when chronic cholesterol is the cause, lecithin helps to emulsify and loosen fatty wastes in the arteries. Check for a lymphatic rosary across the body structure because it may indicate arthritis. Check the gland area for incorrect calcium balance. An imbalance can cause further calcium build-up and hardening of the arteries." (Taken from *The Essentials of Iridology* by LaDean Griffin).

It is felt by some iridologists that the white rosary beads can indicate a lazy metabolism. It could also accompany a slow pituitary and thyroid function and also increase weight gain to one degree or another. It would be very hard to lose weight no matter what diet is used until the glands are cleaned, fed and nourished. The glands indicate that their function is slower than they should be and cannot keep up with the cleansing process. Exercise is indicated. Helpful herbs are gentian, rosehips, yellow-dock and dandelion. (These are iron herbs. Iron quickly burns up rubbish and excess toxins in the body.) Kelp, echinacea, sarsaparilla, lobelia, black walnut, red clover, licorice, chaparral and pau d'arco are also beneficial. These herbs will help regulate and balance body functions. After the glands are cleansed and nourished, the body will thank you!!! At this time, the body will be able to more readily shed unwanted pounds if a proper diet is followed. Also, with balanced glandular health, energy is increased and you will want to stay on a weight loss diet.

The powerful job of the lymph glands is to collect day-to-day rubbish which accumulates in the cells. If this has collected over the years without being eliminated from wrong eating habits, air pollution, preservatives, etc., the lymph glands can very well be loaded with toxins.

If you do not perspire easily or not at all, you need to improve skin function. This could be causing lymphatic clogging just underneath the skin area which is able to breathe. This keeps the toxins from being eliminated from the skin, the largest organ of the body. Skin brushing is indicated if this is the problem. A natural brush fiber should be used just before a shower or bath to tone up lymphatic circulation. Physical exercise or a sauna will help speed up sluggish lymph circulation throughout the body. Remember that the lymphatic circulation needs constant stimulation and movement as much as the arteries and veins do.

The type of person who may have lymphatic clogging is the somewhat overweight, slow thinking, slow-moving individual who does very little physical exercise. This type of person needs to gather all the energy he or she can to enable the body to withstand the mental and physical exercise necessary to reach lymphatic health. When people in this category start on a cleansing diet, using the herbs suggested above and start exercising, the change is noticed very quickly. Enthusiasm and energy is achieved where it was not apparent before, and now they want to do more mental and physical work. Lymphatic clogging can be a stumbling block in your life. It can make your body think its tired. If you think you have lymphatic clogging, look for the tell-tale rosary beads which appear in the circulation zone on the iris of the eye. If they are present, this indicates that your health can be improved.

Another tip that might be a problem in lymphatic congestion is the lack of mineral assimilation. Minerals must be digested properly and assimilated if the glands are to be cleansed and nourished. Minerals need an acid condition in th stomach for proper assimilation. Hydrochloric acid and digestive enzymes are valuable in achieving mineral assimilation.

Babies can be born with lymphatic congestion due to acquired infections and drug contamination. This is usually manifested as poor resistance to infections and constant colds, runny nose and ear aches.

Constipation can also keep the body from achieving lymphatic health. The lymphatic vessels are numerous in the colon. The excess water in the colon is absorbed by the lymphatic vessels. If water is lacking in the colon area, the job of the lymphatic vessels cannot continue to eliminate the toxins. At the same time it will cause constipation.

Lymphatic health can be achieved if highly refined foods are avoided, and wholesome natural foods are eaten. Use a good mineral balance, green drinks, and lots of raw fruits and vegetables.

HEALTH TIPS & HEALTH THREATS

AGING AND AGE SPOTS —

No one wants to talk about age these days-at least not in our society. We want to live as long as we can, but we often make two serious mistakes: our life styles don't bring longevity and we wouldn't know what to do with the extra years if we had them! What causes aging? Why can't we all live to be 100? What can we do to live longer or at least live healthier with the years given us?

All the systems of the body need proper food and stimulation in order to function at high levels and to prevent depletion of organ reserves. The nervous system need to be fed, the skeleton needs the proper exercise and nutrients. The kidneys need proper fluid intake, the liver needs correct nutritional supplements, and the vascular system need strengthening through regular aerobic exercise.

One situation in which the elderly find themselves trapped, is becoming dependent upon social and medical support system and losing control of their own life. Studies have indicated that these changes have a negative consequence on the person's belief in the value of their life. This puts stress, worry, and a feeling of doom which increases risk of illness.

Drs. Philip Scharz and Ralph Bircher, both European scientists, report that the aging process is intensified by amyloid, a by-product of protein metabolism. This by-product is then deposited in our bodies' connective tissues and causes tissue and organ degeneration, leading to premature aging, as well as a number of age-related diseases. Many forward-looking nutritionists now agree that Americans eat twice as much protein as they really need and this includes both animal and vegetable protein.

It has been found that the low protein diets of the Hunzakuts of Pakistan, the Bulgarians, the Russian Caucasians, the Ucatan Indians and the East Indian Todos have enabled them to have average life spans of 90 to 100 years. On the other hand, the high protein diets of Eskimos, Greenlanders, Lapplanders, and Russian Kirgis tribes make for a life expectancy of 74 years. Longevity in the U.S. is further hampered by radiation pollution from electronic sources which can cause cell mutation and speed the aging process.

Jeffrey S. Bland, Ph.D., said in an article in his November/December 1986 issue of *Complementary Medicine Magazine*, "A connection has recently been found between Down's Syndrome and Alzheimer's disease. Dr. Melvyn Ball of the University of Western Ontario is following 400 Down's patients, studying their brain anatomy, neurochemistry and family histories. He is searching for microscopic signs of aging-plaques formed by clusters of deteriorating nerve endings called neurofibrillary tangles, which may come as a consequence of accelerated free radical damage in the central nervous system of these children. These symptoms also occur in normal aging, but the brains of Alzheimer's patients show up to 100 times as many of these tangles as normal aged brains. Alzheimer's disease patients and those with Down's syndrome also share another common trait-similar, fingerprint patterns. The difference between Down's syndrome and Alzheimer's disease could be the rate at which these fibrillary tangles and other degenerative processes occur in the nervous system and might be tied to specific genetic risk factors. The extra chromosome in Down's syndrome children, for example, carries the gene for increased synthesis of superoxide dysmutase, an enzyme that traps superoxide, but does not contain the gene for increases synthesis of catalase, the enzyme that traps hydrogen peroxide. It has been proposed then that the Down's syndrome brain is exposed to higher levels of superoxide, which is chemically converted to hyrdoxyl radical without being quenched, and which increases the rate of peroxidative damage."

Environmental factors can amplify these

genetic risk factors, such as aluminum which may increase the rate of neurofibrillary tangle formation in the brains of individuals susceptible to Alzheimer's disease. Other toxins that may do damage are: cadmium from cigarette smoke, lead, mercury, air pollution from industrial plants, and many other pollutants in the air.

Motivation to live longer will increase longer life. Have something to do in your late years. Keep the brain stimulated by reading, thinking and even attending adult education classes. Memory loss is a symptom of both normal and abnormal aging of the brain. You should not be alarmed if you misplace something, such as your glasses, but you might worry if you forget that you wear glasses. Try not to depend on drugs as you get older. Use natural food, supplements and herbs to stimulate brain function. Exercise, proper rest and recreation are essential for proper brain function. You don't have to be old to lose proper brain function.

Age Spots

Age spots have also been called liver spots. They are the brown spots that appear on the body, and are often seen on the hands of the elderly. They are considered a by-product of free radical damage. These spots are an accumulation of waste material in the cells. Free radicals in the body are caused by rancid oils, poor liver function, poor diet, autointoxication, and lack of exercise.

Natural Therapy - Purify the blood, keep the bowels open, and nourish the glands. Exercise physically as well as mentally. A positive attitude protects the immune system. Increased supplements are needed along with digestive enzymes and hydrochloric acid to assure assimilation of food and supplements.

Foods to Heal - High quality protein and amino acids. Grains and sprouts are high in amino acids. Millet and buckwheat contain protein and are easy to digest. Eat raw vegetables, fruits, seeds, grains, nuts, sprouts, broccoli, cabbage, cauliflower and eat a lot of fiber foods. Psyllium is great for healthy bowels.

Vitamins and Minerals - Vitamins A, C, and E along with the mineral selenium are all natural antioxidants and destroy free radicals and protect against toxins, viruses and bacteria, smog and radiation. Vitamin D increases absorption of minerals in the bones, especially calcium. B-complex (deficiencies are seen in the elderly), especially B6, pantothenic acid, folic acid and B12. Vitamin C (essential for the production of interferon, that destroys viruses), protects cells and heals wounds. Vitamin E increases resistance to disease and free-radicals. Selenium protects against cancer and improves antibody production. Zinc is seen lacking in the elderly. It builds the immune system, and is healing for wounds. All vitamins and minerals work together. Calcium can be obtained from an herbal calcium formula. Minerals, can be found in herbs such as alfalfa, kelp and dulse.

Single Herbs to Benefit Aging - Alfalfa, cayenne, damiana, dong quai (strengthens all female organs). Eyebright (cleans and protects the eyes), false unicorn, garlic (protects the veins ad immune system), gentian (protects the digestive system), ginkgo (strengthens blood vessels, increases blood flow to the brain), ginseng (strengthens whole body, prevents senility), gotu kola (improves memory and brain function), hawthorn (builds heart muscles and dilates blood vessels), hops (feeds and nourishes the nervous system), horsetail (contains silicon which increases absorption of calcium and other minerals), ho-shou-wu (improves health, stamina), kelp (rich in minerals, chelates metals), lady's slipper (strengthens nerves), licorice (increases energy), lobelia (keeps the stomach clean, and helps other herbs absorb), oatstraw, papaya, pau d'arco (protects the liver), red clover (cleans the cells), sarsaparilla, Suma (immune system booster), yellow dock (rich in iron), yucca (cleans deep in the cells).

Supplements - Bee pollen and spirulina (RNA-DNA, protected against aging), evening primrose oil, fish oil lipids, salmon oil, lecithin (choline and inositol), royal jelly (dilates and strengthens the blood vessels, tissue rebuilder, and feeds the glands), whey powder (helps joints remain limber and prevents calcium deposits), blue-green algae (provides oxygen to the cells and builds the immune system).

Avoid - Rancid oils (which would include old nuts and seeds), processed foods, coffee, tea, cocoa, caffeine drinks. Alcohol (dilates the bloods vessels and causes weak veins), excessive consumption of soft drinks can deplete calcium, with their high content of phosphorus and increase bone problems such as osteoporosis. Chlorinated water speeds the aging process. Avoid salt, fats and sugar. Also avoid tobacco, red meat, alcohol, and fried foods.

HAY FEVER
Relief with Herbs

Hay fever is an inflammation of the nasal mucosa. Healthy mucous membranes protect all the organ linings from invasion by bacteria. When this healthy mucus is not being produced, the membranes are vulnerable to irritation by germs or any air borne irritant, and this irritation results in an increase of mucus flow which is out of control.

The cells of the mucous membranes are completely renewed every thirty days. We are able to have some control on this system and can take the proper means to protect hay fever from invading our body.

Hay fever is an allergic reaction to substances (foreign material) in the air such as pollen that enter the blood through the mucous membranes, by breathing. This reaction is manifested in five systems in the body.

1. The Adrenals-Tiny glands above the kidneys have the job of producing hormones which render foreign proteins harmless.

2. The Liver-When the liver is healthy and not overloaded, it detoxifies the foreign toxins, preventing harmful reaction.

3. The Digestive System-When digestion is inefficient, built-up protein substances causes an allergic reaction in the bloodstream.

4. The Mucous Membranes-When they are healthy and working efficiently, they do not allow foreign proteins to enter the bloodstream.

5. The Nervous System-This system works with the immune system. You cannot have a healthy immune system, which protects the body from foreign material, without a strong nervous system. We will discuss these five systems later.

Millions of Americans suffer untold allergic reactions each spring and summer. It manifests itself in watery eyes, itching nose and eyes, runny nose, blurred vision, headaches, sinus aches and pains and a head that feels as big as a balloon. Red swollen eyes and difficulty in breathing are both common in hayfever. Tickling in the nose and throat are very irritating. Hay fever is like a very severe cold without any relief, continuing day after day and usually grows worse year after year unless natural methods are used to help nature eliminate it through normal channels.

Hay fever, chronic rhinitis, bronchitis, bronchial asthma, and sinusitis are all different manifestations of chronic catarrh of the air-passages. Chronic catarrh of the middle ear can build-up and cause partial or complete deafness with involvement of the mastoid cells. It can be serious if not taken care of.

Hay fever and all other allergic reactions are acute catarrhal symptoms. The pollen of weeds and flowers are accused of causing these allergic

191

reactions. An allergy is a disease of the mucous membranes of the nose. It is an elimination of toxins by way of the mucous membranes. It is also nature's way of cleaning the body of toxins and protecting the body from further harm.

Before hay fever develops, there is catarrh of the stomach, due of overloading the stomach with overeating, wrong combinations and wrong kinds of food, too much rich food and feeling anger, hate or negative thoughts. Protein acids, starch acids, acids from over-consumption of fried and rancid oils, hate and anger acids build up in the body. These all create irritations and inflammations of the stomach lining. This creates a chronic gastric fermentation. The gas from this fermentation is passed directly by way of the stomach and also builds up in the lungs. Conditions such as hay fever are primarily caused by the irritations from gas elimination (toxic gas) that is being generated in the stomach.

When the body is overloaded with too much of these toxins, and is trying to eliminate them from the natural eliminative organs, (the kidneys and colon), the stress is then put on the nasal membranes. In trying to eliminate, chronic catarrh and hay fever develops. If the mucous membranes are weak, the process may have started in childhood.

The catarrhal mucous membranes are very sensitive. If the tendency to have hayfever is inherited, and it starts from early childhood, it doesn't have to develop unless we continue the habits of wrong eating and living that will cultivate this disease. If hay fever is suppressed with drugs, overeating as well as eating rich foods while the body is attempting to eliminate, toxins can develop into more chronic types of disease later, such as pneumonia, typhoid fever, bronchitis, gastric or duodenal ulcers or even cancer.

Hay fever is a symptom which gives giving the body signals to eliminate and let nature take its course. This hypersecretion is made possible because of toxins wanting to leave the body. These toxins cause inflammation and irritation of the mucous membranes and the underlying tissues. When these secretions are suppressed by drugs and overeating, they become thick and hardened

membranes as the tissues decompose and ulcerate. There is no difference between a cold, hay fever, asthma or bronchitis except in the degree of complications.

Eating aggravates all acute diseases (cold, flu, fever, childhood diseases, hay fever and etc.) until distress becomes unbearable and help is sought out with any drug to get some relief. The relief may come with drugs but it suppresses the diseases of elimination (remember this is the cure) to manifest itself again or in another chronic disease later in life.

When the stomach is kept in constant turmoil with foods beyond the body's needs such as too much meat, fried foods, refined starch, fats, sugar, bread, cake, candy, pie, eggs, and dairy products, hayfever develops. This overstimulates the stomach and creates a toxic state of the blood, and causes the nervous system to be over-sensitive. Therefore any dust, pollen perfumes or odors will cause the hay fever to continue until steps are taken to help nature eliminate the toxic build-up.

Henry G. Beiler, M.D., one of our pioneers in nutrition, said in his book *Food Is Your Best Medicine,* "Hay fever develops after there is an atrophy of the nasal and sinus mucous membranes. These membranes when catarrhal, are extremely sensitive to irritating pollens, dust, animal exhalations, smog and/or chemicals which often cause violent sneezing and coughing when they come in contact with the sensitive, inflamed membrane. But the inflammation comes first and irritation follows. When there is no catarrhal state, there is no hay fever, no matter what irritant is inhaled.

Here again is seen the process of vicarious elimination with a definite salty background. Hay fever sufferers, with few exceptions, have overindulged in table salt. This explains the popularity of silver applications as a cure, just as silver nitrate is used as a spray or swab in the treatment of cold. But not only excess salt eliminated but also toxic products of starch and protein indigestion. The high vitamin content of the fresh spring and summer fruits often stimulates the endocrine glands to overactivity and produces a crisis which we call hayfever. That explains why it is so prevalent in those times of the year when the pollen count is highest, but remember that the irritants inhaled at these times do not cause hayfever unless the mucous membrane is already inflamed. (A speck of dust or other foreign body can cause a much more violent irritation in a sore eye than in a normal eye.).

Using less salt, abstaining from toxemia-producing proteins and starches and exercising greater care in the selection and amount of fresh fruit ingested comprise the first step in controlling the toxemia that causes the disease. Nor must the endocrines be forgotten, for heat stimulates the adrenal glands. These glands, when overactive, reciprocally stimulate the thyroid gland through the sympathetic nervous system. Then the thyroid causes vicarious elimination through the mucous membranes, thus aggravating the hay fever symptoms. Therefore, hay fever sufferers often find relief in colder climates. But if the adrenals are weak and the thyroid still strong enough to cause vicarious elimination when toxemia exists, the victim will not benefit by moving to a colder climate."

FIVE SYSTEMS OF PROTECTION FROM HAY FEVER

1. **The Adrenals:** A healthy body can neutralize toxins; the adrenal cortex destroys white blood cells and thus inhibits inflammation. A hormone called aldosterone fights stress and prevents fatigue. Certain nutrients are required in order for the adrenals to produce hormones. When these nutrients are under supplied for a long time, the adrenals atrophy and must be rebuilt.

   Potassium is essential to strengthen the adrenals. Magnesium is called the anti-stress mineral. It assists in the absorption of calcium, phosphorus, sodium, potassium, B complex, C and E. It is an activator of enzymes in the use of protein and vitamins. Protein is essential for the adrenals. Using more grains and beans, and brown rice along with fresh

vegetable salads will fortify the adrenals. B vitamins are necessary for the general health of the adrenals, and can effectively guard against allergic reactions. Pantothenic acid is directly related to the production of natural cortisone. It is one of the B complex vitamins. Pantothenic acid requirement is increased under stress, rapid growth, illness or exposure to toxins, which include pollens, dust and etc. A formula to use in high stress situations: Taken from *Vegetarian Times/ Well-Being Issue #45*, by Bhavani Worden, "Use when an allergic or hay fever attack is beginning to occur: 1,000 mg of high quality vitamin C with bioflavonoids, 300-6-- mg sustained release pantothenic acid, 1 amino acid chelated calcium-magnesium with 200 mg. Calcium, 100 mg. magnesium. This combination gives immediate support to the adrenals in their attempt to produce cortisone, and to the entire system in its detoxification effort." Bhavani Worden suggests that, "If the system is already slowed down by the time you get around to taking this formula, i.e., the allergic reaction has begun, the mucous membranes are inflamed, the digestion has slowed, the blood sugar level has dropped, and fatigue, irritability, headache or depression have set in then it would be wise to crush the tablets and mix them with yogurt to ensure their efficient digestion."

Essential fatty acids are needed to produce adrenal hormones, as well as to synthesize pantothenic acid in the intestines. They are found in Evening Primrose Oil, Black Currant Oil, Fish Oil Lipids and Flaxseeed Oil. Iodine is necessary to produce thyroid hormone, which keeps the rate of metabolism, controlling the speed of body activities. The lack of thyroid hormone results in exhaustion, of a feeling of coldness, and susceptibility to acute diseases. Kelp, Dulse and sea salt, are all high in iodine. A sodium-potassium balance is essential in treating hay fever. When the adrenals are under-nourished, the adrenal cortex hormone, aldosterone, is not produced and fatigue and exhaustion accompany every stress. Herbs that are high in potassium and will help in the sodium-potassium balance are: Alfalfa, blessed thistle, capsicum, chickweed, comfrey, dandelion, garlic, ginger, hops, horsetail, kelp, licorice, parsley, red clover, safflower, scullcap and yarrow.

2. **The Liver:** The liver's job is to detoxify poisonous material, even when it's produced in the body. It produces an enzyme called histaminase. If the liver is congested with fats or accumulated toxins, it cannot produce this enzyme. Cleaning the liver is essential. An excellent herbal formula to clean the liver is: red beet, dandelion root, golden seal root, yellow dock, bayberry, oregon grape root, and pan pien lien. Vitamin C and E help to reduce the production of histamine under stress. Histamine is a toxin to the liver and can provoke an allergy attack and hay fever.

3. **The Digestive System:** Improper digestion can be one of the main causes of hay fever. Undigested protein and starch can enter the bloodstream and cause hay fever. Protein digestive aids and food enzymes will help in digesting food left in the intestines. Changing the diet is essential. Stay away from additives, artificial food colors or flavors, chemically grown food, processed oils, refined flour and sugar. Stay away from stimulants such as alcohol, coffee, or soft drinks containing caffeine. These foods overstimulate the adrenals and lower resistance and deplete energy. Eat sprouts, millet and buckwheat. Use high quality natural food.

4. **The Mucous Membranes:** Healthy mucous membranes protect all the organ linings from invasion by bacteria. Since the cells of the mucous membranes are completely renewed every thirty days, we can start now to protect from allergies and hay fever. The healthy cell membrane prevent toxins from entering into the blood stream. If the membranes are weak

and do not prevent the germs from entering, it will poison the cell, and foreign proteins such as pollen, dust and any foreign matter will gain easy access to the center of the cell where they can do much damage and trigger asthma, allergies and hay fever. Vitamin A is essential to strengthen and protect the mucous membranes. Some experts suggest taking 100,000 I.U.'s daily with vitamin D during the hay fever season. Use both the Beta Carotene and Fish oils to get your vitamin A. Vitamin E should be used along with A to protect it from destruction. Vitamin C is vital, it binds foreign proteins and carries them out of the body. It can bind any toxin, even the toxins produced by incomplete digestion of food. It cannot be stored in the body, so high amounts are needed before the pollen season begins. Vitamin C is also essential for the production of cortisone and histiminase, as well as for cell membrane permeability. Herbs to help the mucous membranes are mullein and comfrey. Mullein strengthens the mucous membranes, glands, bowels and inflamed nerves. Comfrey is an herb to soothe, nourish and heal the mucous membranes. One excellent combination for cleansing and nourishing the mucous membranes is: Comfrey, Fenugreek, Yerba Santa, Hyssop and Wild Cherry. Single herbs are: aloe vera, capsicum, comfrey, fenugreek, garlic, hops, lobelia, mullein, scullcap, slippery elm and yarrow.

5. **The Nervous System:** This system is closely linked with the immune system. The nervous system controls and coordinates all of the functions of the body, including that of the pituitary gland. This gland masters the entire endocrine network. An excellent herbal combination for the nerves is: Extract of Scullcap, Chamomile, Valerian, Passion Flower, Kava Kava, and Catnip. Single herbs excellent for the nerves are: gotu kola, hops, kelp, lady's slipper, lobelia, passion flower, scullcap, and red clover.

In the book, *The Ultimate Healing System*, by Donald LePore, N.D., he says, "In stressful situations, the adrenal glands must send various hormones to organs that counteract stress. This accelerated pace, caused by stress, cannot be maintained for a long period of time without exhausting the supply of nutrients that feed the Adrenal glands. In our research we have found that when Adrenal glands become exhausted, the person immediately becomes allergic to citrus fruits (lemons, limes, oranges, grapefruits, tomatoes, pineapple, cantaloupe, and all bioflavonoids). The nutrient that corrects this condition is Vitamin B-5 (Pantothenic Acid), at least 2000 mgs. In my practice I use a product called "Royal Jelly," which is a natural source of Pantothenic acid and niacin (Vitamin B-3). One 1000 mg. capsule of Royal Jelly has the potency of a 500 mg. Pantothenic acid pill, and a 500 mg. Niacin pill (without the "flush" of Niacin)."

Another problem that may occur when the adrenals are exhausted, is a sinus condition. To check this out, place a finger on each side of the nose about 3/4 inches away from the nose with one hand while extending the other arm to be "pumped". If the extended arm goes down when pressed, this is an indication that the sinuses are inflamed. Inflamed sinuses in this case are caused by a citrus allergy, because of stress and exhaustion of the adrenal glands."

We have many natural methods in helping us to overcome and prevent hay fever. We need to educate ourselves to the herbs, natural vitamins and minerals, and supplements along with natural foods, exercise, and the right mental attitude in order to overcome our allergies and hay fever.

Single Herbs For Hay Fever

Black Walnut - Natural antihistamine, antiseptic to clean all toxic blood conditions.

Boneset - Reduces fever, relives stomach congestion.

Burdock - Purifies blood, aids in lymphatic system congestion.

Cayenne - Stimulates mucous secretions to relieve congestion.

Chickweed - Natural antihistamine.

Echinacea - Purifies blood, and acts as a digestive tonic, cleans the glands.

Elder Flowers - Contains bioflavonoids, anti-catarrhal.

Ephedra - Natural cleanser and antihistamine.

Eyebright - Detoxifies nasal cavities, relieves eye, nose and throat irritations. Excellent for hay fever and allergies.

Garlic - Natural antibiotic and antihistamine.

Golden Seal - Natural antibiotic, cleans stomach congestion.

Kelp - Supplies natural iodine for an antiseptic, cleans the mucous membranes and balances minerals in the system.

Marshmallow - Heals and soothes irritated mucous membranes.

Mullein - Relieves sinus congestion, reduces swelling and inflammation.

Parsley - Eliminates excess mucus and acts as a decongestion.

Peppermint - Soothing to the stomach and mucous membranes.

Psyllium - Cleans colon to prevent toxic waste to enter the blood stream.

Red Raspberry - Eliminates mucus from the system, aids digestion and provides iron and calcium to the body.

Slippery Elm - Nourishes and soothes the mucous

membranes in recovery from all diseases. Relieves constipation and diarrhea. The tea is excellent for coughs and bronchitis when used with natural cough remedies.

Wood Betony - Natural antihistamine, relieves aches and pains.

DEPRESSION AND DISEASE

Depression can affect the health of the cardiovascular system as well as the ability of the immune system to protect the body. After the holidays, many people find themselves in a sate of depression. This could result from many causes. It could come from fatigue, diet of rich sugar products, or a lonely feeling after the family leaves and the house is quiet.

It is normal for all of us to feel the minor ups and downs of mood swings. We have days when we feel especially good and other days when we feel lousy. There are days when we feel particularly unhappy or depressed. Maybe a song or a word will trigger an unhappy event in our past which reminds us of an unhappy experience and dumps us into a depressed state. The ordinary blue days are usually short and self-healing. It is the long, stressed out depression that we need to be concerned with.

Depression is manifested in many forms. It is much more than just one thing. It is different things to different people. It is seen as discouragement, despondency, self-depreciation, gloom and a mental state of sadness. It can leave a hollow feeling within. It can reveal a morbid condition of emotional dejection and withdrawal. It can show in a sadness greater and more prolonged than that warranted by any objective reason.

Depression, stress and prolonged grief have an effect on the physical/chemical response of the immune system. It is now widely accepted that stress and depression and our perception of the world we live in can actually suppress the immune system. Depression prevents the central nervous system to adapt to environmental input. In all the experience I have had with depression, the nervous system has to be built up and this strengthens the immune system. An old journal by Priddy Meeks, an early Herbalist from Utah, says order the heading *As New Theory About The Hysterics In Women and The Hypochondria In Men*: "Now the learned doctors of the day says that only women has the hysterics, while men has the hypochondria. Now I aim to show their mistake. It is the same complaints in both sexes. Nothing different. Symptoms and characteristics is exactly the same in both sexes is not denied by anyone, and I say the same cause produces the complaint in both sexes alike, and I shall call it the "hippo" or the blues, which is caused by nothing less than the drying or shrivelled up of the nerves. And no wonder he has the blues, (depression) for the whole man is perverted, and everything seems to be wrong and foremost, which throws the whole phenomenon of nature into confusion double as bad on some individuals as others. Some has been transformed in their feelings and mind that they would actually look at everything ina wrong light. Their organs of sense would be so deranged that they would see sorts of forms which it does not see. The smell would detect odors which do not exist. The touch demonstrates to the brain objects with which it does not come in contact with. The taste is perverted and disordered to an extent which seems to an uninterested observer, impossible. And the ears convey imaginary sounds of the most perplexing and terrible character, and this is not half the symptoms resulting from the shrivelling up of the nervous system. Every authority I have examined very readily admits that such a state of those symptoms is the cause of the derangement of the nerves. But I hold it as settled truth that the drying up or shrivelling up of the nerves according to the law of old age is the primary cause of all those symptoms." Priddy Meeks practiced herbal medicine in Utah and used Thompsonian course of medicine for every complaint. He said, "it was the safest and surest plans for success that ever was derived by man, as he thought, and it proved to be true." He used lobelia and cayenne in his practice with excellent results. He used lobelia for depression and found that it removed obstructions and strengthened the nerves.

DEPRESSION AND HEART ATTACKS

Depression or stress is often followed by heart attacks. The story of Paul "Bear" Bryant, the winningest college football coach in history, is one example. It is well known that retirement is one of the most major of life changes, and may put some persons at increased risk for illness. Within 37 days of his retirement, he was dead from a heart attack. He had said to his friends just a day before his death that there were "no more Saturdays," and that he had nothing more to which he could look forward. Edgar Bergen, the ventriloquist, known and loved by all of us for years for his performance with "Charley McCarthy," died from a heart attack just two weeks after officially putting Charley in a box and retiring from show business. We all need to prepare ourselves mentally and nutritionally for the life style changes in our live that we all will face.

Depression is often caused by numerous nutritional deficiencies. If a person is depressed and nothing specific has actually happened to cause this feeling and discussing it does not help, it could be nutrition deficiency. If the body is depleted of minerals, it is more likely to absorb toxic metal pollutants. Severe depression is the usual symptom of chronic lead poisoning in adults. It prevents concentration, and can cause hallucinations and paranoid thoughts.

Bromine salts, advertised for the relief of acid indigestion, when used excessively can cause toxicity, and one of the signs is depression.

HERBAL COMBINATION FOR DEPRESSION

The following combination has been found to be very useful when under stress, for anxiety, as a relaxant, for the nerves, and for the treatment of nervous breakdowns.

Valerian Root, Scullcap, Hops, Thiamine Mononitrate, Riboflavin, Nicotinamide, Calcium Pantothenate, Pyridoxine, HCL, Ascorbic Acid, Choline, Bitartrate, Inositol, Para-aminobenzoic Acid, Schizandra Chinesis, Piper Methysticum, Folic Acid, Cyanocobalamin, and Biotin.

STRESS AND CIRCULATION

Stress plays havoc with many organs of the body, most notably the heart and entire circulatory system. With heat attacks and strokes claiming thousands of lives each year, we cannot ignore the importance of PREVENTION.

Diet, stress-management, and exercise are three key elements involved in protecting the heart and ensuring that it does not give out before its time.

When a person is tense and uptight, the blood vessels become constricted and the heart is forced to pump wildly in order to circulate the blood adequately. This places an undue burden on the heart and overworks it. In time, it becomes weakened to the point that one day the stress placed on it is too much for it to handle. It then stops....hence, a heart attack.

A stroke can be caused by several factors. One of the most common is blockage in one of the main blood vessels. When circulation is stopped or impeded, oxygen to the brain is diminished. Cells in that particular malnourished area die of "asphyxiation." Sometimes it is in the area of the brain that controls speech, sometimes in the area that dictates muscular reflexes.

Clots will often form and obstruct circulation

197

to the brain or heart. Sometimes plaques of cholesterol will adhere and collect on the walls of the blood vessels. Compare this to pipes in a house in which hard water deposits minerals as it flows through them. Over a period of time, the pipes become clogged. When pipes are blocked, plumbing goes haywire. It is the same with our 'life-line' pipes, our blood vessels. They are our vital links to LIFE.

The American Heart Association advises us to reduce blood cholesterol by increasing intake of fresh fruits, vegetables and lean meats. It suggests that intake of fatty meats and dairy products be reduced. However, the human body needs a certain amount of cholesterol, and if not supplied through diet, will manufacture its own. From *Vitamin Bible* by Earl Mindell, we read: "At least two-thirds of your body's cholesterol is produced by the liver or in the intestine. It is found there as well as in the brain, the adrenals, and nerve fiber sheaths. And when it's good, it's very, very good:" *Cholesterol aids in the metabolism of carbohydrates. (The more carbohydrates ingested, the more cholesterol produced.) *Cholesterol is a prime supplier of life-essential adrenal hormones, such as cortisone, and sex hormones.

New research shows that cholesterol behaves differently depending on the protein to which it is bound. Lipoproteins are the factors in our blood which transport cholesterol. High-density lipoproteins (HDL) are composed principally of lecithin, whose detergent action breaks up cholesterol and can transport it easily through the blood without clogging arteries. Essentially, the higher the HDL, the lower your chances of developing heart disease. It is worth mentioning that though the egg consumption in the United States is one-half of what it was in 1945, there has not been a comparable decline in heart disease. Although the American Heart Association deems eggs hazardous, a diet without them can be equally hazardous. Not only do eggs have the most perfect protein components of any food, but they contain lecithin, which aids in fat assimilation. Most importantly, they raise HDL levels!

If a person is prone to developing blood clots,

raising their daily intake of Vitamin E may be the solution. Vitamin E thins the blood, helps increase oxygen in the body, and strengthens the heart. It is also a 'vasodilator', which means it opens up blood vessels for better circulation. The weakening of blood vessels over a length of time can result in an "aneurism," or ballooning of the fragile blood vessel wall. Often, due to high blood pressure, it is debilitated to the point that it gives way or bursts, and a hemorrhage ensues. This can be fatal, especially if it is in the brain area.

Hawthorn Berry has been used for centuries as a "heart" herb. Regular use strengthens the heart. Louise Tenney states in "Today's Herbal Health": "Hawthorn Berry has been used in preventing arteriosclerosis and in helping conditions like rapid and feeble heart action, heart valve defects, enlarged heart, angina pectoris and difficult breathing owing to ineffective heart action and lack of oxygen in the blood. Some herbalists recommend Hawthorn to use against disease before actual symptoms are manifest."

High blood pressure is a circulatory disorder definitely related to stress and diet. Supplements which have been very effective in controlling this disorder are calcium/magnesium and garlic oil. Of course, one cannot rely solely on a pill to magically disperse the affliction. Conscientious effort must be employed in order to alleviate this problem, through diet, exercise and relaxation. Salt has been indicated as one of the major dietary culpritis contributing to high blood pressure, when ingested in excessive amounts.

Do you experience heart palpitations, blurred vision, ringing or pain in the ears? These are some of the body's danger signals in reaction to stress. It is sending the message: "SLOW DOWN...CALM DOWN!" Stress management begins with attitude. If you can't change the stress-causing circumstance, or remove yourself from it, then you must change your outlook toward it. A useful motto is "Act...Don't React!" We are familiar with this prayer by St. Francis of Assisi from centuries ago, yet still applicable today: "Lord, help me to accept the things I cannot change, to change the things I can, and the wisdom to know the difference."

Sometimes we have no control over the stress in our lives. Without initiating it, frequently problems are literally dumped upon us all at once, when we are unprepared. We feel a surge of energy at first, as nature provides us with the 'fight or flight' response. The adrenal glands send us an abundance of *adrenalin* to cope with the situation. When this happens often, the adrenal glands become exhausted and can predispose one to ailments like hypoglycemia or Addison's Disease. Many other diseases have been linked to stress, among them, cancer.

Exercise is an integral part of the stress-management picture. Studies have been conducted which prove exercise to be a sedative and relaxant to the body. It will help tone-up the entire circulatory framework, so that when heavy stress *does* occur, your system can take the shock. Bicycle riding, swimming and brisk walking are excellent forms of exercise. Jogging is not advised for many people because it puts a burden on the joints and tendons. It places an extreme hardship on the heart when it is weak, and also the internal organs. This is especially true if the sport is conducted on hard pavement.

Remember, the best way to protect the heart and blood vessels and assure a long and disease-free life is to have a proper attitude, eat a healthful diet and exercise daily. HERE'S TO A *HEARTY* LIFE!!

COPING WITH STRESS

Stress should not be considered all bad as long as we are capable of handling situations that we are confronted with. It can be a good force to challenge and motivate us to do things we do not think we are capable of. All people have stress. It is how we handle this stress that is important. Stressful situations can build up over the years and take a toll on our physical and emotional health if we do not fortify our bodies. We need to teach ourselves to avoid stress we cannot handle and how to handle stress we cannot avoid. Stress

can be controlled by improving our ability to cope with situations that cause the stress. We can strengthen our nerves, build up our immune system and learn the art of relaxation as well as become involved in some type of exercise. We need to look at our eating habits and improve them, if necessary, as well as add vitamins, minerals and herbs to strengthen our bodies.

Nutritional doctors are finding that people in stressful situations are not emotionally unstable people. They are often very deficient in essential nutrients, such as vitamins and minerals. They find that the use of caffeine causes many to have exaggerated emotional feelings. Ted Flicke D.C., Ph.D., says in *Bestways* June 1986 page 58, "Caffeine acts directly upon muscles to increase their tension, stimulate the adrenal gland to produce adrenalin, and irritates the nervous system into unproductive, frantic activity. The physiological and biochemical events produce the universally recognized symptoms of caffeine - irritability, anxiety, nervousness, insomnia and inability to concentrate. Many victims of chronic stress-related muscle tension find that their problems are completely resolved once caffeine is eliminated from the diet." Lack of exercise also contributes to stress. The muscles and joints can tense up, and is often seen in people with stress. The physical, emotional and nutritional needs are necessary to overcome extremely stressful situations. The most dramatic change is seen with changing the diet and adding supplements such as vitamins, minerals, herbs and amino acids.

There have been many studies done on the correlation between emotional/physical ailments. It has been well established that the nervous system and the immune system are connected and when one goes the other goes. One such study was conducted by a group of researchers in Wisconsin. ("Specific Attitudes in initial interviews with Patients Having Different Psycholosomatic Diseases", by Dr. David T. Graham, M.D., *Psychosomatic Medicine*, Vol. XXIV, No. 3.)

The Study Revealed

ACNE: a feeling of being nagged or picked on, accompanied by a desire to be left alone.

BRONCHIAL ASTHMA: Feeling rejected and unloved; wanting to shut out the rejecting person or situation.

CONSTIPATION: a feeling of being trapped in a negative situation, when there is no way to change.

DUODENAL ULCERS: feeling unjustly treated, and wanting to take revenge.

ECZEMA: feeling thwarted and misunderstood, with no alternative but to take out such frustrations on oneself.

HIVES: having a sense of taking an unfair beating, and being unable to do anything about it.

HYPERTENSION: feeling constantly endangered.

HYPERTHYROIDISM: (overactive thyroid gland), fear of losing a loved one, or a loved object.

LOW BACKACHE: wanting to run away, to escape from an unpleasant situation.

METABOLIC EDEMA: (fluid retention by the body's tissues), a sense of being unduly burdened, and of wanting others to carry their share of the load.

MIGRAINES: feeling driven toward the achievement of some goal or goals; can relax only after the completion of such goals.

PSORIASIS: a constant sensation of gnawing irritation that has to be put up with.

RAYNAUD'S DISEASE: (chronic constriction and spasms of blood vessels of the toes, fingers, tip of nose, etc.) a feeling of hostility.

RHEUMATOID ARTHRITIS: (a specific type of arthritis involving inflammation of the joints resembling symptoms of rheumatism), feeling constrained and restricted.

VOMITING: guilt for some wrongdoing on the patient's part.

The psychoanalysts say that the symptoms the patients suffer from symbolizes their inner feelings. This may be true, but we need to understand that stress does not cause disease, it only puts a burden on the weakest part of the body. Stress puts a burden on the body and makes it more susceptible to disease.

I personally feel that when the body is fed and nourished properly the emotional problems go away. I do not believe our hostilities cause the disease, but I do believe they will put such a burden on the body to trigger symptoms of the disease.

SYMPTOMS OF EMOTIONAL STRESS

1. Situations are magnified with emotional stress.

2. Inability to retain information, short-term memory is difficult.

3. Concentration is difficult, the power to focus and concentrate long enough to deal with a problem is lost.

4. Thinking and concentrating on ideas is difficult because of the uncontrollable speed they race through the mind.

5. Negative thoughts are always in your mind, especially when trying to relax or sleep.

6. Becoming stubborn, feeling that if you don't people will take advantage and make you feel you can't make decisions.

200

7. Critical attitude is developed because of negative thoughts. Positive thoughts are hard to develop.

8. You feel you are a victim and cannot accept personal responsibility in dealing with problems.

9. Losing your sense of humor, you cannot see laughable situations because of negative thoughts.

10. Feeling that you need to control people and become very demanding.

11. Responsibilities become difficult to control and fulfill. Planning becomes impossible because of the inability to deal with present emotions and problems.

12. It becomes more appealing to escape into a fantasy world. The grass is always greener on the other side.

TOXEMIA

Toxemia and enervation (lowered resistance) are the underlying causes of all diseases. Chronic disease is the beginning of the end of the slow poisoning caused by constitutional toxemia. Conditions of toxemia and enervation make secondary infections possible by preparing the soil upon which germs and viruses (microbes) feed, multiply, and flourish. Toxins can be passed on from the prenatal environment and they can also accumulate from infancy throughout life.

What is intestinal toxemia? It describes a toxic condition in the intestinal tract, and it has many causes. When we eat the wrong kinds of foods, and in the wrong combinations and amounts, bacteria in the bowels will feed on them and produce toxins, which will next be absorbed into the bloodstream. Health experts believe all sickness begins in the colon. Before World War II, doctors understood this concept and treated illness by giving enemas and colonics. This was before drugs and surgery became the supposed universal antidote to disease. If food is not digested properly, the amino acids can be converted by the microbes into powerful toxic substances. These can cause symptoms such as fatigue, nervousness, gastrointestinal upsets, skin problems, headaches, insomnia, glandular and circulatory system disturbances and others.

At the turn of the century, Dr. J.A. Stucky, M.D. made this observation, "That blood is poisoned through absorption of toxic material from the intestinal canal more frequently than from any other source, I think will not be questioned."

Toxins, due to disturbed body chemistry, are manufactured daily in the intestinal canal and remain in the system. The result is a protest from the irritated nerves and poisoned cells, which manifest in rheumatic pains, asthmatic attacks, vertigo, obscure neuroses of eye, ear, nose and throat, neuralgias and periodic headaches.

Medical literature has published reports over the years which support the theory of toxemia and disease:

- One doctor studied over 450 cases of allergies and found that the allergies cleared up when intestinal toxemia was eradicated.

- Another doctor, after observing patients for 23 years, stated that toxemia is the root cause of the condition and the "the results of treatment justify my position."

- It has been found that approximately half of all cases of inflammatory arthritis can be greatly improved by removing the toxins formed in the intestine.

- About one-fourth of all cases of 'irregular heart beats' responded well to elimination of toxemia.

- "Several hundreds of cases" of ear, nose, and throat diseases reported in the scientific literature were from autointoxication.

• Toxemia in pregnancy many times stems from eating a high-protein diet, in conjunction with constipation.

• Many cases of eye diseases and problems were improved when intestinal toxins were removed from the body.

• At an annual meeting of the AMA (American Medical Association) in 1917, a scientific report was shared that stated 517 cases of mental problems were relieved by eradicating intestinal toxemia. These symptoms ranged from mental sluggishness to hallucinations. More recently, schizophrenia has been added to the list of mental disorders which improve when the toxemia is eliminated.

Norman W. Walker, D. Sc., Ph.D., has lectured and written about toxemia. In his book, *Colon Health*, he says: "If a person has been eating processed, fried and overcooked foods, devitalized starches, sugar and excessive amounts of salt, his colon cannot possible be efficient--even if he should have a bowel movement two to three times a day! Instead of furnishing nourishment to the nerves, muscles, cells and tissues of the walls of the colon, such foods can actually cause starvation of the colon. A starved colon may let a lot of fecal matter pass through it, but it is unable to carry on the last of the digestive and nourishing processes and functions intended for it. The bulk, which is so essential for the proper and complete digestion of our food, is needed in the colon just as much as the small intestine. Such bulk, however, must be composed of fibers or roughage of raw foods. When these fibers pass through the intestines they become, figuratively speaking, highly magnetized, and in this condition are very helpful in the functions involved in the various parts of the intestines. In addition to receiving the residue of that part of our food which is not digested, the colon also accommodates itself to fiber--the roughage--in the food upon which it depends for its intestinal broom."

HOMEOPATHY

A study performed by reputable scientists working in Canada, France, Israel and Italy confirms the healing effects of homeopathy. The research was published in *Nature* magazine (Vol. 333, issue No. 6176, June 30, 1988, p. 816-818). The research concluded that the homeopathic remedies are both safe and effective in healing the body. Though the reason they work is often not known, the fact that they do work in extremely low dosage is now proven.

Many major newspapers and periodicals published articles on this amazing experiment. *The Washington Post* and *The New York Times* along with major magazines were among the first to print articles on the subject. Homeopathy is gaining respect throughout the world, and evidence is mounting supporting the benefits of this method.

Homeopathy is not a new idea. It has been around in the western world since the early 1800s. A German physician, Samuel Hahnemann is credited with its rediscovery and use. Anciently homeopathy was used in the Eastern culture. It may date back as far as 3000 B.C. It is an important part of Hindu medicine and is used throughout India.

Hahnemann, while experimenting with medicines, discovered that overdoses of the drug quinine in a healthy individual caused symptoms very similar to malaria. Quinine was known to cure malaria. This lead him to study the effects of giving patients drugs which normally cause the problems they were experiencing.

Hahnemann experimented on himself and others. He discovered that diluted and safe amounts of drugs that produce symptoms of a disease in a healthy person could cure the disease without dangerous side effects. This lead him to the theory of the law of similars. Similia similibus curentur, ("Let likes be cured with likes").

The law of similars states that any substance which can cause symptoms of an illness when given to a healthy person can heal an individual who is suffering from similar symptoms. The theory is that the same anatomy of the cure and the illness are brought together to heal.

Conventional medicine has also practiced the law of similars. In immunizations, small amounts of the disease are given to immunize a patient against that disease. The theory is good but vaccinations are not prepared using homeopathic methods and may cause side effects. Allergy sufferers are often given injections with small dilutions of the substance they react to in order to build up a tolerance. Cancer patients are given radiation treatments and radiation is known to cause cancer. These modern common medical practices are similar to the ancient homeopathy. The do not however, obey the major principle of homeopathy. This includes the treatment of the person as a whole physically and psychologically using one single medicine.

Modern medicine has sought to cure the symptoms of a disease. This often leads to covering up an illness. Homeopathy as taught by Hahnemann and his observations conclude that symptoms are the body's response to the stresses it is undergoing. Therefore, instead of curing the symptoms, treatment should help stimulate the body's own defense system.

The body makes great steps to heal itself, but sometimes it is not strong enough. This is when homeopathic medicine in very diluted amounts can help the body to free itself of disease. Conventional treatments suppress symptoms and are often temporary. For instance, antibiotics can kill harmful bacteria but they also kill the good bacteria which can leave the body susceptible to other illness.

In homeopathy, only one medicine is given at a time. Even though there may be many symptoms there should be only one cure. Whether the condition be chronic or acute one medicine should stimulate the body into action. While using just one medication, the effect of the treatment can be monitored and changed more easily if necessary. Many chronically ill patients are given different medications at one time. This can lead to dangerous side effects and problems with the drugs interacting.

Dr. Hahnemann began his research in Germany. In 1820, Hahnemann was not allowed to practice medicine by the German Government. His methods were unorthodox and therefore unaccepted. He moved to Paris in 1835 and continued his research and practice.

Homeopathy is becoming more accepted in the western world. Western Europe has been very receptive. The Royal family in England are well known users of homeopathic medicine. Queen Elizabeth has her own personal homeopathic physician on her medical staff. Homeopathy is widely used in the Hindu religion and throughout India.

The U.S. has been less receptive of homeopathy, but more medical doctors are using homeopathic medicine along with traditional treatment. We are seeing an awakening of homeopathic medicine in America.

Certainly traditional medical practices can be life saving. Antibiotics can save lives when a serious infection of vital organs is involved. Most illnesses however, are not life threatening and can be healed with homeopathic medicines. Homeopathy is a growing field and is finding its place in the medical community.

HEALTH THREATS

AIR POLLUTION

Threat To Our Lungs

Our lungs are being threatened daily with the huge amount of chemicals that are being thrown into the air. It is believed that impure air is one of the greatest causes of illness. There are a wide range of chronic symptoms resulting from sensitivities to substances in the air. Doctors cannot always pinpoint the causes of these symptoms. Symptoms from toxic air range from mental confusion, anxiety, fatigue, headaches, depression and personality changes to hyperactivity, joint pain, breathing difficulties and numerous allergies. As long as we are exposed to chemicals, dust, pollen, molds, carbon monoxide, lead, cadmium, aluminum, and many other toxins, we need to become acquainted with our lungs, learn their function and how to protect them. The lungs can be protected from the threat that is constantly hanging over us. We need to use supplements of herbs, vitamins, minerals, amino acids and other essential nutrients such as CoQ10, fish lipids and germanium. These added nutrients and an immune diet can protect our lungs from damage.

These pollutants carry particulate matter from industry in processing and burning fuel, especially coal. These pollutants can carry heavy metals and cancer-causing matter deep into the lungs. Children are particularly vulnerable along with the elderly and persons who have lung ailments. Children are more vulnerable to breathing contaminated air because before the ages of eight to ten children lack fully developed immunity system to combat respiratory pathogens in the air.

Contaminated air also accentuates the danger of maternal smoking. Dr. James Metcalfe a spokesman for the American Heart Association says, "when levels of carbon monoxide are high as they are in the blood of smoking women during pregnancy, adverse effects from carbon monoxide can be recognized by retarded fetal growth and persistent behavioral defects after birth."

The danger continues after birth too, Janice Cram, director of the Sudden Infant Death Syndrome (SIDS) project center at Portland State University, told a hearing that, "the adverse effects of carbon monoxide are enhanced by anemia; a condition common among premature and low birth weight infants. These babies are at increased risk for sudden death syndrome, which is characterized by a sudden cessation of breathing or asphyxiation called apnea."

Among adults who have arterial disease to one degree or another have a higher risk from breathing carbon monoxide, and other pollutants. There are approximately eight million Americans with cardiovascular disease.

In Steubenville, Ohio, investigators found a direct correlation between particulate levels and increased hospital emergency room admissions for respiratory disease. The investigators say that for each hospital case there are necessarily a larger number of people made ill enough to seek out a doctor, miss work and suffer pain.

The cancer-causing particles of sulfates formed along with sulfuric acid from burning coal, are the most widespread and dangerous. Lead pollution is also widespread and dangerous. A survey by the National Center for Health Statistics showed that four percent of United States children under five, almost a half million preschoolers, are lead poisoned. The most profound effect of lead contamination is brain damage. But it is more commonly seen as mental retardation or hyperactivity.

Lead is found in the soil and dust near highways which comes from airborne lead from automobile exhaust. Some children eat dirt deliberately or accidentally get into their mouths from their hands. It can also be in the child's diet. The lead from the air settles on the ground and is absorbed by a food plant's roots. Lead can also be in the animals raised for food when they eat the contaminated plant. An infant fed on formula made from a soldered can of evaporated milk would get much more lead than a breast-fed baby. In fact, breast feeding is the best protection against contamination from the air.

Appearing on television on the east coast following radiation leaks at Three Mile Island, La Leche League International President Marian Thompson cited evidence from the British Medical Journal, *Lancet*, "Absorption, Excretion, and Retention of Strontium by Breastfed and Bottlefed Babies," that breastfed babies excrete more strontium (a radioactive substance) then they ingest. If born with five milligrams of strontium (or strontium 90) a breastfed baby would be free of the material within three months. However, the bottlefed baby would have twice as much strontium as he was born with after about one month. The difference was attributed to the high content of strontium in cows' milk and the low phosphorus content of human milk. When phosphorus was given to breastfed babies, the excretion of strontium was reduced. Thus, the likelihood is that strontium would not be retained by babies as long as they are fully breastfed.

Dirty air seems destined to be part of our environment for years to come. The environmental Protection Agency's studies found that almost all United States citizens carry within them one or more toxic chemicals. Many of these toxic chemicals have been shown to accumulate and remain in the body for long periods of time if our immune level is down. These toxins are stored in lipid deposits, but can be removed with a cleansing program. The threat that is hanging over us from our polluted air can be eliminated with the proper breathing exercise and those nutrients that protect the lungs.

LUNG PROTECTION ———

Incomplete digestion and poor nutrition, along with free radicals and rancid fats, can result in particles of matter which gradually close the "pores". The lungs then lose their elasticity. Constipation is a threat to the lungs. When the kidneys cannot eliminate properly, the lungs try to take over the job of elimination and become a poor substitute for them. This causes irritation to the lungs and brings on asthma, bronchitis, pneumonia and other lung diseases.

VITAMIN A - Releases an enzyme called proteolytic which tends to soften the matrix of the cell tissues. It strengthens the lungs, protects against infections and toxins. At the beginning of a cold, some people respond by taking large amounts for about five days.

B COMPLEX - Strengthens the lungs, nourishing and healing.

B6 - Reduces the severity of asthma and lung problems.

BIOTIN - Helps to prevent lung infections.

VITAMIN C with bioflavonoids - Needed every day, helps to rebuild the capillaries and cells of the lungs. Also builds up immunity against lung diseases.

BARLEY WATER - Cook barley in pure water, strain, drink liquid with lemon. Contains hordenine which relieves bronchial spasms.

CAYENNE - Useful to add to soups to loosen up mucous.

CALCIUM - Necessary for healthy lungs.

CHLOROPHYLL - Liquid or green drink, blood purifier, rich in vitamins and especially iron. Necessary for healthy lungs.

COMFREY - Soothes and heals the lungs, removes mucus, heals inflamed tissues.

CRANBERRY JUICE CONCENTRATE - One teaspoon at a time in water. This contains natural citric, malic and benzoic acids, acting as an intestinal antiseptic and aids in digestion.

DANDELION - Blood cleanser and purifier, strengthens the lungs and expels phlegm.

ESSENTIAL FATTY ACIDS - Increases the oxygen-carrying capacity of the blood, thus reducing the need for oxygen.

EXERCISE - Deep breathing fresh air has a vital effect on all parts of the body.

VITAMIN E - Antioxidant that guards against toxins. Enough vitamin E in the body can utilize more available oxygen. Vital in protecting the lungs against air pollution.

ELECAMPANE - Expectorant, good for chest colds. Helps lungs and bronchi.

FENUGREEK - Dissolves mucus, contains natural dehydrating properties, cleanses the kidneys.

FLAXSEED - Cleans mucus from bronchial tubes; cleans bowels.

GARLIC - Clears congestion and mucus from the nose and chest. Cut cloves in water and heat, add fresh lemon juice.

GOLDEN SEAL - Expectorant, soothes inflamed mucous membranes. Good for infections of nose, sinuses and throat.

HORSERADISH - Used with lemon juice very good for the lungs.

IRON - an essential nutrient to lung tissue; use natural because inorganic iron oxidizes or burns up vitamin E.

JERUSALEM ARTICHOKES - Contain vitamins A, B, B2 and C. Feeds the lungs and helps to relieve lung conditions; best to use grated, raw in salads and soups.

KELP - Rich in iodine and is needed for healthy lungs. Contains all the essential minerals for healthy lungs.

LICORICE - Builds the body's resistance to allergies. Aids adrenal functioning.

MARSHMALLOW HERB - Soothes irritated tissue of lungs, removes hardened phlegm and relaxes bronchial tubes.

MULLEIN - Calms nerves, relieves pain and is rich in potassium. A lack of potassium can cause asthma.

ONIONS - Sliced with garlic and honey and soaked overnight. Use this honey morning and night to strengthen the lungs.

PAPAYA - Aids in digestion for better assimilation.

PINEAPPLE JUICE - Fresh, sip slowly for sore throat.

RED CLOVER - Builds the body's resistance to allergies.

ROSE HIPS - Supplies the body with easily assimilated source of vitamin C.

SUNFLOWER SEEDS - Easily assimilated protein.

VEGETABLES - Especially green leafy, contain vitamin A, necessary to maintain elasticity in lung membranes. Contain both vitamin E and iron.

WHEY - Mineral food, high in calcium and natural phosphorus. Aids digestion, stops intestinal fermentation, holds calcium in solution for limber joints.

YOGURT - High in protein and easy to digest. Replaces enzymes that are destroyed by air pollution and antibiotics.

Sodium chloride (table salt) and starch are toxic to person with lung problems. It would be better to eliminate those from the diet as well as milk, eggs, chocolate, sugar and white flour. Too much animal phosphorus foods can damage the lungs and kidneys. The kidneys and lungs have the job of expelling the largest percentage of built up phosphorus. If too much phosphorus is consumed over a long period of time, the lungs and kidneys can lose their efficiency. The oxidation in the blood and tissues is upset when our bodies have toxic by-products of phosphorus.

ARTIFICIAL SWEETENERS

G.D. Searle, the company which markets the sweetener, aspartame, has launched a comprehensive advertising campaign. In their ads, they extol the 'benefits' of using products containing this substance. The reason the firm is making these efforts is because of recent adverse publicity regarding aspartame.

NutraSweet® and Equal® are the trade names for this sweetener. Everywhere you turn, NutraSweet® pops out at you on product labels.

Let us examine some of the advertising statements made by Searle regarding NutraSweet®. Then we will share with you some of the latest research pertaining to each statement. Searle: "If you eat, you've eaten what's in NutraSweet® brand sweetener. It's made from two building blocks of protein (amino acids, in more scientific lingo). They're just like those found in fruits, vegetables, grains, meats and dairy products. And your body treats them no differently than if they came from a peach or tomato."

In *New Age Journal*, 12/85, we read: "The problem is, no matter what Searle implies, NutraSweet® is far from a natural construct. It is composed of two amino acids, phenylalanine and aspartic acid, that are found abundantly in nature, but nature never intended these compounds to be isolated from the up to eighteen other amino acids they normally keep company with. And because NutraSweet® contains only these two compounds, it delivers them in a much more concentrated form than the body is used to."

Searle: "NutraSweet® was put through over 100 separate scientific studies. Proving itself in test after test. That took time. In fact, while it might seem like a recent discovery, NutraSweet® is twenty years old this year."

N.A.J.: "Last year the National Center for Disease Control reviewed more than five hundred reports of dizziness, headaches and mood changes from among roughly six hundred complaints that had been filed by people who associated these symptoms with their use of aspartame."

Searle: "Science can't explain why some things are sweet and some aren't. The protein components in NutraSweet® aren't sweet by themselves. But when you put them together, they're 200 times sweeter than sugar."

Dennis Remington, M.D., a specialist in treating obesity, and Direct of the Eating disorder Clinic at Brigham Young University in Utah says, "Artificial sweeteners are hundreds of times sweeter than table sugar, so researchers are guessing that the taste buds are tricked into signaling that the body is getting a huge amount of sugar. Metabolic processes adjust, leaving the dieter tired and hungry and often eating something sweet to pick up his energy a few hours later. This may be the reason that in a study conducted by Searle, the people using aspartame complained more about weight gain than those who didn't."

Searle: "The Food and Drug Administration has given NutraSweet® its blessing. So has the American Medical Association. In the large part, because NutraSweet® is nutritive."

In the *New Age Journal*, there are more facts: Richard Wurtman, a physician who is director of the clinic Research Center at the Massachusetts Institute of Technology says aspartame-containing products may, in fact, affect the brain. That is because aspartame contains the amino acid phenylalanine, which can impair the production of several brain neurotransmitters. Neurotransmitters are the molecules by which nerve cells communicate with each other—one nerve cell releases a particular neurotransmitter, and the adjoining nerve cell receives it and whatever chemical message it's carrying. Wurtman has shown that when rats are fed a large dose of aspartame the level of phenylalanine in their brains skyrockets. In other words, high doses of aspartame changed the chemical composition of the rat's brains...it changed the brains levels of some amino acids and thereby affected the production and release of some neurotransmitters. These changes, Wurtman says, are likely to affect numerous brain functions, (such as control of blood pressure and appetite) and various aspects of behavior (such as sleepiness and mood changes).

William Pardridge, associate professor of medicine at UCLA, says that whatever chemical changes take place, they will have the most pronounced effect on children and fetuses, whose brains are still developing. Certain 'genetically predisposed' women who consume large quantities of aspartame...say, a couple of liters of Diet Coke and a pack of NutraSweet® flavored gum a day...while pregnant, could lower their babies IQs by as much as 10 percent, he says. These women are carriers of a gene that makes it difficult for them to metabolize phenylalanine. People born with two of these genes have phenyldetonuria, a rare disease that can quickly lead to severe mental retardation if phenylalanine consumption is not tightly restricted from birth. Aspartame is absolutely off-limits to people with PKU, and there are labels on every NutraSweet® containing product to warn them. But at least four million Americans have one of these genes and don't know it. These people don't have to worry about the phenylalanine found in meat and dairy products, but scientists say they might have trouble handling large concentrated doses of the compound. Women with one PKU gene who consume large amounts of aspartame may endanger their unborn children, and children with one PKU gene are also at risk. Searle, in fact, suggests in its promotional literature that parents of children with one PKU gene "consult their physicians or dieticians" before using the sweetener, but it does not mention that most PKU carriers have no way of knowing about their condition.

In spite of these hazards associated with the consumption of aspartame, Searle admits: "America isn't the only place you find NutraSweet®. It's approved as a sweetener by the World Health Organization and the health organizations of over 40 countries around the world, from England to Switzerland to Hong Kong. In Canada, it's the only low-calorie sweetener allowed in food and beverages."

Are you willing to take risks with your health by ingesting a product which has been shown to produce side effect and altar brain chemistry?.....THE CHOICE IS YOURS.

ASPIRIN

You may have seen ads lately touting the "benefits" of aspirin. "An aspirin a day keeps heart attacks away" seems to be a popular idiom. While aspirin may contain blood-thinning and anti-inflammatory properties, the adverse effects outweigh the positive.

Excessive aspirin causes bleeding of the mucous lining of the stomach. This can predispose one to ulcers and perhaps even to stomach cancer. Some people may be allergic to aspirin, yet be unaware of it. Allergies to this drug can manifest themselves in the form of respiratory difficulties. Doctors tell their patients who feel sick, "Take a few aspirin, drink lots of fluids and stay in bed."

Aspirin used to be routinely prescribed for children with fevers. Now it has been linked to the fatal disease, Reye's Syndrome.

Aspirin destroys nutrients in the body. It kills vitamin C, which is essential to repair cells, including those of the skin and connective tissues. Vitamin C deficiency can lead to scurvy. Aspirin can cause a loss of potassium in the urine which can lead to electrolyte imbalances.

Betty Kamen, Ph.D., writes *Health Freedom News* (4/86), "Problems With Aspirin": "(Doctors) issue the caveat that aspirin crosses the placenta and can cause hemorrhage in the newborn, and that the effect of aspirin on the risk of placental abruption (premature detachment of the placenta) is not known. Without doctors' encouragement aspirin already takes first place as the drug most commonly taken during pregnancy. There is increasingly epidemiologic evidence that aspirin is associated with spontaneous abortions and teratogenic effects (fetal malformations) in test animals. In addition, aspirin persists in fetal blood; when women take as few as two aspirin tablets two weeks prior to delivery, the blood of their newborns has shown reduced platelet clumping and gastrointestinal or other bleeding. More extensive use of aspirin results in stillbirths (especially when taken later in pregnancy, as recommended in this study), to anemia and prolonged labor..."

Natural alternatives to aspirin, without dangerous side-effects, seem to be the best choice. They include White Willow, Yucca, Vitamin E. White Willow is the "original" aspirin. It is valued as a nerve sedative because it works like aspirin but is mild on the stomach and is natural. The properties of Yucca help in arthritis and rheumatism, due to the plant's high content of steroid saponins, (precursors to cortisone). Vitamin E has blood-thinning abilities and is useful in preventing blood clots. Pain killing herbs include Wood Betony, Scullcap and Lady's Slipper. However, when your body gives you warning signals such as pain or circulatory problems, it is time to "consider the source."....and get to the heart of the matter!

CHEMICAL ADDITIVES —

Americans eat approximately nine pounds of chemical food additives a year. Chemical additives have doubled during the past twenty years. America's food industry puts 800 million pounds of chemical additives into our food. They are classified as stabilizers, colorings, flavorings, chemical preservatives and other artificial substances and have not been completely determined as safe for human consumption. Hundreds of additives have never been tested and may never be. When these additives are tested, they are done one at a time. The real harm can

come when these hundreds of chemicals are combined, and when we ingest more than one of these products, our chances are increased of having health problems. These chemicals can build up in the body and the combined results are very harmful and can cause cancer, heart disease or deformities to our future children after twenty years of ingesting these products.

What has happened to The Delaney Clause---- "No additives shall be deemed safe if it is found to induce cancer in humans or animals."

Today, there have been appeals by the powerful food industry. They have a lot of power. After all it means money to them, why should they care that their food additives could cause cancer in human beings. Cobalt 60 is used to preserve food and is claimed to be harmless. One scientist asked his fellow scientists if they would eat food that contained cobalt 60, and all but one told him no. The one exception said he would only eat it if there was nothing else left to eat.

The center for Science In The Public Interest has issued warnings that citrus red dye #2, Red #40, Yellow #5, BHT, brominated vegetable oil, caffeine, sodium nitrite and saccharin (to name a few) can be harmful to your health. Even if the warranties banning additives by the FDA are in our best interest, it still takes at least eight more years for something to be done. In the mean time millions of innocent people are being subjected to poisons in their seemingly innocent food, without any clue of what it can do to their bodies.

We have already discovered that hormone and antibiotics fed to cattle and hogs can cause side effects. An epidemic of early puberty was discovered in Puerto Rico in 1984. In an article by Ameila A. Morella, she says, "An epidemic of early puberty in both males and females is sweeping through Puerto Rico. In various parts of the continental United States health authorities are also reporting enlarged breasts in pre-teen children. Epidemiologist studying the problem stress the possibility that hormones in meat and chicken may be implicating factors. Puerto Ricans eat more chicken per capita than any other people in the Americas. The Puerto Rican doctor, Saenz de Rodriquez, Director of Pediatrics at De Diego Hospital, San Juan, also implicates milk as a possible source of estrogen overload. She has been recording cases of premature puberty for several years. When she started finding the number of cases increasing, she became convinced that the children were being contaminated with estrogen. Four and five-year-old girls were suffering from enlarged breasts and ovarian cysts. In Puerto Rico, Dr. De Rodriquez noted, many forms of estrogen compounds are available to farmers. Any farmer with a skinny cow can fatten it up quickly with these synthetic drugs at very little cost. No one has raised the question in the continental United States."

We in America are supposed to not question the effects that drugs have upon the population. I think we should do a lot of questioning. Amelia A. Morella goes on to say, "Much of what we consider healthful growth in our youngsters could be similar to the fattening process the ranchers now use for their cattle. We should not, however, underestimate the time-bomb that is present in those skyrocketing sales figures for fried chicken and hamburgers among young people."

Have you ever wondered why fruits and vegetables in the stores seem to keep fresh for days? These are shipped all over the country. Chemical Science now sprays apples with one or more of the following: shellac, ammonia, propylene glycol. Cucumbers, peppers, tomatoes and other vegetables are almost forever preserved with hot spray most often consisting of petroleum jelly and paraffin. Oranges, like most fruits, are picked while still green, then placed in a special room containing ethylene gas, which stimulates an enzyme in the skin of the fruit, which turns the oranges to yellow in about four days. Then the oranges have to be treated with red citrus dye #2, then the oranges are heated to complete the oranges turning to their original color orange.

Red potatoes are colored with Red Dye #40. And many other products are treated with this red coloring. There are regulations on these additives but the FDA admits that it cannot adequately enforce it. They continue assuring us that the waxing and coloring are harmless. That is what they said about vinyl chloride, which was what they once coated citrus fruit with. The vinyl chloride was banned because it was cancer causing.

Let's take a look at the foods that contain BHA, BHT, preservatives and other additives that increase the shelf life of supposedly foods. Fresh pork and pork sausage, crackers, potato chips, vegetable oils, many dry cereals, cake mixes, frozen pizzas, instant teas, drink powders, punches, doughnuts, shortenings, steak sauces, vegetable packs with sauces, breakfast drinks, potatoes (packaged), nuts, canned puddings, toaster tarts, gelating desserts, dry yeast, dry soup mixes, are just a few.

BHA and BHT are petroleum products and found in lard, chicken fat, butter, cream, shortening, bacon, potato chips, processed meat, fish and pastries. They are suspected of causing cancer and liver ailments. They are forbidden in food in Great Britain and other countries. They may also cause allergic reactions. They are also suspected to cause metabolic stress, growth retardation, weight loss, liver and kidney damage and fetal abnormalities.

NITRITES and NITRATES are used as preservatives for curing and coloring. They are found in bacon, frankfurters, sausages, frozen pizzas, smoked fish, baby foods, smoked and processed meats (ham, bologna, salami, tongue, corned beef and pastrami). They are considered TOXIC, and overdoses have caused fatalities. They combine in the body with other chemicals to form cancer-causing compounds. Banned in fish in Canada, they also cause possible reproduction problems. The FDA is supposed to be studying this. CARMAL coloring is used for coloring and flavoring. It is found in soft drinks, breads, pizzas (frozen), instant teas, candies. This has been on the FDA's high priority testing. It could cause genetic defects and possible cancer causing factor. EDTA (Calcium Disodium) is used in preservatives for flavorings. It traps metallic impurities produced in processing. It is linked to kidney disorders, intestinal upsets, cramps and skin rashes. It is used as shellac solvent. The United States Government has a study in progress at this time.

HYDROXYLATED LECITHIN (Lecithin without being hydroxylated is all right). It is used for mixing ingredients to keep them together. It is used in ice cream, margarine, soup mixes, candies, baked goods, mayonnaise, and artificial flavors.

LACTIC ACID, an acidity regulator, is used for preservatives. It is used in pizzas (frozen), processed cheeses, gelatin and pudding desserts, olives, beer, carbonated beverages and frozen desserts.

MODIFIED FOOD STARCH. A thickening agent and cheap filler in many foods. It's found in baked beans, canned corn (cream style), beets (in jar), dry-roasted nuts, ravioli, drink powders, frozen pizzas, pie fillings, baking powder, frozen fish (packaged), soups and bottled gravies. There is an alkali used in making it. It is sodium hydroxide and is suspected of causing vomiting and lung damage. On the FDA's top priority list as needing further study. MSG (Monosodium Glutamate), is a flavoring agent which used to be in baby food to please the parent's taste until October 1969. It is used in salad dressings, canned soups, processed cheeses, frozen pizzas, beer, broths, chinese food, dry roasted nuts, soup mixes, vegetables (packaged with sauce), canned meats, croutons, tomato sauces, bouillon cubes, bread crumbs, meat tenderizers, frozen spinach packages, seafood (packaged), tomato pastes, and frankfurters. It can cause headaches, tightness in chest, burning sensations in forearms and back of neck. It effects the nerve cells, and could effect the fetus. Pregnant women should restrict MSG intake.

PROPYGALLATE is a preservative. It is used in pickles, chewing gum, vegetable oils, vegetables (packaged with sauces) and meat products. It could cause damage to the liver and birth defects.

POLYSORBATE 60, 65, and 80. It is used for creaminess as an emulsifier. It is used in ice cream, frozen custard, bread, sherbet, soft drinks, whipped toppings, cookies, cakes and mixes, pies, shortening and vegetable oil, milk substitutes, gelatin desserts, chocolates, pickles, doughnuts, cake icings and fillings. It has been known to cause diarrhea. The FDA has determined that more adequate study is essential.

RED DYA 40: It is used for coloring. It is found in red pistachio nuts, frankfurters, gelatin desserts, chewing gum, cereals, candies, soft drinks, and baked goods. It is suspected of causing cancer, and may be possible birth defect factor. It is under FDA investigation as a health danger.

TANNIN (Tannic Acid), used for flavoring. found in coffee, tea, cocoa, beer, and wine. Used in artificial flavorings as in butter, caramel, fruit, brandy, maple flavorings and in nuts. It is connected with liver damage and tumors and may be a cause of cancer. It is used in leather tanning. Further testing is needed as to its safety.

SACCHARIN, a cheap substitute for sugar. It is used in soda drinks, frozen desserts, breakfast drinks, sugar substitute in many products and in diet food. It is linked as a possible cause of tumors and bladder cancer. It is under close U.S. government scrutiny and study. A DANGER warning is now required on all packages. It has also been known to cause allergic responses and toxic reactions affecting the skin, heartbeat and gastrointestinal tract.

These are just a few of the food additives that we should be aware of. We need to protect our bodies. We need to learn to read labels.

ELECTROMAGNETIC RADIATION AND YOUR HEALTH

Leukemia linked to strong electrical fields

Modern technology offers us many opportunities previously unimagined in past decades. However, along with sophisticated knowledge there comes an element of danger. Whatever can be used for our benefit and good, can also be turned around and used against us. Recently, there have been many articles written on electromagnetic radiation and how it affects our immune systems. Dr. Andria Puharich, M.D., has researched this topic and tells us that "extremely low frequency magnetic fields (range: 1-100 cycles per second)...can affect biological systems. In spite of their ultra weak power they are capable of affecting the human biological system in a most profound way, one which can be a blessing or a curse. The only beneficial frequencies are in the range of 7-9 Hz. or cycles per second. This frequency is related to the 8 Hz. magnetic fields from the sun and also the 8 Hz. frequency of the earth."

In September 1988 issue of *Let's Live Magazine* we read: "A study by C. Byus, S. Pieper, and Dr. W. Ross Adey was published in the October 1987 issue of *Carcinogenesis*. The researchers found greater enzyme activity in tumor cells exposed to certain frequencies, which is a step toward understanding the statistical association of leukemia, brain tumors, and miscarriages with proximity to power lines."

"Strong electrical fields at power-line frequencies are known to increase the division rate of certain kinds of cells." In 1979, two researchers from the University of Colorado Medical Center in Denver published a study of childhood cancer and power lines. After careful analysis, the scientists concluded that the death rate from leukemia, lymph node cancer, and nervous system tumors among children from high-current homes was more than twice that from the low-current homes. A Swedish study linked childhood leukemia with 200-kv power lines running within 200 yards of the stricken children's homes. And S. Milham from Washington State published an article in the *New England Journal of Medicine* on the high incidence of leukemia among workers exposed occupationally to strong electromagnetic fields.

"Much information on the hazards of electronic pollution can be gleaned from the excellent books by Dr. R.O. Becker and Gary Selden, *The Body Electric* (New York, William Morrow, 1985). The potential hazards are by no means limited to power lines: Dr. Becker points to increased cancer incidence among people living in the corridors between microwave towers, for instance. Dr. Becker's book is a trove of information on the new science of electronic biology, a fledgling field from which much future benefit can be expected."

U.S. Navy discovers adverse effects

The authors of *The Body Electric* state: "The...immune system is geared to fight tangible invaders—bacteria, viruses, toxins, and misbehaving cells of the body...It includes a system of circulating antibodies, by which specialized cells recognize the intruder.

The cells controlling this phase then select appropriate defenders...each programmed for a certain function...Electromagnetic energy isn't consciously perceived, however. It tricks the immune system into fighting a shadow. Thus, we can predict that just like the fire company answering a false alarm, the body will be less able to fight a real fire."

The U.S. Navy, in conducting secret testing for seven years, discovered the following: electromagnectice radiation can...**alter behavior of cells, tissues, organs and organisms; alter hormone levels; alter cell chemistry; alter the time perception in animals and humans; inhibit or enhance bone growth; inhibit or enhance RNA synthesis and processes; affect immune processes; destroy and rupture cells; entrain brain waves; cause defects and alterations in embryos; cause up** to six times higher fetus mortality rate in lab animals than in controls; cause sterility in male animals; and many other side effects.

Sources of electromagnetic frequencies

We are bombarded daily with electromagnetic radiation from such diverse sources as microwaves, computer terminals, garage door openers, refrigerators, cellular phones, power lines, microwave ovens and other technical equipment. Sometimes the effects are not felt immediately and sometimes they are manifest in ways that may be misinterpreted as something else. Some of the more subtle reactions to electromagnetic radiation are excessive fatigue, neckaches, irritability, headaches, cramps, stress, prolonged jet lag, diminished reflexes, auto sickness, sexual dysfunction, loss of memory and dizziness. The constant bombardment of electromagnetic radiation has been called "electronic smog."

Dr. Puharich has found that one E.L.F. frequency can cause cancer in rats in 2 days. Another frequency can reverse the process! One frequency can cause depression, another can cause anxiety and another can stimulate mob behavior, etc. This can be produced from E.L.F. fields which originate on the other side of the world and directed as specific areas. It seems to be the latest "war weaponry," from which no one can hide.

Stress on the brain and the body

Dr. McBirnie tells us the "E.L.F. signals generate tiny, unfelt, vibrations inside various brain parts, which shake loose the barrier, creating leaks in it...They also reduce the ability of brain cells to hold calcium, a vital element in the action of nerves...The electrical signal can move ions (such as sodium or calcium) across the membrane of a cell, unleashing a chain of chemical reactions within the cells itself, which may ultimately lead to the unraveling of DNA (component of a cell which transmit hereditary traits).

"Weather modification expert and author Lowell Ponte wrote in the January, 1980 *Reader's Digest*: 'The earth's magnetic field and other naturally occurring...fields influence the way all living things synchronize their internal clocks...(Artificial electromagnetic pollution) alters our natural biological rhythms, the internal clocks that regulate waking and sleeping and thousands of more subtle body processes...(Humans) respond by adjusting (their) biological rhythms to the pulse (frequency) of the electric smog...(which generates) stress on the body."

"When under stress, an organism activates certain areas of the brain that prepare it to meet the challenge. This is fine for short-term situations. But when the stress is prolonged, effects linger, and a series of hormonal reactions increase blood sugar, speed up the metabolism and suppress the immune system."

"In short, general resistance breaks down, allowing a person to fall prey to diseases that he otherwise would have fought off. Many doctors agree that stress plays a role in at least 40 diseases (including viral infections), and may even influence every physical illness."

"Stress more directly impairs the immune system by immobilizing key cells called lymphocytes, which help clear the system of bacterial intruders. Hence, the subsequent lack of lymphocytes allows toxins to multiply and take hold."

Nutrients and herbs to help

Electromagnetic impulses have similar effects on the body as that of radiation. They target the central nervous system, (especially the brain), and when the delicate signals go awry, the glands become affected, (especially the reproductive system). The entire immune system is affected.

Herbs and nutrients which benefit these areas include:

Central Nervous System: Calcium, Magnesium, B-complex, Ho-Shou-Wu, Wild Yam, Blue Vervain, Lady's Slipper, Lobelia, Rosemary, Red Clover, Mullein, Hops, Valerian, Scullcap, Passion Flower.

Brain: B-complex, Gotu Kola, Ginseng, Dong Quai, Blessed Thistle, Sage.

Glands: Ho-Shou-Wu, Kelp, Dandelion, Alfalfa, Ginseng, Sarsaparilla, Golden Seal, Licorice, Echinacea, Bee Pollen, Gotu Kola.

Reproductive System: Vitamin E, Ginseng, Scullcap, Damiana, Saw Palmetto, Sarsaparilla, Rosemary.

Immune System: Germanium, CoQ10, Yellow Dock, Echinacea, Golden Seal, Bee Propolis, Vitamin C, Vitamin A, zinc, Garlic, Pau D'Arco, Chaparral.

Our bodies are constantly having to fight off the onslaught of injurious substances from land, sea and air. While we can't always control our exposure to adverse elements, fortifying and strengthening our bodies to the best of our ability will help mitigate the potential harm.

INDOOR POLLUTION ____

And you thought that working indoors saved you from air pollution! Here are some recently discovered problems which may require environmental protection indoors--home, office, or factory:

1. Excessive use of methyl alcohol in cleaning products. Daily exposure can cause everything from headaches to vertigo. Watch all household detergents.

2. Lack of proper ventilation leads to toxic levels in offices from a combination of formaldehyde, photocopier fumes and cigarette smoke.

3. Asbestos. 30 million tons have been used since 1900. Health problems may not show up for 30 years.

4. Radium in brick and concrete.

5. Use of formaldehyde in home insulation.

6. Nitrogen oxides emitted from gas stoves can cause respiratory diseases.

7. Air conditioners have been suspected of promoting fungus growth and spreading organic matter through the air. Watch humidifiers as well.

These matters are just beginning to come to the attention of the public. You are bound to hear of more in the future. (*Current Comments*, 13, March 30, 1981, by Eugene Garfield).

IRRADIATED FOODS ____

Nuclear Radiation is something which we take great pains to avoid. We go out of our way not to expose ourselves or our families to unnecessary x-rays. We also try to eat fruits and vegetables which are not heavily contaminated with herbicides or pesticides.

Now comes the NUCLEAR NEWS...a real **bomb** to our health. The Food and Drug Administration has okayed commercial irradiation of fruits and vegetables, herbs and spices. In fact, there are 47 herbs and spices which have been authorized for irradiation since July 1983! McCormick, a major herb and spice company sells irradiated food products NOW.

On April 18, 1986, the FDA passed a law which will triple the amount of radiation allowed on these herbs and spices. This will escalate the radiation bombardment to 3,000,000 rads. (A rad is a physical unit for absorbed radiation). The maximum amount on other foods is 100,000 rads.

There has been widespread information published in the health field on the irradiation subject. From the IV issue of *The American Herb Association Quarterly Newsletter*, volume IV, by Svevo Brooks and Kathi Keville, we read:

"Proponents of food irradiation, especially the military, private industry and commercial growers, argue that irradiation will reduce our dependency on toxic chemicals currently being used to keep food from spoiling, make more food available to world countries, and provide a safe and effective way of disposing of nuclear waste. In general, it will reduce spoiling and prolong shelf life.

Opponent of food irradiation claim it has not been proven a safe procedure. (Of 413 studies reviewed by the FDA, 344 were considered inconclusive and only 5 clearly support safety.) They also point out that because food irradiation uses more nuclear waste than is being produced, the procedure will greatly enlarge the entire industry. Furthermore, opponents say studies show that irradiation changes the chemical composition and nutritional value of food. Some of the possible problems studies have indicated include testical and kidney disorders, abnormal white blood cell development, chromosome changes and genetic damage in children."

Further facts uncovered are alarming at the least. In the July 1986 issue of *The American Chiropractor* by Kathleen M. Power, D.C., states: "The process of irradiation involves exposing food to electron or x-ray beams, or sources of gamma ray emission, either cobalt-60 or cesium-137. At doses of 100,000 to 3,000,000 rads, the new FDA limit, ripening and sprouting is delayed, and insects, as well as microorganisms of spoilage and disease, are destroyed. The major purpose, therefore, is to extend shelf life and control some pathogens. ANOTHER PURPOSE IS TO HELP THE DEPARTMENT OF ENERGY RID ITSELF OF ITS BURDEN OF RADIOACTIVE WASTE MATERIALS FROM NUCLEAR WEAPONS PRODUCTION BY LEASING IT TO IRRADIATION FACILITIES.

At prescribed doses the food does not become radioactive—unless the equipment is improperly calibrated, poorly monitored, or malfunctioning—but its molecular structure is altered. Gamma rays knock electrons out of orbit; this initiates a series of chemical reactions in the food. The process is very different from microwave cooking; microwaves do not possess enough energy to ionize molecules.

What happens to the nutritional quality of food subjected to ionizing radiation? The effects are well summarized in a publication entitled *Food Irradiation: Issues and Answers for Elected Officials*. It states, "Exposure of any food to gamma or ionizing radiation produces either deleterious or uncharacterized effects on nutrients: essential nutrients such as fat-soluble vitamins (A, E, and K), water-soluble vitamin (C, B1, B3, B6, and folic acid), essential amino acids (cysteine, methionine, histidine, and tryptophan), nucleic acids, and enzymes are either depleted or destroyed...; further, unsaturated fatty acids are converted to toxic, peroxidized lipids."

The industry hopes to solve part of this dilemma by adding a few synthetic vitamins to the food after it has been treated with radiation. However, the potency of vitamins are unstable when added to irradiated food.

The FDA certainly does not have the welfare of the consumer, in mind. "Destruction of nutrients," it has stated, "is not a concern of this rulemaking."

We find more startling information in the same issue of *The American Chiropractor*. "The depletion of nutrients and the breakdown of vital food components is disconcerting enough. But there is another disturbing consequence of irradiating food. This is the creation of an entirely new class of chemicals, the unique radiolytic products (URP's), the end products of molecular disintegration and recombination in irradiated foods. At doses of 100,000 rads, these are formed in the concentration of approximately three parts per million. They vary with each type of food. Only a few of these have been identified; these include benzene, formaldehyde and hydrogen peroxide." Dr. Walter Herbst, of the Radiologic Institute in the University of Freiborg explains;

"These free-radical mediated chemical by-products have neither been adequately characterized nor tested for their long-term, latent toxicity...Foods that have been exposed to gamma or ionizing radiation may also contain a wide variety of 'economic poisons' (herbicides, insecticides, pesticides, and fungicides) added to foods by growers, processors, and distributors. When these 'economic poisons' are irradiated they will also be converted to .....URP's (of) unknown toxicity. Processed foods frequently contain a wide variety of GRAS listed additives: colorants, steroids, preservatives and stabilizers which will also be converted to...URP's...of unknown toxicity."

Some people have difficulty digesting their food. Irradiation generally reduces the digestibility of food even **more**. There are even more severe and grave health problems associated with irradiated food:

• Rats fed irradiated pork showed an increased enzymatic activity in liver tissue.

• Dogs fed such food showed spleen enlargement and congestion.

• When malnourished children in India were fed freshly irradiated wheat, their white blood cells began to become leukemic (showed beginnings of leukemia). The same thing happened to monkeys and mice fed on the wheat.

• Mice fed irradiated chicken demonstrated an increase in testicular tumors, immune kidney disease, lowered survival rates, offspring death and other distressing results.

• Two studies in Russia showed kidney and testical damage in rats fed irradiated food.

• Canadian studies showed animals who ingested irradiated food developed an extra set of chromosomes.

• A Cornell University study found that *eating irradiated sugar produced the same genetic changes as exposure to radiation itself.*

The American Chiropractor article continues: "A Japanese doctor, Takahashi Kosei, reviewed the studies upon which the World Health Organization based its approval of irradiation. He found in re-analyzing the data, that: irradiated potatoes caused arterial problems, higher mortality, mutations and increased organ weights; irradiated wheat caused white blood cell changes; irradiated onions caused higher death rates and ovarian and testical changes; and irradiated rice caused disturbances in the pituitary, thyroid, heart and lungs, as well as tumors. His report cast grave doubts in he reliability or scientific activities of international authorities such as...WHO.

Perhaps the most convincing evidence against the safety of irradiation was a review of 1,223 studies by Dr. Jozsef Barna of Budapest, Hungary, published in 1979. The study results were classified as neutral, adverse or beneficial. Since the studies could address more than one issue, each study could have several outcomes. Dr. Barna found 1,414 adverse effects, 185 beneficial effects and 7,191 neutral effects. 278 different foods were reviewed. Here is an example of the adverse effects of just one food, **corn**: reduced digestibility, reduced weight of offspring, increased frequency of lymphoblastoma in the liver, kidney, thymus, lung and spleen."

There are many other problems concerning irradiated foods, of which the public should be aware. Botulism spores can withstand 100,000 rads by producing rad-resistant spores. The radiation destroys the organisms which help keep 'clostridium botulinum' in check. Aflatoxin production increases up to eighty percent in some irradiated foods and this natural 'mold' is one of the most potent cancer causing agents there is.

The American Chiropractor Magazine warns: "Radioactive emissions from the 1,000 planned radiation facilities will add to the burden of radioactivity already carried in our bodies from fallout and nuclear power plants. These have been linked to fatal and neonatal mortality, childhood leukemia, learning disorders, respiratory disease, and cancer. There is also the increased risk of environmental contamination by cesium-17, which as cesium chloride, is as water-soluble as sodium chloride, in the event of an accident during transportation and handling. There is also a potential for mutation of organisms exposed to radiation. The FDA says this is "an inevitable consequence of irradiating foods...(but)...many mutations will only be temporary." What about those which aren't? Consider the consequences of mutant strains of pathogenic organisms being distributed throughout the country from centralized sources."

Svevo Brooks and Kathi Keville, in the AHA Newsletter, further voice their concerns, (as should each of us, by writing letters.) "While the controversy about the safety of irradiated food will likely continue for many years, the appearance of irradiated food in the world marketplace seems a certainty. With the official support of the UN Food and Agricultural Organization and the World Health Organization, food is already being irradiated in over twenty different countries. The U.S. Department of Energy has appropriated funds from the nuclear budget to build irradiation facilities, including mobile units which will be used on site in agricultural areas."

NOTE: Instead of the original "Picowaved" term, irradiated products will be labeled with "Treated With Radiation" or "Treated By Radiation," and the symbol of the tulip. After two years, only the symbol will be used. HERBS, SPICES AND IRRADIATED FOODS THAT ARE PROCESSED AND COMBINED WITH NON-IRRADIATED FOODS IN THE PREPARATION OF PROCESSED FOODS LIKE MIXES AND TV DINNERS ALREADY **DO NOT REQUIRE LABELING**.

Herbs Authorized For Irradiation

Allspice	Marjoram
Anise	Mustard Seed
Basil	Mustard Flour
Bay Leaves	Nutmeg
Caraway Seed	Onion Powder
Black Cumin	Orange Petals
Cardamon	Oregano
Celery Seed	Paprika
Chamomile	Parsley
Chervil	Pepper
Chives	Red Pepper
Cinnamon	Peppermint
Cloves	Poppy Seed
Coriander	Rosemary
Cumin Seed	Saffron
Dill Seed	Sage
Dill Weed	Savory
Fennel Seed	Sesame Seed
Fenugreek	Spearmint
Garlic Powder	Star Anise Seed
Ginger	Tarragon
Grains of Paradise	Thyme
Horseradish	Turmeric
Mace	

MILK. . .the IMperfect Food –

Milk...from the time you could remember, has been your comfort food. The perfect food. The wonderful gift from cows which helps your bones, your teeth, your nerves, the ultimate provider of calcium. "Drink four glasses of milk daily," your parents and teachers have always told you. Indulge in yogurt, ice cream, cheese...as long as it is made from milk, you will get your nutrition.

However, old myths die hard. The udder truth is sometimes a bitter pill to swallow. That which is worshiped and white has now tumbled from its throne. It is quite a shock to find out that something you though pure and wholesome is actually quite indecent and detrimental to your health. Consider the following facts:

Heavy metals, detergents, antibiotics, cancer viruses, polio viruses and other toxins have been found in milk. Heavy metals can originate from cows grazing in contaminated areas and detergent residues can result from the milk machinery cleaning process. Pathogens come from animals which have been weakened and diseased and then treated to fight their infections. People who are sensitive to certain antibiotics should be very concerned. Many veterinary drugs are used legally and illegally on dairy farms. Residues of drugs found in milk include the following list: Chlorampehnicol, Clorsulon, Ivcermectin and Thiabendazole, Nitrofurazone, Penicillin, Streptomycin, Tetracyclines, Aminoglycosides and Sulfonamindes, Sulfamethzine, Sulfadioazine and other Sulfa drugs. Shockingly, diseases from animals to humans have been linked to the milk supply. ("Some Diseases of Cattle Transmitted to Man Through Milk" *Journal of the American Veterinary Medical Association* 78:500-505, 1931) Diarrhea in babies has been traced to diarrhea in cows, from transmission of the same virus. Live viral substances have been found in white blood cells of normal and leukemic cattle, as well as in milk, and tissue and cell cultures from the cows. (A Multiple Share of Myeloma. *Medical World News*, May 16, 1969. p. 23)

The three major components of milk have the potential of causing the strongest allergic reactions. These substances are: butter fat, milk protein (casein) milk sugar (lactose). Milk can cause allergic reactions ranging from nasal congestion, hay fever, asthma, middle ear disorders, croup, headaches, dizziness and seizures, to vomiting blood, colitis, bedwetting, skin allergies, and a myriad of other seemingly unrelated symptoms. Cow's milk is high in protein and is designed to nourish calves, not people. Human milk is relatively low in protein and is ideal for the growth of babies. Some breast-fed infants can indirectly develop colic from cow's milk. Babies can develop a sensitivity to the protein in the milk that the mother drinks. If the mother stops drinking milk, this type of colic usually goes away. It is estimated that over thirty million Americans lack sufficient amounts of the enzyme lactase to process the milk sugar lactose. Cases of "lactose intolerance" have been misdiagnosed as nervous or ulcerative colitis, or spastic or irritable bowel syndrome. Symptoms range from diarrhea, nausea and cramps to vomiting and abdominal pain.

Milk contains an imbalance of nutrients. It offers a high quantity of sodium, and a low quantity of vitamin C and iron. This disparity can contribute to the formation of kidney stones and can also lead to iron deficiency anemia if milk products become a major source of nutrition in comparison to fruits, vegetables, grains, and other wholesome foods. Calcium and phosphorus are needed to build strong bones and teeth. However, cows milk contains ten time the amount of calcium and three times as much phosphorus as human milk. This percentage actually causes the calcium to be leached from the bones and can lead to weakening of the bone structure and osteoporosis. ("Milk Has Something For Everybody?" *JAMA* 232(5)539, May 5, 1975) High quantities of vitamin D can create a deficiency of magnesium in heart muscle. It is believed that this condition can lead to heart problems in some individuals. Vitamin D is added to commercial milk. (Marie Krause. *Food, Nutrition, and Diet Therapy*. Philadelphia:

W.B. Saunders, 1972, p. 127)

High amounts of xanthine oxidase, an enzyme which is believed to lead to cardiovascular disease, is found in commercial milk. As a result of homogenization, xanthine oxidase is absorbed through the gastrointestinal tract in the fine particles of fat. It proceeds to abrade artery walls and this injury makes it possible for fats to plaque or adhere to the sides of blood vessels.

Synthetic hormones have been used to quickly fatten cattle and are linked to premature puberty in children, especially those who ingest a high amount of animal products. Synthetic hormones are also administered to cows to make them produce more milk. The latest of these is BST (bovine somatotrophin), also called BGH (bovine growth hormone). It is marketed under the name Posilac and is designed to supplement the growth hormone that cows naturally produce on their own. In the works of several years, Monsanto Co. has released this genetically-engineered hormone that is supposed to stimulate milk production in cows. The FDA formally approved its use on November 5, 1993. However, due to consumer outcry, a 90-day moratorium was implemented until February 3. Agencies like the National Institutes of Health, the Office of Technology Assessment, the American Medical Association, the American Dietic Association, American Farm Bureau Federation and the Grocery Manufacturers of America support its use.

Opponents of the use of BST include the Consumers Union (publisher of Consumer Reports), the Humane Society, the Consumer Federation of America. They cite the fact that safety data has not been established, except in one study on rats. BGH could also very well lead to a very serious growth disorder in humans. One FDA report entitled Bovine Growth Hormone: Human Food Safety Evaluation was quoted in the August 24, 1990 issue of Science magazine. It states: "Recombinant BGH treatment produces an increase in the concentration of insulin-like growth factor-1 (IGF-1) in cows milk." Health experts cite the fact that high levels of IGF-1 can cause acromegaly (gigantism), a condition in which

the hands, feet, nose and chin become greatly enlarged. When owners of small dairy farms were surveyed, 80 to 90 percent expressed concerns and stated they wouldn't use BST. They agree that more research should be conducted on this hormone. As of the printing of this article, milk which contains BST is not required to be labeled, so consumers will not know if their milk contains it or not. Several companies which market milk and milk products will try to monitor BST. These companies include the supermarket chain Kroger's and ice cream makers Ben & Jerry's Homemade Inc.

One may ask, "If we can't drink milk, what can we use instead?" For those who wish to retain the taste of milk, there are whey-based products on the market. Whey is the nutritious portion of milk which is removed during the cheese-making process. It is easily assimilated protein in the form of lactoglobulin and lactalbumin. You can receive many nutritional benefits from whey.

Non-dairy foods which contain a significant amount of easy-to-assimilate calcium include carrot juice, the herbs alfalfa and kelp, beans and nuts (especially almonds), dark leafy greens and sesame seed butter (tahini). Some vegetarians rely on almond milk. You can make this by taking an amount of raw almonds that you select and whipping them together in a blender with pure water. Additional nutrients found in the above foods can even assist the absorption of calcium by the body. (If calcium is not used properly, it can cause health problems such as bone spurs, arthritis, kidney stones, and even hardening of the arteries).

Investigate alternative sources for your calcium. Experiment with a variety of tastes and foods.

Homogenized Milk and Atherosclerosis

Since pasteurization and homogenization have invaded our country degenerative diseases are at epidemic proportions. We will continue to see an increase of circulatory diseases as long as we continue consuming large amounts of homogenized dairy products. It is almost considered child abuse if we neglect to see that each of our children don't receive a quart of milk a day.

Atherosclerosis was not a common disease before 1900, yet these people consumed large amounts of dairy products. It is the unnatural process of homogenization and pasteurization that is creating our problems. This altering of our milk is the cause and not the cholesterol concept.

One tribe in East africa, called Masai, are cattle herdsman. Their diet consists of nothing but meat, milk and blood. This would be considered an extremely high fat and cholesterol diet in the United States, but atherosclerosis is practically unknown among these primitive people.

The process called homogenization is when the fat particles of the cream are broken up. The fat is strained through tiny pores under great pressure. This results in the fat staying in suspension, and this causes the cream to be evenly distributed throughout the milk.

The normal fat globules are too big to go through the gut wall and into the blood stream, but homogenization causes them to pass through easily. The fat passes through the intestinal walls unaltered and is not digested properly. The reason so many people are allergic to milk is that the bloodstream has undigested milk fat in the system.

Research conducted by Dr. Kurt Oster, Chief of Cardiology at Park City Hospital, Bridgeport, Connecticut, explained why the tiny undigested fat fragments of homogenized milk pose a serious health problem. One element of milk is xanthine oxidase (XO), an enzyme that attacks heart arteries, leading to deterioration of heart function. Dr. Kurt Esselbacher, chairman of the Department of Medicine at Harvard Medical School, agreed with Dr. Oster's findings, saying "homogenized milk, because of its XO content, is one of the major causes of heart disease in the United States." When milk is raw or merely pasteurized, leaving the fat globules their normal size, XO does not pass through the intestinal walls. Failing to reach the bloodstream, it is harmlessly excreted. ("The Truth About Milk," *Healthview Newsletter*, No. 14.)

This is the beginning of fatty deposits called plaque, that collects in the smooth inner artery walls. In time, fatty deposits can thicken and grow hard resulting in a narrowing of the passageways through which blood travels. Elasticity of the arterial wall is lost. Circulation becomes impaired and calcification deposits accumulate and harden.

Atherosclerosis may not appear until the disease is well advanced. It is only when the oxygen supply to a given area of the body is cut off, that pain as well as other symptoms occur.

When oxygen fails to reach the heart, then chest pain known as ANGINA PECTORIS is experienced. If the blockage is severe then a HEART ATTACK may occur. If the blockage affects the brain then a STROKE can develop. There is a condition called RENAL ISCHEMIA when there is constriction of the arteries supplying the kidneys. If the arterial blockage to the legs occur, it can cause ULCERATION or even GANGRENE. CATARACTS can develop if the eyes lack enough arterial supply.

Let's take care of our arteries and do something about our health before its too late.

STEROID VERSUS HERBS AND NUTRITION

What will make you stronger and bigger in the fastest amount of time? Youth are looking to steroids for this answer. Especially those in competitive sports. There are one million users of steriods and one half of those are under the age of eighteen. Youth who are not in sports are using them so they can develop sex appeal.

In the olympics many athletes have been tempted to cheat. There is no honesty and integrity in some youths in the sports field. Some are looking to drugs for performing ability instead of their own performance.

Ben Johnson was one of those caught using steroids. The U.S. Olympic Committee has regarded steroid use as a form of cheating and have outlawed them. In the *Deseret News*, Salt

Lake City, Utah, Monday October 10, 1988 ran an article titled, *Runner Confesses She and Johnson took Steroids.* Angella Issajenko says, "I just don't care any more. I'm fed up with all the bull. Ben takes steroids, I take steriods. Jamie (Astaphan) gives them to us, and Charlie (their coach) isn't a scientist but he knows what's happening." She says, "Cocaine, heroin, LSD, what ever they can do to win, they'll do it."

Steroids are used in epidemic proportions. Teenagers are turning to steroids and do not care about the side effects. A twenty-two year old started taking steroids at the age of thirteen. He now admits that there is always a price to pay for abusing your body. He has had lingering effects of steroids and now has heart problems and is taking heart medication.

WHAT ARE STEROIDS?

Androgenic-Anabolic Steroids are drugs that were originally developed to treat arthritis, anemia and various bone and skin disorders. They resemble male hormones both chemically and functionally, (the meaning of androgenic). In people with hormone deficiencies they promote growth, accelerate bone maturation and cause weight gain (this tissue-building effect is what anabolic means).

Steroids force the body to build tissue and add weight, and therefore are appealing to athletes and their coaches. There are conflicting results of increase in strength and improvement in performance. The American College of Sports Medicine having studied all the available evidence, came to the following conclusions: 1.) Medically approved doses of steroids don't improve strength, endurance, muscle mass, or body weight. 2.) The evidence that larger doses-the kind that most athletes take but that no doctor could ethically prescribe-work better is inconsistent and inconclusive. 3.) Contrary to a common belief among athletes, high-protein diets don't make steroids work more effectively than regular diets.

Most users of steroids feel that the beneficial effects in strength occur only when accompanied by heavy workouts-usually weight training. The International Federation report points out "credit should probably go to the heavy training which itself builds strength, rather than to steroids-which do not work if you don't."

Women suffer more obvious side effects as seen in many female former East German athletes. They look like men, they stop menstruating, their voices are deeper, they grow facial hair, and their clitorises enlarge. They are also much more likely to become sterile or to bear defective offspring. Most of the damage is irreversible.

Prolonged use of steroids by athletes will certainly have a harmful effect, as stated by Dr. Bernd Friedlander, a specialist in sports medicine. He conducted a study among 12 athletes who were regular high-dose users of steroids. He looked at the biochemical indicators of blood, hair and urine. He said, "the results showed evidence of a definite strain on the liver as well as biochemical evidence of some damage to kidneys and heart." He added, "there is a tendency among female users to develop larger muscles, a deeper voice and hair on the face. Men may be prone to impotency."

Steroids create a deceptive surge of physical energy and sense of overwhelming power. The athlete feels so good he or she often overstrains and severely stresses the body causing serious injury. Withdrawal from steroid use is another problem and often causes soreness throughout the body. There is a tendency to suffer more injuries during this time, such as stress fractures and aggravated hamstring muscles. Steroids can also create a weakness factor both physical and mental, because of the prior dependency.

Dr. Friedlander is health oriented. He tells his athletes to eat fresh fruit, vegetables, poultry or fish, eggs, whole grains cereals and drink spring water and herb teas. He tells them to avoid refined carbohydrates, processed foods, coffee or black tea, alcoholic beverages. He also advises them against dairy products and red muscle meat. His nutrition program also includes vitamin and mineral supplements, bee pollen, octacosanol, glandulars, and amino acid supplementation. Amino acids increase mental and physical work

221

capacity. They help break down fats for energy use, strengthen the body's connective tissue against injury, improve mental alertness and reflexes, promote a positive mood, and build the immune system and prevent illness.

SALT FACTS

Salt, which is a chemical combination of sodium and chloride is an essential part of our life. All body fluids contain salt, and without it the fine balance of body fluids can not be maintained. Sodium chloride is responsible for the homeostasis of the body fluids which help with the flow of blood, the heart, some enzyme formations, and nerve transmissions. Sodium makes up 40% of the salt combination. The other ingredient is chloride. The two work together and separately to perform important life functions. Chlorine helps with the process of forming hydrochloric acid which is essential in the gastric digestion of proteins. But the amounts of salt needed by the body to function properly are low, and excessive salt can be harmful to the body.

We really need not add salt to our diet to meet the body's daily requirements. The 500 milligrams needed by the body can be found naturally in the food we eat. The average American consumes nearly 20 times the amount of salt needed physiologically.

Excessive amounts of salt in the diet can be extremely dangerous. It can lead to high blood pressure, heart disease, kidney problems, stroke, premenstrual tension as well as other problems. But how much do we really know about the salt we ingest? And how can we control our salt intake?

We can refrain from adding salt to our food and remove the salt shaker from the dinner table. But that is just the beginning. The real problem is in the hidden salt added to processed and prepared foods. High amounts of salt are added to canned goods, frozen foods, cheese, ice cream, cereals, crackers, and baked goods.

Salt is used by the food industry to preserve and process foods. These chemical compounds contain sodium. Some of the common compounds include monosodium glutamate (a flavor enhancer), sodium saccharin (a sweetener), sodium phosphates (emulsifiers), sodium caseinate (a thickener), and sodium nitrate (a preservative). These all can cause problems for the body systems. Salt is added to canned vegetables to enhance flavor. Canned fruits are often dipped in a sodium substance to prevent discoloration and make peeling easier.

Sea salt can be used in small amounts for those who cannot give up the salty taste. It is a natural compound. There are also natural salt substitutes available which usually contain potassium chloride. There are also many low sodium products available.

There are many ways to eliminate or cut down on salt without eliminating taste. Use fresh foods when possible. Lemon juice and natural spices can add to and enhance the flavor of foods. There are some excellent spices available.

Basil is great in soups and salads. It has a warm flavor and is used in many Italian foods. Chives is a member of the onion family, but it has a softer flavor. It can be used in salad dressing and sauces. Dill has a sharp taste and smell. A small amount is delicious with salads, eggs, fish and poultry. Rosemary either fresh or dried is a wonderful spice added to meat stews and soups. Spices are great as a salt substitute.

In the book *Shake the Salt Habit* by Dr. Kermit R. Tantum he lists the sodium content of many different foods. Here are a few.

Table salt, 1 tsp	1,850 mgs
Cheddar cheese, 1 oz	176 mgs
Mozzarella cheese, 1 oz	106 mgs
Milk, 1 cup	122 mgs
Canned Tuna in oil, 3 oz	303 mgs
Canned Tuna in Water, 3 oz	288 mgs
Garlic powder, 1 tsp	1 mg
Orange juice, 1 cup	5 mgs
Apple juice, 1 cup	5 mgs
Egg, 1	59 mgs
Chili con carne, 1 cup	1,194 mgs

Chicken breast, 1/2	69 mgs
Beef broth, 1 cup	1,152 mgs
Chicken noodle soup, 1 cup	1,107 mgs
Whole wheat bread, 1 slice	132 mgs
White bread, 1 slice	114 mgs
Broccoli raw, 1 cup	23 mgs
Carrots raw, 1	34 mgs
Carrots (canned), 1 cup	386 mgs
Corn cooked, 1 ear	1 mg
Corn (canned creamed), 1 cup	671 mgs

The best way to control salt intake is to become an educated consumer. Look for the salt information of products purchased. Stick to home cooking whenever possible. Eat a lot of fruits, vegetables, and whole grains, and avoid adding additional salt. Use herbal spices instead.

ARE YOU DRINKING SAFE WATER???

Drinking water from the tap may be hazardous to your health. Once we thought we were insulated against water contamination, but our nation's rural areas are now being threatened by unsafe water. Recently, Cornell University in New York released a study indicating that approximately 39,000,000 rural citizens were drinking unsafe water. It seems that our drinking water could be an invisible threat to our health. There are over 35,000 toxic chemicals in use today and more than 500 new chemicals are developed each year. Most of these chemical residues end up as a by product in our drinking water. These chemical wastes are entering our ground and surface waters, and this trend will only increase in the future.

In the twelve years between 1961 and 1973 over 50,000 incidents of sickness linked to drinking water were reported. In Florida some years ago, 97 cases of typhoid were reported at a migrant work camp. During the 1960's there were about 130 reported outbreaks of disease of poisoning traceable to the drinking water. Twenty people died. About 375 became ill. How many illnesses of this kind go unreported. Diseases such as hepatitis, cholera, salmonella, polio, tetanus and numerous viruses deadly to humans have been traced to water pollution. One of the serious problems is fluoridation. Over 100 million Americans drink water that is artificially fluoridated. Some scientists and doctors believe that fluoride inhibits the action of enzymes in the human body that would normally promote repairs in genetic material and other cells. By retarding such repairs, it is believed fluoride leads to cancer and genetic damage.

The 1983 *U.S. Pharmocopia* volumes on drug information, list the following diseases that can occur among people taking tablets containing one-half to one milligram of fluoride per day (this is the amount of fluoride found in one or two pints of fluoridated water).

BLACK TARRY STOOLS
BLOODY VOMIT
DIARRHEA
FAINTNESS
NAUSEA AND VOMITING
SHALLOW BREATHING
LOSS OF APPETITE
STOMACH CRAMPS OR PAIN
TREMORS
UNUSUAL EXCITEMENT
UNUSUAL SALIVA INCREASE
WATERY EYES
WEAKNESS
CONSTIPATION
PAIN & ACHING OF BONES
WEIGHT LOSS
SKIN RASH
SORES IN MOUTH & LIPS
STIFFNESS
TEETH DISCOLORATION

The cumulative effect of fluoride causes enzyme inhibition, collagen breakdown, genetic damage and disruption of the immune system. (read *Fluoride The Aging Factor*, by Dr. John

223

Yiamouyiannis) Fluoride slows down and weakens the body's immune system. When minor infections invade the body, it takes longer to throw the infections off and more serious illnesses invade the body such as cancer.

If you feel you are getting pure drinking water when you turn on your tap at home, chances are in most cases this is not true. Most of the nation's water treatment plants are obsolete. (read *Your Water and Your Health* by Dr. Allen E. Banik with Carlson Wade) They were developed to cope with the water problems years ago. Their aim at that time was to cope with danger of bacteria and suspended solids. We have a much larger problem today with dangerous chemicals, viruses, metals and many other toxins now present in our drinking water. These inorganic materials cannot be properly handled by the body without side effects.

Toxins Found in Water

ALLERGENS
ARSENIC
ASBESTOS
BACTERIA
CADMIUM
CHEMICAL CHLORINE
COLIFORM
DETERGENTS
DIOXIN
FLUORIDE
GERMS
HERBICIDES
HUMAN WASTES
INORGANIC MINERALS
LEAD
MERCURY
NITRATES
POISONOUS HEAVY METALS
PESTICIDES
RADIOACTIVE PARTICLES
TOXIC CHEMICAL WASTE
TRICHLOROETHYLENE
URANIUM, AND VIRUSES

When COLIFORM is present in the water it indicates the presence of fecal matter and possible disease-bearing organisms. CHLORINE has been linked to heart disease and other human illnesses. Chlorine can react with organic material in water to produce trihalomethanes, which are substances known to produce cancer in mice. CHLORINE as a natural occurring mineral in herbs, fruits and vegetables is vital to your health. The body needs chlorine. It cleans the bloodstream and washes wastes from the body. Chemical chlorine is put in drinking water as a disinfectant which the body cannot utilize, and it will accumulate in the system. It suffocates and kills. If you can smell it in your water, that is the time to purify your water. DETERGENTS in the water could promote cancer by acting on the lining of the digestive tract changing the tissues so that they more easily absorb dangerous chemicals. TRICHLOROETHYLENE is the nations most popular solvent for stripping grease from metal parts, dry cleaning clothing, industrial operations and decaffeinating coffee. Long exposure can cause dizziness, nausea, fatigue, facial paralysis and psychotic behavior.

Next to oxygen, water is the most important factor for survival of humans and animals. We can do without food for several weeks but we can only survive a few days without water in some form. Water is essential in the regulation of body temperature. It is essential to the excretion of soluble wastes through lungs, skin and kidneys. Water lubricates your joints and acts as a cushion to protect the body from injuries resulting from impact and shock.

The kidneys are our "filtering system" that help in the removal of toxins and by products carried by the blood to the kidneys. The kidneys can only do their job properly if the body takes in pure water. When bad water is taken into the body, there is inadequate flushing out of waste products from the kidneys as well as poor oxidation. Pure water actually helps the kidneys dissolve toxic poisons that accumulate in the system. Pure water will help eliminate intestinal bacteria and germs in the blood to help us avoid disease.

WORMS AND PARASITES —

Worms and parasites are becoming a real problem in the United States. We believe our country is highly sanitized; the best in the world. The infestation of parasites are causing many diseases that have baffled doctors. Physicians receive little training in diagnosing and treating parasitic infections. Sanitation measures have been breaking down and people have ingested contaminated food, water or dirt. The body under normal circumstances would destroy worms and parasites if the hydrochloric acid was functioning properly. They would be destroyed along with the larva, but the body has to be free from toxins. The diet of the American people encourages worms and parasites. A diet rich in fat, starch and sugar provides food that parasites and worms live on. A clean, well nourished body would provide an environment that they could not thrive on.

Major Problems of Parasites

One current problems is a parasite that causes intestinal infections that is sweeping across the country. It is called Giardia Lamblia, a parasite that has now become the No. 1 cause of waterborne disease in the United States.

Tapeworm infections are increasing by leaps and bounds. It is felt that this is linked with American's increasing fondness for raw and rare beef.

The most deadly parasite is Amebiasis. There have been reported deaths from Amebiasis. It is usually passed from person to person.

Baiantidium parasite comes from pigs and causes intestinal infections in humans. This is a good reason to leave pork out of the diet.

Dr. Henry Lindlahr said, "Parasites and head lice peculiar to other parts of the body live on scrofulous and psoric taints. When these are consumed, the lice depart as they came. The microzyma theory furnishes the solution to this and similar problems. This is confirmed by the fact that these noxious pests do not remain with all people who have been infected with them, only with those whose internal or external conditions furnish the parasites with the means of subsistence."

Dr. Lindlahr said, "In a number of instances we have seen healing crisis take the form of lice. At that time the patients were living in the most cleanly surroundings, taking various forms of water treatment every day, so that infection was practically impossible.

In each of these cases the patient recalled having been infested with parasites at some previous time, and remembered that sulphur and molasses, mercurial salves or other means of suppression had been applied.

We prescribe for the removal of lice only cold water and the comb. Even antiseptic soaps should be avoided. The forgoing statements, more than any other portions of this volume, have brought down upon it violent criticism and condemnation. However, many of our patients who have developed, under natural treatment, such parasitic crisis will testify to their reality." (*Philosophy of Natural Therapeutics*, Volume 1, by Henry Lindlahr, M.D. 1918).

Dr. Lindlahr said, "As I am writing this, one of our guests is just recovering from one of these parasitic crisis. Before this woman came to us she had lived for many years in her own luxurious home and since she has been with us during the last four months she has not left our institution. She has occupied a room alone and has received several water treatments, including head bath, every day, so that infection was impossible. Still, four weeks ago, the attendant who gives her treatment discovered he scalp covered with nits which within a few days developed into swarms of live. The lady was very much alarmed and shed tears of mortification, until she better understood the nature of the phenomenon. I showed her original examination report which, in the section devoted to diagnosis from the iris, had the entry "psora positive, several itch spots", indicating suppression of itchy, parasitic skin eruptions. When told that the psora taint on which these parasites live is the soil of tuberculosis and cancer, she encured her itchy crisis with great equanimity. The pesky little visitors remained about three weeks and then suddenly disappeared as they had come. Nothing was used to combat the parasites except fresh, cold water and the comb."

Parasites and worms are scavengers and organisms that live within, upon or at the expense of another organism, known as the host, without contributing to the survival of the host.

Parasites take on the vibration of the host they invade. They are therefore very hard to detect.

Parasites and worms feed off toxins and waste material of the body. If the body is clean then the scavengers have nothing to live on. The danger of having them in the body is that their waste is extremely poisonous to us. Many parasites produce toxic substances harmful to the host. Other parasites act as foreign-body irritants in the tissues of the host and call forth a chronic inflammatory reaction. Some worms rob the host of serious amounts of blood and large tapeworms deprive it of digested food.

Parasites vary in their effect on their host. Sometimes they seem to be harmless. The parasites considered dangerous are called "pathogens." The parasite which causes malarial fevers in an example of this. Many protozoans (one called animals) are parasites, such as a certain type of amoeba which can destroy the lining of the intestines of humans. They produce a painful and serious disease called "amoebic dysentery." It can cause the body to become dehydrated and eventually cause bleeding and ulceration in the bowel.

Flatworms and roundworms are parasites that can cause serious damage and can often kill their hosts. There is one type of flatworm called "fluke" which lives and grows quite large in the intestines, liver, lungs or blood of animals and man. The tapeworm is another parasite which matures in the intestines, attaching itself to the intestinal wall with what appears to be suckers or hooks. The tapeworm absorbs digested foods from its host, but the hookworm is the most harmful. It lives in the intestines and feeds on the blood of the host.

Some forms of external skin parasites are ticks and mites. The skin is irritated by such bites, but the spread of disease is far more serious than the bite. Ticks are blamed for spreading Rocky Mountain spotted fever, yellow fever, African sleeping sickness, typhus fever and Lyme disease.

Trichinosis is a disease from eating infected or undercooked pork. The trichina is a tiny worm that infects pigs. The larvae, after burrowing into the intestinal wall of the pig, then enters its blood vessels. The blood carries the larvae on the muscles where these tiny worms spread into the muscle fiber and live. Then when humans eat the pork, the cycle begins again in the human body. Symptoms of trichinosis are headaches, fever, sore muscles, swollen eyes, and even painful breathing. These symptoms are similar to other diseases so people do not even realize that they could have internal worms.

Salmonella is a microscopic organism which can spread throughout the body cause a person to become acutely sick with what is commonly called cholera. It is felt that many people today have the intermittent fever of cholera but are given antibiotics and never told what their problem has been.

Bacteria are one-celled organisms. There are three main types of bacteria: 1.) Bacilli is rod-shaped, often grows in long chains. 2.) Cocci is spherical and grow in grape-like clusters and 3.) Spirrila is spirally curved.

Bacteria is involved in contagious diseases such as diphtheria, chicken pox, measles, mumps, scarlet fever, whooping cough, tetanus, pneumonia, gonorrhea, tuberculosis, typhoid fever, syphilis, leprosy, meningitis and plague.

The host can also feel pressure effects produced by parasitic cysts especially if they are situated in the brain, spinal cord, eye, heart or bones.

Obstruction effects are produced by large ascarids migrating into and blocking the pancreatic ducts and even the intestines.

It was discovered that cancer may also be caused by a parasite. Dr. Virginia Livingston-Wheeler, M.D., in her book the *Conquest of Cancer*, calls the parasite the progenitor cryptocide. This parasite begins as the lepra or tuberular bacillus and changes form to become the cancer parasite. She says that, "This microbe is present in all of our cells, and it is only our immune systems that keep it suppressed. When our immune system is weakened, either by poor diet, infected food or old age, this microbe gains a foothold and starts cancer cells growing into tumors." (Page 12, *The Conquest of Cancer*).

Strengthening the immune system is the most important thing you can do for your body in preventing parasite and worm invasion.

Life cycle of the Hookworm:

Step 1: Eggs exit the human with the feces. The eggs are so small they can enter the host with the air in the form of dust.

Step 2: Eggs hatch in the warm, moist soil into larvae.

Step 3: The larvae become attached to the skin and burrow through it into the blood.

Step 4: Larvae travel via blood or lymph to the lungs after spending a period of time in the different parts of the body.

Step 5: Larvae burrow through the alveolae in the lungs and climb up the windpipe and then fall into the stomach. They are now adult size.

Step 6: In the small intestine the larvae attach to the mucosa with hook-like teeth, mostly in the jejunum, undergo sexual reproduction, the female laying 10,000 eggs a day. The worms have a lifespan of 2-3 years.

Possible Problems Caused by Parasites and Worms

ALLERGIES
ARTHRITIS
BACK PAIN
BRUSIM (GRINDING OF TEETH)
CANCER
COLITIS
FATIGUE
DIABETES
FULLNESS IN STOMACH
HEADACHES
HYPOGLYCEMIA
INDIGESTION
INSOMNIA
LUPUS
MINERAL IMBALANCE
NAUSEA
NECK PAIN
SINUS TROUBLES
THYROID IMBALANCE
VOMITING

The body is a wonderful machine and when nourished and treated properly, will not harbor these scavengers. When there are sufficient amounts of healthy bile in the intestines and the body is free of toxins, the bile contains all its normal required elements to keep it in healthy working order. Then the parasites and worms cannot continue to prosper or even to survive. When there are sufficient amounts of healthy bile, the parasites and worms, their larvae and eggs, are neutralized and evacuated rapidly out of the body.

We need to provide an environment that will not allow scavengers to survive. We need to live and eat the proper food so they will not want to invade our bodies. Parasites and worms do not like a clean body. They especially do not like minerals. Herbs have high amounts of minerals and other elements that will help the body eliminate them.

Sometimes people become discouraged when they try to live a cleaner, more wholesome diet or try to go on a cleansing purge. It is hard for them to stay on it because the parasites within are crying for the kind of junk foods upon which they live and grow. It is probably wise to clean the body of the parasites first. Since the parasites cling on to the mucus in which they live, the body cannot be made well even in a fasting or semi-fasting situation.

After eliminating the parasites, a total change of diet is essential if a person expects to maintain healthy and free of them. Try to eat quantities of organically grown fruits and vegetables if possible. Eat raw nuts and seeds.

Herbal Formulas for Parasites and Worms

1. Black Walnut, Wormwood, Sage, Fennel, Senna, Male Fern, Distilled Water, Glycerine.

An extract that helps rid the body of parasites, toxins, worms and used externally for ringworms.

Black Walnut - kills parasites, burns up excessive toxins and fatty material. It is rich in iodine with antiseptic and healing properties.

Wormwood - is used in this formula to help with constipation and indigestion. It helps with an acid stomach.

Sage - is used for disolving toxins.

Fennel - has a gentle diuretic effect and helps in eliminating toxins.

Senna - increases intestinal peristaltic action and helps eliminate parasites and worms.

Male Fern - is used for expelling tapeworms and parasites.

Food and Herbs Beneficial to Eliminate Parasites and Worms

Black Walnut: kills worms and parasites, especially effective in the head area. Rich in iodine.

Burdock & Black Walnut: use equal parts for purging out parasites and worms.

Chaparral: kills parasites and harmful bacteria. It is a strong blood cleanser.

Dulse: It is rich in minerals. It strengthens the immune system to prevent worms and parasites. Kelp absorbs toxins from the body fluids.

Echinacea: It improves lymphatic filtration and drainage, and helps remove toxins from the blood. It is considered one of the best blood cleansers.

Garlic: is one of the best herbs for pin worms. The sulphur content in garlic and onions helps to kill worms and parasites.

Golden Seal: kills worms and parasites. It heals and cleans the intestinal tract, and is effective in killing giardia.

Horsetail: kills parasite and worm eggs, and larva. It is rich in silicon and calcium.

Kelp: It is rich in minerals, cleans the blood and destroys toxins in the body.

Pau D'Arco: is an excellent blood cleanser, protects the liver and builds up the immune system.

Pumpkin Seeds: grind and use the seeds often on cereals. It kills worms and parasites, and is especially beneficial for children.

Senna: is beneficial for ridding and eliminating worms and parasites from the colon.

Wormwood: destroys and removes parasites and worms from the body.

Yellow Dock: kills live parasites and worms. Rich in iron and other essential minerals for a healthy body.

Beets: Eat beets raw and grated. They can effectively kill worms.

Carrots: can be scrubbed, washed and eaten with skin left on. They are rich in organic minerals and the sugar acts as a worm killer.

Figs: figs, and fig juice paralyze any worms. White figs are excellent.

Hydrochloric Acid: is an aid to help kill worms.

Papaya Seeds: are effective for expelling worms.

Pomegranate: kills worms.

THE NEW AND OLD GERMS

Life-threatening, obscure illness have emerged throughout the world causing panic and concern in African villages as well as in suburban communities in the United States. With world travel common place, germs are easily transported from nation to nation across miles of ocean or land. A strep bacteria resistant to antibiotics, the hantavirus, hepatitis and tuberculosis are some of the new and re-emerging plagues.

Plagues have been around since the beginning of time. The Black Death spread through Europe nearly killing a third of its population during the fourteenth century. The Spanish Flu spread through America during 1918-19 killing many individuals. Polio left its mark on the world population. Smallpox killed many in the second century. Scientists around the world are beginning to show great concern over the new developments of deadly diseases. Philip E. Ross in an article in *Scient & Technology*, says the following: "It is a matter of biological chance that human immuno-deficiency virus, the bug that causes AIDS, is not very contagious. It it were as easy to catch as the common cold, we might all be dead now." (Phillip E. Ross, "A New Black Death?" *Science & Technology*, September 12, 1994, p 241.)

Medical researchers now believe that this is just the beginning. They think that a new, even more serious germ will emerge. Someday, another great plague will probably appear though no one can predict where or what it will be. "Once considered well within management by drugs and vaccines, life-threatening germs had been shoved to the back burner. But now we may be paying a price for letting down our collective guard. Experts admit that we no longer have the threat of infectious diseases in check. "The range of diseases is increasing, and an alarming number of these germs are resilient," says Ralph Bryan, M.D., project coordinator at the National Center for Infectious Diseases, at the Centers for Disease Control and Prevention, in Atlanta. (Sherry Helms, "The New Germs You Must Know About, *Ladies Home Journal*, September 1994, p 52.)

Trying to make sense of all this information can be extremely confusing. Why this is happening is another concern. There are various reasons according to some experts.

ANTIBIOTIC THERAPY

First of all, just about everyone agrees that antibiotic therapy has been misused. Infectious disease which were thought to be under control, are not. Bacteria are able to develop a resistance to antibiotics. The problem stems from individuals going to the doctor and wanting a cure. They don't feel the visit was worthwhile if they don't leave with a prescription for antibiotics. A prime time news show did a study on this problem. They sent a well woman to four different doctors asking for antibiotics because of a sore throat and cold. Three of the four doctors gave her the prescription even though there appeared to be no problem at all. One doctor justified her prescription by saying that she felt in order to keep patients, she needed to give them what they want. Well, an over use of antibiotics has resulted in their ability to become resistant to the cure. Also, individuals who are on antibiotics need to take the full course in order to kill all the bacteria responsible for the infection. If not, the strongest will survive with the ability to resist future antibiotic treatment. Increasingly, researchers are being confronted with microbes that have learned to become resistant to drugs. One example is that forty years ago gonorrhea could easily be treated with small doses of penicillin. Now, it requires massive doses to kill the organism. Antibiotics should be used only as a last resort.

NEW TERRITORY

Another problem is in the tropical jungles. With humans making contact with previously unknown organisms, there will most certainly be problems. "As a result of the green revolution and medical advances, the human population is growing, concentrating, linking up by air, mixing, and coming unprecedented contact with the richest reservoirs of parasites in the world: tropical jungles," says Philip e. Ross.

"It is in this lush greenery that we ought to look for the coming viruses," concluded a 1992 study by the Institute of Medicine in Washington, D.C. "There, in these places so beloved by romantic environmentalists, lie seething cauldrons of diverse species, each with its own army of parasites, each one of which must be eyeing the growing mountain of succulent human flesh. The bug that can sink its teeth into that flesh wins the jackpot." (Ross, p 242.)

LIVING CONDITIONS

Unsanitary living conditions promote the growth of germs. This is prime transmission territory for any number of diseases. Rodents coming in to contact with humans also contribute. Individuals in crowded living space can easily transmit germs from one to the other. Poor nutrition also is a key factor. These living conditions are prevalent throughout the world in developing nations as well as in areas of the more prosperous nations.

INVASIVE GROUP-A STREP

This is an extremely serious form of the streptococcus bacteria that causes strep throat. It is very dangerous and sometimes fatal. It is thought by some to be a return of a bacteria that caused scarlet fever, which a century ago resulted in thousand of deaths and then disappeared. Infections appear to occur in cycles. It can cause a drop in blood pressure as well as organ failure. It is also responsible for the cases of necrotizing fascitis which is a secondary infection that eats away at the muscle, fat, and flesh. The seriousness lies in its quick progression. The infection can spread as rapidly as one inch per hour.

Toxins released by the strep bacteria poison the skin and surrounding muscle tissue along with internal organs. This causes the immune system to

quickly fail. This is similar to the way the hantavirus produces a toxin that rapidly breaks down capillary walls in the lungs causing its victims to drown in their own fluids.

If caught early enough, it can be treated with penicillin. Fortunately, this is not an antibiotic resistant strain of bacteria. If tissues have died, antibiotic therapy has no way to treat the area because blood flow has ceased. Sometimes surgery is required to remove large pieces of affected tissue and even amputation of affected limbs may be necessary. These infectious microorganisms are spread primarily through open wounds or cuts in the skin. The fatality rate is approximately 28 percent among those who contract the flesh eating symptoms.

HANTAVIRUS

This mysterious illness surfaced in the Southwest United States in May of 1993. This illness has brought to the attention of the average citizen that infectious diseases are not under control. Researchers were already studying the increases in the rodent population in New Mexico. When the virus was identified, the rodent researchers were able to identify the deer mouse as the carrier of the hantavirus involved. It infects as people breathe tiny particles of infected rodent feces, urine and saliva that get into the air. It is clear now that the Southwestern rodents are not the only carriers. A Florida man's illness has been traced to the cotton rat. The virus has also been found in chipmunks and squirrels. The disease does not appear to spread from person to person, but it does seem to affect seemingly healthy individuals.

"During the Korean War, approximately 3,000 U.S. trrops were stricken with an illness that caused high fever, hemorrhages, and kidney damage. Although they were acutely ill, the majority of patients recovered from what later turned out to be infection with hantavirus. Over the past 40 years, four strains of hantavirus have been blamed for periodic outbreaks of illness characterized by flu-like symptoms, fever, and kidney problems.

They new hantavirus is different and more deadly. The Muerto Canyon virus, as the altered form that arose in the Southwest is now called causes a fast-moving, deadly pneumonia that physicians now call hantavirus pulmonary syndrome. Although patients with this disease are 10 times more likely to die than those with other hanta-related illness, many of their symptoms and signs are the same. These include fever, blood cell abnormalities, and cardiac arrhythmias." (Ann Guidici Fettner, "New But Not So Novel," *Harvard Health Letter*, volume 19 number 11, September 1994, p 2.)

This new strain causes death by breaking down capillary walls in the lungs causing its victims to drown in their own fluids. Earlier symptoms before the lungs become involved are often hard to detect. Some believe this is due to an over reaction of a strong immune system.

HEPATITIS B AND C

The viral infection known as hepatitis is on the rise. It has been around for sometime but is being seen in greater numbers. It causes an inflammation of the liver and can cause chronic liver disease. The liver is essential in clearing toxins from the body.

"About 5 to 10 percent of Hepatitis B cases, and as much as 70 to 90 percent of Hepatitis C, are chronic conditions for which there is no definite cure. (Hepatitis A is still another form of the virus, but it is typically carried in contaminated food and water, not blood. It is less prevalent and threatening than the two other kinds.) (Helms, p 90.)

Hepatitis B and C are both transmitted through infected blood and through sexual intercourse the same as AIDS. It is often seen in intravenous drug users. It is treated with a natural protein known as interferon. Some patients do not seem to respond to this drug.

TUBERCULOSIS

Tuberculosis was a serious life threatening illness during the turn of the century. It was no longer considered a threat, however until the last few years. "From 1985 to 1992, there was a 20 percent jump in the number of overall cases reported in the U.S., with a 35 percent jump among children. (There was a slight turndown in 1993.)"

This bacterial infection affects the lungs. It is transmitted in small drops of sputum in the air of infected individuals. It can spread from the lungs to other parts of the body. It causes scar tissue to develop and damage to the lungs.

Some of the most virulent strains of this disease are resistant to antibiotic therapy. Some individuals carry an inactive form of the disease without developing a full blown case. Immigration is thought to be a part in the rise of T.B. cases in the United States. It is widespread in some of the developing nations throughout the world. It is seen in a number of AIDS patients probably because of their low immune system response, which makes them more vulnerable to infection.

PREVENTION

These volatile germs can be extremely frightening. There are ways however, to protect ourselves. Strengthen the immune system. Good nutrition and exercise will help the body protect itself. Cleanliness is essential. Wash hands regularly especially when preparing food and handling babies. Keep a distance from individuals who are ill. If you feel your resistance is low, take some time to rest and eat well. Keep living areas clean.

BUILDING THE IMMUNE SYSTEM

Each time a foreign substance enters the body the immune system goes to work. Factors that contribute to a low immune system include certain drugs, viruses, chemicals, pollution, parasites, antibiotics, stress, depression, lack of sleep, alcohol, smoking, poor diet including fats and refined products, fried foods, and caffeine drinks.

The best way to protect the body is to strengthen the immune system and use natural methods of healing, such as herbs, when needed.

1. Exercise

We hear over and over again about the important of exercise. It is believed that exercise can improve the white blood cell count in the body which fights germs. It stimulates the lymphatic flow and blood circulation which allows for the blood flow to increase to the brain and all areas of the body. It can help release hormones that actually help you to feel good. Exercise can help relieve built up anxiety and stress in the body. It can help increase energy and an overall sense of well being.

2. Vitamin and Minerals

- Calcium is helpful in healing the body.
- Chromium is needed in small amounts and is important in fighting germs and foreign bodies.
- Iodine helps the thyroid gland in producing thyroxine which aids in the absorption of vitamin A.
- Magnesium produces properdin, which is a blood protein that fights invading viruses and bacteria.
- Manganese helps activate enzymes that work with vitamin C. As a team, they fight toxins and free radicals.
- Selenium may help reduce cancer risk.
- Zinc helps produce histimine, which dilates the capillaries to aid the blood in fighting infection.
- Vitamin A helps increase the body's resistance to infection.

- Vitamin E helps deactivate free radicals that promote cellular damage and malignancy.
- Vitamin C helps with the formation of connective tissue. It also helps in deactivating free radicals which can cause havoc in the body. It aids in killing viruses and bacteria.
- B-vitamins help protect the immune response and help the body when under stress.

3. Herbs For The Immune System

- Garlic is considered a natural antibiotic and effect against viruses as well as bacteria. It is also being explored and used to lower cholesterol levels and reduce the risk of heart disease. Various studies seem to support these claims.
- Alfalfa is rich in vitamins and minerals. It can help remove poisons from the body which can inhibit the immune system.
- Echinacea helps stimulate the immune response. It is a natural antibiotic.
- Burdock is known as a blood purifier which can help rid the blood of impurities leading to disease.
- Catnip helps increase circulation in the body.
- Kelp helps the thyroid function as well as the lymph glands. The lymph glands aid in building the body's immunity against infection.
- Parsley can help increase the body's resistance to infection and disease.
- Prickly Ash can help increase the circulation throughout the body.
- Pau D'Arco is used as an antibiotic and contains viral killing properties. It is thought to attack the cause of disease and help the body fight infection.
- Red Clover helps build the immune system and strengthen the liver.
- Comfrey helps promote the growth of strong cells and rid the body of waste.
- White Oak Bark helps tone and strengthen the entire system including the cells.

NUTRITIONAL SUPPLEMENTS

VITAMINS

Vitamins are complex organic substances needed by the body, often in small amounts, for good health. They are in fact necessary for life. Vitamins work with the body to perform life giving functions.

Vitamins must be obtained from our diets. They are contained in the food we eat, herbs and supplements. Vitamins are used in the body constantly and must be replaced daily.

Vitamins help the body use other nutrients. They contribute to the breaking down of protein, carbohydrates, and fats into useable forms. The body must have a balance of vitamins to function properly.

Vitamins are either water or fat soluble. Most fall into the water soluble category. This means they combine with water in the body to function and then are excreted in the urine. These vitamins only remain in the system for two to three hours and must be taken regularly whether in the food we eat or as a supplement.

Vitamins A, D, E, F and K are considered fat soluble. They remain in the body for a longer period of time. They combine with fats to be absorbed in the body.

Vitamins should be taken before meals for proper absorption in the body. Vitamins work together in the body and should be combined for the most benefit.

The following lists some information and benefits of essential vitamins.

Vitamin A

Vitamin A is fat soluble which means it requires fats to be absorbed properly. It can be stored by the body but in extremely high doses can be toxic. It helps maintain and repair healthy tissue, fights infection, counteracts night blindness, treats skin problems, and aids in the growth and maintenance of healthy bones, skin, teeth, and gums.

Vitamin A is found in fish liver oil, liver, green and yellow vegetables, eggs, milk, carrots, apricots, and sweet potatoes.

Some herbs which contain vitamin A include Alfalfa, Blessed Thistle, Capsicum, Fenugreek, Passion Flower, Parsley, Slippery Elm, Ginseng, Scullcap, Papaya, Saw Palmetto, Rose Hips, Red Raspberry, Uva Ursi, Peppermint, Comfrey, Catnip and Chaparral.

Vitamin B1 (Thiamine)

Vitamin B1 is water soluble and needed by the body in only small amounts on a daily basis. It helps the body metabolize carbohydrates. It is known to help strengthen the nervous system.

It is found in whole wheat, oatmeal, peanuts, sunflower seeds, rice bran, wheat germ, millet, brewer's yeast, and blackstrap molasses.

Herbs which contain vitamin B1 include Barberry, Burdock, Kelp, Gotu Kola, Alfalfa, Ginseng, Scullcap, Papaya, Peppermint, Slippery Elm, Sage, Parsley, and Feverfew.

Vitamin B2 (Riboflavin)

Vitamin B2 helps the body digest and assimilate fats, proteins, and carbohydrates. It is water soluble and must be replaced daily. It is essential for proper enzyme formation, normal growth, and tissue formation.

It is found in almonds, dry hot red pepper, wheat germ, wild rice, dried peas, liver, fish, white beans, millet, parsley, and sesame seeds.

Some of the herbs which are high in vitamin B2 include Alfalfa, Barberry, Gotu Kola, Parsley, Kelp, Hops, Ginseng, Sarsaparilla, Papaya, and Peppermint.

Vitamin B3 (Niacinamide)

Vitamin B3 is thought to promote good physical and mental health. It helps the body produce cortisone, thyroxine, insulin, and female and male hormones. The body can usually produce enough on its own if vitamins B1, B2, and B6 are present in a high enough amount.

Rice and wheat bran, sesame seeds, sunflower seeds, liver, kidney, fish, eggs, white meat, avocados, whole wheat, and prunes all contain vitamin B3.

Herbs which contain this vitamin include Butcher's Broom, Kelp, Horsetail, Hops, Gotu Kola, Feverfew, Red Raspberry, Red Clover, Peppermint, Parsley, and Papaya.

Vitamin B5 (Pantothenic Acid)

This vitamin helps produce various hormones. It is found in every living cell in the body. It helps with digestion.

Some foods which contain this vitamin are brewer's yeast, molasses, egg yolks, soybeans, peanuts, wheat germ, whole grains, chicken, green vegetables, tomatoes, and potatoes.

Barberry, Parsley, Kelp, Hops, Gotu Kola, Papaya, Peppermint, Ginseng, Slippery Elm, and Spirulina all contain vitamin B5.

Vitamin B6 (Pyrodixine Hydrochloride)

Vitamin B6 is essential for proper chemical balance in the body. It is also helpful in the conversion of fats and proteins into useful energy. It helps with the production of red blood cells.

Foods which contain this essential vitamin include brewer's yeast, wheat germ, blackstrap molasses, honey, liver, egg yolks, almonds, carrots, spinach, liver, milk, bananas, and leafy green vegetables.

Herbs which contain this vitamin include Alfalfa, Ginseng, Peppermint, Papaya, Parsley, and Kelp.

Vitamin B9 (Folic Acid)

This water soluble vitamin is helpful for the entire nervous system. Recent studies have shown that women who take folic acid early in their pregnancies have a greater chance of having babies without certain birth defects.

Foods which contain vitamin B9 are green leafy vegetables, fresh mushrooms, sprouts, liver, brewer's yeast, eggs, yogurt, whole wheat, vegetables, and carrots.

Herbs with folic acid include Barberry, Ginseng, Kelp, Hops, Gotu Kola, Parsley, Peppermint, Slippery Elm, and Papaya.

Vitamin C (Ascorbic Acid)

This water soluble vitamin is essential to the body. It helps prevent infection by increasing and speeding up activity of white blood cells and aids in destroying viruses and bacteria. It aids in the formation of collagen which is essential for good teeth, bones, and growth of children.

Citrus fruits, vegetables, broccoli, cauliflower, berries, cantaloupe, potatoes, and peppers are good sources of vitamin C.

Herbs which contain vitamin C include Catnip, Ginseng, Hops, Hawthorn Berries, eyebright, Rosehips, Parsley, Passion Flower, Juniper Berries, Lobelia, Aloe Vera, Burdock, Dandelion, Horsetail, and Bayberry.

Vitamin D (Calciferol)

This important vitamin is responsible for regulating mineral and vitamin metabolism including calcium, phosphorus, and vitamin A. It is produced naturally by the action of sunlight with oils on the skin. This vitamin is fat soluble and is stored in the skin, brain, liver, and bones.

Foods rich in vitamin D include dairy products, fish liver oils, egg yolks, spinach, tuna, sardines, and salmon.

Herbs which contain vitamin D include Fenugreek, Eyebright, and Alfalfa.

Vitamin E (Tocopherol)

Vitamin E is fat soluble and needed in small amounts. It is activated by vitamin A. Selenium increases the effectiveness of vitamin E. It helps control the unsaturated fats in the body and is thought to reduce cholesterol. It is helpful when applied to wounds to lessen the growth of scar tissue.

This vitamin is found in wheat germ, vegetable oils, peanuts, lettuce, spinach, whole grains, egg yolks, and corn.

Herbs which contain vitamin E include Alfalfa, Blue Cohosh, Dulse, Kelp, Dong Quai, Eyebright, Spirulina, Ginseng, and Scullcap.

Vitamin F (Unsaturated fatty acids)

This vitamin is fat soluble. It is essential for healthy function of the adrenal and thyroid glands. It is aided in its absorption when taken with vitamin E.

It is found in all unsaturated vegetable oils. It is also found in oats, rye, nuts, avocado, whole raw milk, and cod liver oil.

Some herbs which contain vitamin F are Alfalfa and Irish Moss.

Vitamin H (Biotin)

Vitamin H is essential for normal growth of all body tissue and cells. It is helpful in the utilization of B-complex vitamins.

Foods which contain this vitamin include brewer's yeast, egg yolks, liver, milk, wheat germ, sprouts, molasses, and yogurt.

Alfalfa and Barberry are herbs which contain vitamin H.

Vitamin K

Vitamin K is a fat soluble vitamin which is well known for its blood clotting abilities. It is essential in the formation of prothrombin which is a blood clotting chemical. With vitamin C, it is useful to stop bleeding after surgery.

Foods which contain this vitamin are yogurt, green leafy vegetables, carrots, potatoes, turnips, alfalfa, safflower oil, kelp, whole grains, legumes, and egg yolks.

Herbs which contain vitamin K are Alfalfa, Cornsilk, Irish Moss, Kelp, and Shepherd's Purse.

Vitamin P (Bioflavonoids)

Vitamin P increases the effectiveness of vitamin C. The two work together to strengthen connective tissue and capillaries.

It is found in citrus fruits, apricots, blackberries, cherries, grapes, plums, rose hips, buckwheat, and spinach.

Herbs which contain this vitamin are Paprika, Black Currants, and Rose Hips.

Vitamin T

This vitamin is not very well known. It seems to assist in normalizing blood coagulation and forming of platelets.

It is found in sesame seeds, tahini, and egg yolks.

Vitamin U

This vitamin was recently discovered. It is high in chlorophyll.

It is found in cabbage juice, sauerkraut, and raw celery juice.

THE IMPORTANCE OF MINERALS

Many laboratory experiments have been done regarding the importance of minerals in the body and determining what part they play in healthy development. The body certainly needs small amounts of many minerals to function normally. These minerals need to be supplied on a daily basis to maintain and regulate necessary body functions. These can either be supplied by a nutritious diet or through supplements. Minerals aid the body in assimilating vitamins. The body needs minerals, vitamins, water, protein, carbohydrates and fats to survive. Minerals can help keep the body young and healthy. They are necessary for the nervous system, normalizing the heartbeat, improving the brain and mental abilities, fighting fatigue and increasing energy, electrolyte balance, and aiding the metabolic process.

Most minerals cannot be used by the body in their free state. They need to be taken in a combined form for them to be of benefit to the body. This combination allows them to be broken down into a more digestible form. This process is called chelation. Minerals may be purchased in chelated form which eliminates the body's need to break them down and makes better use of the minerals.

There are two different categories of minerals. These include major minerals and trace minerals. Both are equally important, but the major minerals are those required by the body in large amounts. The trace minerals are only needed in small amounts, and in fact can be toxic if used in large quantities.

Minerals help regulate the delicate balance of body fluids. They are essential for all mental and physical functions. Minerals aid in the process of osmosis which includes emptying the body of waste and bringing oxygen and nutrients to the cells. They help equalize the fluids in and out of the cells.

It is thought that 28 minerals are found in the human body. 14 of these are considered trace minerals because they are found in such small quantities. Studies are on going as to the part each mineral plays in the body process. The minerals are tested to see what harm a deficit may cause. From the studies done, it appears that iron and iodine are the most important trace minerals. Zinc, copper, manganese, fluorine, and chromium are also essential to good health. Of lesser importance seem to be molybdenum, selenium, cobalt, nickel, tin, vanadium, and silicon.

The following are the functions of some of the minerals found in the body.

Calcium

Calcium is the most abundant mineral found in the body. And that is a good indicator of just how essential it is. Most of the calcium in the body is located in the bones and teeth. It is necessary for the transmission of nerve signals. It is important for smooth functioning of the heart muscles and muscular movements of the intestines. To function efficiently calcium must be in combination with magnesium, phosphorus, vitamins A, C, and D as well as zinc.

Herbs that contain calcium are: Alfalfa, Blue Cohosh, Chamomile, Capsicum, Dandelion, Horsetail, Irish Moss, Kelp, Mistletoe, Nettle, Parsley, Plantain, Pokeweed, Pumpkin Seeds, Raspberry, Rose Hip's, Shepherd's Purse, Yellow Dock and Watercress.

Phosphorus

This mineral has many important functions in the body. Phosphorus is found mainly in the bones and teeth. Phosphorus and Calcium work together. It helps with the formation of strong bones and teeth, aids the pH balance of the blood, helps metabolize fats, aids in activating the oxidation of carbohydrates, and is required for the production of body energy.

Phosphorus is found in the following herbs: Alfalfa, Blue Cohosh, Caraway, Capsicum,

Chickweed, Dandelion, Garlic, Irish Moss, Kelp, Licorice, Parsley, Raspberry, Rose Hips, Watercress, and Yellow Dock.

Potassium

Potassium works with sodium to regulate fluids and the flow of nutrients in and out of the cells. It is involved in the maintenance of regular heart rhythm. It helps stimulate the kidneys and helps with normal function of the adrenals. It is important in stimulating the nerves impulses which cause muscle contraction.

Herbs that contain potassium are: Alfalfa, Blue Cohosh, Chamomile, Comfrey, Dulse, Dandelion, Eyebright, Fennel, Irish Moss, Kelp, Mistletoe, Nettle, Papaya, Parsley, Peppermint, Plantain, Raspberry, Shepherd's Purse, White Oak Bark, Yarrow, and Wintergreen.

Sodium

Most of the sodium in the body is found in the fluid surrounding the cells. Sodium works with chlorine to regulate the pH of the fluids in the body. Potassium and sodium work together to regulate the flow of nutrients in and out of the cells. Excess sodium can cause serious health problems including hypertension and edema. It is a valuable mineral but can usually be supplied in the foods we eat without a supplement.

Sodium is found in Alfalfa, Dandelion, Dulse, Irish Moss, Kelp, Parsley, Shepherd's Purse, Willow, and Yarrow.

Chlorine

Chlorine is essential for the production of vital gastric juices aiding in digestion. It is rarely lacking in the diet because of the chlorination of drinking water.

Herbs containing chlorine, include: Alfalfa, Dandelion, Kelp, Parsley, and Raspberry.

Iron

Iron is a mineral that most people are familiar with, yet many people suffer from a deficit of iron in their diets. It is not easily absorbed by the body. For proper assimilation, an adequate amount of hydrochloric acid must be present in the stomach with vitamins C and E. Iron is known as the anti-anemia mineral because of its aid in the oxygenating of cells and combining with protein to form hemoglobin.

Iron is found in the following herbs: Alfalfa, Burdock, Blue Cohosh, Capsicum, Dandelion, Dulse, Kelp, Mullein, Nettle, Parsley, Pokeweed, Red Beet, Rhubarb, Rose Hip's, Strawberry Leaves, and Yellow Dock.

Manganese

This is a trace mineral essential for the proper function of the pituitary gland as well as the healthy function of all the body's glands. It is found in many enzymes in the body. It aids in the utilization of glucose. It also helps in reproduction and in normal functioning of the central nervous system.

Magnesium

Magnesium is an essential part of the enzyme system. It is poorly assimilated by the body and should be taken daily. It is a major regulator of cellular activity including the maintenance of DNA and RNA. It is considered an anti-stress mineral. It assists in the absorption of calcium, phosphorous, sodium, potassium, and vitamin B-complex, C and E.

Herbs which contain magnesium include: Alfalfa, Blue Cohosh, Capsicum, Dandelion, Kelp, Mistletoe, Mullein, Peppermint, Primrose, Raspberry, Watercress, Willow and Wintergreen.

Iodine

Iodine is a trace mineral needed only in very small amounts. It is part of the thyroid hormones thyroxine and triodothyronine.

Iodine is found in the following herbs: Black Walnut, Dandelion, Dulse, Garlic, Irish Moss, and Sarsaparilla.

Fluorine

This is considered an essential trace mineral, but it has been the subject of much controversy because of it's presence as an additive to drinking water in many states. It is known to increase the absorption of calcium to create stronger bones and teeth.

Herbs containing fluorine include: Alfalfa and Garlic.

Copper

Copper is an important trace mineral. It aids in the absorption of calcium, the assimilation of iron and the formation of red blood cells. It is part of every body tissue. It helps the body oxidize vitamin C.

Copper is found in Kelp, Parsley, and Watercress.

Cobalt

This trace mineral is essential for human nutrition. It aids in the assimilation and synthesis of vitamin B12 and stimulates many enzymes in the body. It aids in the building of red blood cells. Cobalt is present in all animal and most dairy products.

Chromium

Chromium is a less known trace mineral but equally important. It is essential for the synthesis of fatty acids and the metabolism of glucose for energy. It is also known to increase the efficiency of insulin.

Zinc

This trace mineral performs may vital body functions. It helps with the absorption of vitamins in the body. It helps form skin, hair and nails. It is an essential part of many enzymes involved in digestion and metabolism. Zinc is essential to the growth process. Vitamin A must be present for zinc to be properly absorbed by the body. It helps in healing wounds and burns.

Herbs containing zinc include: Damiana, Ginseng, Ho Shou Wu, Kelp, Licorice, and Marshmallow.

Selenium

This is considered a relatively new trace mineral but is accepted as essential. It is a helper to other nutrients especially vitamin E. It helps the body utilize oxygen and assists in the normal growth function. It may help prevent chromosome breakage which causes birth defects.

Selenium is found in Alfalfa and Kelp.

Sulphur

Sulphur is known to purify and tone the body. It is not considered deficient in the diet because of its concentration in protein. It is involved in collagen formation which helps maintain healthy hair, fingernails and skin. It is an essential component of some amino acids.

Herbs which have sulphur content are: Alfalfa, Burdock, Capsicum, Eyebright, Fennel, Garlic, Irish Moss, Kelp, Mullein, Nettle, Parsley, Plantain, Raspberry, Sage, Shepherd's Purse, and Thyme.

Vanadium

Some believe that this trace mineral may aid in preventing cardiovascular disease. There is not much information available but it is thought to be a factor in normal growth. It is found in some sea foods.

Molybdenum

Molybdenum is a part of some enzymes. It helps with the mobilization of iron. It is thought to inhibit dental caries.

Nickel

Nickel helps activate some enzymes.

Tin

It is thought to be necessary in growth, but it is not known how it works.

Silicon

Silicon is important to normal growth and bone development.

Silicon is found in Alfalfa, Blue cohosh, Burdock, Horsetail, Kelp, and Nettle.

Aluminum

This trace mineral is found in the body but can be extremely toxic. It may play a role in protein synthesis. When aluminum utensils are used in cooking, aluminum may be absorbed in small amounts.

Aluminum is found in Alfalfa and Chlorophyll.

Cadmium

Cadmium is also a toxic trace mineral. It is thought to take the place of zinc in the body if zinc is lacking in the diet. Cadmium is found in coffee and tea.

Lead

Lead can be a very toxic trace mineral. It causes many different problems known as lead poisoning. Smoking and smog are sources of lead and can lead lead to problems.

Mercury

Another toxic trace mineral is mercury. It is found in lakes and streams due to waste dumping from manufacturing companies.

ACIDOPHILUS

Antibiotics are commonly prescribed for all types of infections. Frequent use of antibiotics leads to an imbalance in the body of beneficial and harmful bacteria. The problem arises because antibiotics destroy both good and bad bacteria. This lowers the body's resistance to all types of illness.

With the imbalance of pH and negative bacterial growth, the Candida bacteria flourishes. Vaginal yeast infections often occur after the use of antibiotics. This can spread throughout the body and cause severe problems resulting from a weakened immune system.

Acidophilus is the primary beneficial bacteria in the colon. Antibiotics and poor nutrition aid in the destruction of this bacteria in the colon. The pH is slightly acidic in a healthy colon allowing acidophilus to flourish.

Along with antibiotics, a diet high in meat and protein with few vegetables and fruit can cause the pH to be alkaline. This allows for the harmful bacteria to thrive and acidophilus to be destroyed.

Acidophilus supplements can and should be taken when using antibiotics or when candida is present. The acidophilus must be from human origin. Other forms of acidophilus such as from animals and plants cannot be assimilated by the body and therefore are of no value.

The lack of acidophilus may be responsible for more problems than we realize. Dr. William g. Crook, M.D. in his book *The Yeast Connection* quotes Von Hilsheimer. "Observations of a long series of psychiatric patients disclosed a deficiency of Lactobacillus acidophilus (L.A.) in their stools associated with GI symptoms and other evidences of idiosyncratic responses to food...

Supplementation with high levels of L.A. in the form of freeze dried L.A. in capsules, L.A. cultured milk yogurt or L.A. implanted milk ("sweet acidophilus") resulted in grossly observable changes in stool, increase in stool L.A. and reduction of symptoms associated with food."

It is important to feed the stomach and colon proper food to allow for the acidophilus to prosper. A low protein diet enriched with many vegetables and fruits can help the pH to allow for the growth of the acidophilus bacteria.

> ACNE
> ALLERGIES
> ARTHRITIS
> BREAST DISEASE
> GOUT
> CANCER
> CANKER SORES
> COLITIS
> CONSTIPATION
> DIVERTICULOSIS
> ECZEMA
> HALITOSIS
> HERPES
> LIVER PROBLEMS
> ULCERS

Acidophilus is a valuable supplement to use in your daily diet. The reason it is important is it destroys putrefactive bacteria in the intestinal tract. Putrefactive bacteria liberates histamine, a toxic substance that is the result of undigested protein. Professor Jeffrey Bland, a nutritional biochemist at the University of Puget Sound said, (*Let's Live*, May 1985) "It is estimated that there are more bacteria living in the colon than there are cells that make up the whole body. When these bacteria are living in proper symbiosis (meaning they contribute to us and we provide an environment for them) we have a healthy intestinal tract, efficient elimination of waste materials, and good nutrient absorption. If, however, the intestinal bacteria are in a state of disarray, they may go from being symbiotic to parasitic. In this case, a toxic reaction can develop in the colon, with symptoms of intestinal discomfort, gas formation, constipation, and poor nutrient utilization."

Acidophilus is a cultured milk into which the bacteria of acidophilus has been introduced. Acidophilus milk aids the growth of healthful intestinal flora and also inhibits the growth of unfriendly bacteria. It works like yogurt except it is much stronger. It converts lactose in milk to lactic acid and this supplements the hydrochloric acid in the stomach, easing digestion in a natural, drugless way. It remains in the stomach to provide protection even after it has been eaten and digested. Acidophilus will speed the intestinal recovery from antibiotics which destroy the small intestinal flora responsible for proper digestion and B vitamin production. Acidophilus is good for reducing the amount of histamine liberated by putrefactive bacteria in the intestine. Biotin deficiency is improved with acidophilus. Calcium is more readily absorbed because of the acidic properties of acidophilus.

Adelle Davis in her book *Let's Get Well* points out that vitamin K as well as all of the B vitamins can be synthesized in the small intestine and in the colon by the same lactic acid producing bacteria. She says that the destruction of this friendly bacteria can cause severe vitamin K deficiencies of folic acid and many other B vitamins. She points out the fact that when these products are taken daily, the entire bacteria population of the intestine, which make 80 percent of the solid material of the stools, become exclusively lacticacid organism which destroys the gas-forming, disease and odor-producing bacteria. (*Yogurt and Acidophilus* by Vincent Licata).

Many physicians in Britain feel that bacterial poisons absorbed from the intestine may directly affect almost every chronic disease. This was common thinking in the medical field in the United States before World War II. Using Acidophilus daily would indeed be a wise decision.

ANTIOXIDANTS AND THE IMMUNE SYSTEM

Antioxidants are known for their role as a preventive aid in controlling excess oxidation caused by free radicals in the body. Free radicals are produced when chemical reactions occur in the body that cause oxidation reactions that get out of control. Free radicals are unstable portions of molecules produced from oxygen and fats. The antioxidants are nutrients and enzymes that either absorb the extra energy released or break down the free radicals to prevent them from getting out of control.

Free radicals occur with basic body functions and are usually controlled by the body, but some dietary excesses have been linked to free radical damage in the body. Polyunsaturated fats are thought to be easily converted to free radicals. Salad dressings, oils fried foods, and most junk foods contains high amounts of polyunsaturated fats that have been linked to free radical production and cell damage. Some believe that aging as well as some forms of cancer and heart disease are related to free radical damage to the cells.

The immune system seems to be easily affected by free radical damage. The cell membranes involved in the immune system contain high amounts of polyunsaturated fatty acids which are highly susceptible to oxidation and free radical damage. These membranes are essential in the immune system response.

We can't eat food without ingesting some pollutants. We do not live in a perfect world. Chemical toxins are in some of the food we eat. Most foods unless grown organically will receive pesticide treatment. Even the water used in irrigation, as well as the air, contain pollutants. Meats are often treated with antibiotics and hormones. The antioxidant defense system in the body however, can help protect the body from these environmental pollutants. A diet rich in food sources and supplements of antioxidants can help.

The exact nutrients needed to strengthen the antioxidant defense system has been debated. Most authorities agree that the most important vitamins and minerals needed to aid the system include A, C, E, B-complex, zinc, copper, manganese, sulfur, and selenium.

The best thing to remember is to improve the diet. Eat a diet rich in fruits, vegetables, and whole grains. Take a supplement of vitamins and minerals that can help protect the immune system.

Beta carotene is a water soluble form of vitamin A that can be efficiently used in the body. It has been attributed to helping strengthen the body in many ways. Good food sources include carrots, sweet potatoes, dark green vegetables, spinach, squash, and broccoli. Yellow fruits, apricots, peaches, nectarines and tomatoes are also good sources.

Vitamin C sources include oranges, strawberries, melons, green peppers, grapefruit, broccoli, and brussels sprouts. Adding extra fruit and vegetables to the diet will most certainly increase the body's immune capabilities.

Selenium is found in tuna, ham, poultry, shellfish, and whole grains. The soil may be depleted of selenium and the foods may be lacking. So, a supplement of this and other nutrients is usually recommended.

There seems to be a lot of promise in antioxidants as a defense mechanism for building the immune system. There are many immune related diseases that cause problems for millions of people throughout the world. Increasing The amounts of foods rich in antioxidant properties while adding a supplement may help the body increase its immune capabilities.

FIBER

Fiber has been a big news item in the medical community during the past few years. Fiber has always been important in the natural nutrition world. Advertisers flood the television and magazines with high fiber food products. There is little dispute that fiber in our diets is essential to good health. This is one area where the medical community and the natural health field agree.

There are two different kinds of fiber: soluble and insoluble. Soluble fiber is found in fruits, vegetables, seeds, nuts, beans and whole grains. Insoluble fiber is found in cereals and some wheat products. The ADA recommends we eat 25 to 30 grams of fiber per day. Most Americans eat less than half this amount.

Fiber, for a period of time, was considered non-essential in our diets. In fact, it was removed from foods to make them smooth and more appetizing. Fiber was thought to have no nutritional benefits. But times have changed and more and more people are realizing the healthy contribution fiber can make in their diets.

Dietary fiber consists mainly of the cell walls of foods. Plants are supported by these cell walls that keep them rigid. Every plant cell has a wall of fibers.

Diets low in dietary fiber allow the food to remain longer in the intestines causing toxins to build up and disease to begin. High protein and fat diets are absorbed mainly in the small intestine. This causes constipation problems. Fiber prevents toxins from building up in the colon by keeping the bowels moving.

Oat Bran

Dr. James W. Anderson, M.D. a professor at the University of Kentucky College of Medicine is credited with his research on high fiber diets with diabetics. He noticed that oat bran brought down their insulin requirements as well as their blood cholesterol levels.

The dose of oat bran was very high. He used a diet of 100 g. of oat bran a day which is about one cup of dry oat bran. Blood cholesterol levels dropped about 20% in this study. The patients also lost weight. Practically, this is a much cheaper and healthier way to lower blood cholesterol.

Appendicitis

Patricia Hausman and Judith Benn Hurley in their book *The Healing Foods* suggest how fiber can prevent appendicitis:

"Of all possible dietary explanations for appendicitis, a low fiber intake has been suspected most. The case for a protective effect from fiber rests on the facts such as these. Appendicitis tends to be more common in countries where the diet is low in fiber. During the war, when appendicitis rates fell, residents of Switzerland and the English Channel Islands were eating more fiber (and less fat) than usual. Surveys in African cities by Denis Burkitt, M.D., have shown that appendicitis is ten times more common in whites than in blacks. In Africa, of course, the former are more likely to follow a Western-type diet. Some research shows that children who develop appendicitis eat less fiber. Jean Brender, Ph.D., and associates at the University of Washington School of Public Health reported in 1985 that children who had eaten the diets richest in fiber were only half as likely to develop the disease."

Diabetes

Diabetic control is often made easier if the person is put on a high fiber diet. Eating foods rich in soluble fiber slows the absorption of food in the blood stream. This helps stop the see sawing in blood sugar levels.

Constipation

Adding fiber to the diet will often end constipation problems. Insoluble fiber will add bulk and start intestinal movement. Constipation can be the cause of toxin build-up and disease. So fiber can help keep the colon functioning.

Colon Cancer

Research has shown that low fiber diets can cause food residue to become hard and remain in the colon for long periods of time. If this mass contains some carcinogenic material, it could make contact with the bowel. When a person eats plenty of fiber, the colon flows more uniformly and the food digestion is more rapid. It is sensible to eat a high fiber diet which is low in fat content. The two combined can help reduce the risk of colon cancer. Though nothing is for certain, common sense will tell us to eat nutritional food high in fiber which are often low in fat.

Hemorrhoids

This problem seems to be associated with a low fiber diet. Constipation and straining appear to lead to this problem. The pressure from straining can cause the veins in the anal area to swell and this is known as hemorrhoids. A high fiber diet along with exercise can do wonders for this problem.

Obesity

Individuals put on high fiber low fat diets usually lose weight but at a slow healthy rate. People on a high fiber, unrefined diet absorb less of the energy they take in the form of food. Fiber increases the amount of energy and fat passed in the stools. It may also prevent the complete absorption of food because the fiber foods pass through the bowel more quickly. Researchers are finding that obesity is not so much a problem of how much we eat but of what we eat.

These are just a few of the benefits of a high fiber diet. It is common sense to eat a diet rich in both soluble and insoluble fiber. This can aid in good health as well as slimming down to your ideal weight. By including fiber in our diets and eating less refined foods, we would see less people suffering from colon and bowel disorders. So start today and add some fiber to your life!

GARLIC

Garlic has been known for it's beneficial properties for thousands of years. Its medicinal value was used anciently and continues to be used for both prevention and healing.

The ancient Egyptians used garlic for food and medicine. The Bible, in Numbers, records the children of Israel complaining that they didn't have garlic during their sojourn in the wilderness after leaving Egypt. The ancient Romans believed in the magical power of garlic. Many European countries (especially the Italians and Spanish) have used garlic for over 2,000 years. The Spanish introduced garlic to the new world. The Chinese also used garlic for food and medicine. In many ancient writings throughout the world, garlic is referred to as a cure for many ailments.

The garlic clove contains a very high concentration of sulphur. Sulphur is a mineral that has the ability to carry oxygen to the body. Sulphur carries the oxygen in the body directly to the infected areas.

Medical science discovered that sulphur caused this rapid healing, so in World War II, flowers of sulphur (an inorganic mined-mineral) was substituted for the garlic. In the army, as in other services, sulfa was used for practically every ailment. Wonderful results were seen and doctors were told to use it in ever increasing amounts.

There is an important difference between the healing process of garlic and this inorganic, man-made remedy. The excess of organic materials not used in healing the infection with garlic is easily passed as harmless vegetable fiber from the body. When the man-made sulfa drug is used, however, the inorganic flowers of sulphur remain in the body. This inorganic mineral eventually combines with the urine and forms a substance that cuts up the urinary tract, causing kidney and bladder problems.

Dr. Morton Walker, D.P.M., in his book *The Healing Powers of Garlic*, discusses the healing ingredients in garlic. "The nutritional content of the average-size clove of garlic has been determined by the United States Department of Agriculture. One clove provides 7 calories of energy; 0.31 gms of protein; 0.01 gms of carbohydrates; 1.4 mg of calcium; 10 mg of phosphorus; 0.07 mg or iron; 0.9 mg of sodium; 26 mg of potassium; 0.01 mg of thiamine (vitamin B1); 0.004 mg of riboflavin (vitamin B2); 0.02 mg of niacin (vitamin B3); and 0.75 mg of ascorbic acid (vitamin C). There are also seventy-five sulfur-containing compounds in garlic. They include: allicin, diallysulfide, cysteic acid, methionine, alliin, and the cyrstalline isolates from allium sativum such as S-methyl cysteine and cycloalliin. It also contains seventeen amino acids, including the eight essential ones."

People are often concerned about the offensive breath odor after eating garlic. This certainly can be a problem.

An answer to this problem was discovered in Japan about thirty years ago. A group of researchers found a way to keep the natural healing benefits without the offending odor. This odor-free aged garlic is now available in health food stores, by mail order, and in supermarkets.

This product has the same curative properties as raw garlic but doesn't seem to irritate the stomach and intestinal tract as raw garlic sometimes can.

Moles and Warts: Place a button of garlic slice on top of the growth. Tape it on with a band-aid.

Rheumatic Pains: Massage painful joints and areas with oil of garlic.

Strep and Sore Throat: Take capsules or oil of garlic.

Respiratory Congestion: Use a garlic paste made of grated garlic and vaseline. Apply to the feet and cover.

These are just a few ideas. Garlic is known for it's antibiotic factors so it is beneficial for infections. It can help increase the body's resistance against bacterial infection. Garlic is a great herb to aid the body's own immune system.

CHLOROPHYLL

Fresh herbs can fill the body's need for chlorophyll. If you cannot find local green herbs in your area such as dandelion, chicory, watercress, miner's lettuce or chickweed, you can always grow your own sprouts. The sprouts that I have used successfully are alfalfa, fenugreek, and radish seeds. They are easy to grow and are excellent to use in salads, sandwiches or in green drinks. Using green drinks is an excellent way to start a spring cleanse.

Using chlorophyll in nourishing liquids is very beneficial for the body. You can also use fruit and vegetable juices as a cleansing fast. It can be one day at a time, or for a period of five to ten days or longer if your body can withstand it. You should mentally prepare yourself for a major cleanse.

Green traditionally is part of the spring cleanse and is associated with building and cleansing the body. Green is associated with chlorophyll which is known as "Natures Green Healer." The chlorophyll molecule closely resembles hemoglobin, the red pigment in human blood. Human blood contains a red pigment with a web of carbon, hydrogen, oxygen and nitrogen atoms grouped around a single atom of iron. Chlorophyll is a green pigment with a similar web of the same atoms, except that its centerpiece is a single atom of magnesium.

A research scientist, E. Bircher called chlorophyll "Concentrated Sun Power." He said that "Chlorophyll increases the function of the heart, affects the vascular system, the intestines, the uterus and the lungs." It is considered one of the best tonics for mankind. Liquid chlorophyll is very beneficial for the whole digestive system. It is known to enhance the effect of vitamins and minerals and helps in proper digestion to give the body its full value.

Another discovery of chlorophyll is its antiseptic qualities. An antiseptic strong enough to kill germs and yet soothing and healing to the tissues. Chlorophyll solution was found to increase the resistance of the cells and inhibit the growth of bacteria, therefore preventing the spread of germs.

The daily use of chlorophyll is very beneficial for the prevention of diseases like high blood pressure, arthritis and arteriosclerosis along with other health benefits known to improve these diseases. Chlorophyll has the cleansing ability to help in the removal of toxic material from the walls of the blood vessels.

COENZYME Q10

Coenzyme Q10 is a nutrient that aids in oxygenation within the cells and tissues. It is a vitamin-like supplement that is found in foods like beef, sardines, spinach and peanuts. CoQ10 is considered an essential nutrient that boosts the biochemical ability to activate cellular energy. Many people are deficient in this essential nutrient, however, this is not necessary now. CoEnzyme Q10 is another discovery to benefit mankind and stands along side other vital antioxidants such as vitamin A, E, C, and sulphur-bearing amino acids.

Researchers are finding CoQ10 to benefit ailments associated with its nutrient deficiencies, such as heart disease, aging, cancer and obesity. Richard A. Passwater, Ph.D., in his article Coenzyme Q10: The Nutrient Of The 90's, written in *Health Connection,* April 1987 says, "Dr. Bliznadov's first CoQ10 experiment was on the immune system. He found that CoQ10 doubled the immune system's ability to clear invading organisms from the blood. His research group's next experiment series found that CoQ10 doubled antibody levels. Next, they found that CoQ10 protected against chemically-induced cancer with fewer tumors, smaller tumors and increased survival times. The research group even demonstrated increased resistance to virus infections."

We now have a natural food supplement to stimulate the immune system. We need all the help we can get to protect our immune system. A strong immune system protects us against many diseases, colds, flu, cancer to name a few. AIDS, in epidemic proportions, along with Candida albicans and lupus, Epstein Barr and many immune deficiency diseases can be helped.

Even though CoQ10 is found in some food, scientists found that sufficient amounts derived from food sources declines with age and can actually stop altogether at some point. As more research is conducted on this natural nutrient, we will find more and more diseases being helped. In the meantime, we can use this to protect our immune system and help in the diseases of the heart, in aging, cancer and obesity.

EPA - LIPIDS
Missing Link To Balance Body Chemistry

EPA (eicosapentaenoic acid) is a unique fatty acid found in the high fish diets of Greenland Eskimos. Research by Drs. Bang and Dyerberg revealed that the Eskimo diets were almost the opposite of what was recommended by the American Heart Association. The Eskimos however, do not get heart disease. Their high fish consumption also revealed that they had low levels of blood cholesterol.

Dr. Jeffery S. Bland, Ph.D., says in his article "Fish Oils," In *Complementary Medicine Magazine,* Sept. 1985, "It was first thought that possibly the high polyunsaturate content of the Eskimo diet was responsible for the reduced incidence of heart disease; however, linoleic acid, an unsaturated fatty acid found in high concentrations in the standard American diet did not lower blood cholesterol in the same way as fish oils." This created a missing link to balance body chemistry. After extensive study, it was found that oils such as corn, safflower, sunflower, and soy, which are rich in linoleic acid, were not nearly so effective in reducing blood cholesterol levels as were the fish oils rich in EPA.

This is very revealing, for medical doctors have warned and cautioned us for years about the connection between cholesterol and heart disease.

The American diet, as well as others changed to eating high amounts of animal meat, vegetable oils, and then the diet became depleted of EPA and DHA (docosahexaenoic acid), which increased the risk of cardiovascular disease. Americans listened and their bodies became depleted in the fish that contains these lipids which caused an imbalance in their diets. This made the people worse off than they were in the first place.

Research indicates that heart disease is reduced with high consumption of deep sea fish lipids. Now a new concept makes us understand how a balance of fatty acids is vital to overall health. When we are depleted in just one of the essential fatty acids, an imbalance is created and all kinds of diseases can invade the body. The discovery of fish lipids concentrate has made it possible to obtain these much needed oils. They are called "Omega-3" fatty acids. They are very different from the common fatty acids found in vegetables which are called "Omega-6" fatty acids. "Omega-9" fats are what the typical American diet consists of, which are derived from saturated fats obtained from animal sources such as beef, pork and butterfat. Most health-oriented people realize that the body needs a balance. Now scientists have proven that a balance of fatty acids is as vital to health as a balance in vitamins, minerals and amino acids.

These fish oil lipids not only improve the blood to protect against heart disease, but help protect the immune system. In animal testing they were found to help protect against auto-immune ailments like lupus erythematosus. They protected against kidney damage when the oil was added, as well as prolonged the animals life. Fish lipids are beneficial to enzyme function, glandular health and play a vital role in brain and nerve function. The EPA in the fish oil lipids also controls artery spasms, blood clotting, blood viscosity, lowers cholesterol and triglycerides. Recently they have been found to help in stiffness and aches of arthritis. We are seeing dietary fatty acids in a new light as a source to improve multiple body functions. They help to maintain metabolic processes, a increased proper function of the organs, and keep the blood pure and healthy.

The fish oil (Omega-3 fatty acids) are rich in fat and cholesterol content, but their fat content is unusually different because it has large quantities of long-chain, polyunsaturates. These long chain fatty acids are what gives fish the so called "fishy" odor.

Fatty acids are what scientists describe as the chemical building blocks from which lipids (fats and oils) are made. When the fatty acids are converted from, fats they are either burned for energy; stored to be used later or synthesized into prostaglandins which act like hormones. Richard A. Passwater, Ph.D., says, "The reason that we need the body well stocked with the proper fatty acids is so that it can make as much prostaglandin as it needs. The various human prostaglandins are not readily obtainable in the diet, and if they were, since they are complex molecules, they would mostly be destroyed by the digestive process. Therefore, we should fortify our body's own production of prostaglandins to assure an optimum supply. Because prostaglandins control a multitude of essential functions in the body in relation to such seemingly unrelated disorders as heart attacks, high blood pressure, arthritis, menstrual cramps, allergies, asthma, migraine headaches, fertility, glaucoma, and perhaps, cancer. Prostaglandins are not stored, every tissue makes prostaglandins as needed. Their effect is brief since they are quickly inactivated by enzymes. Some organ systems depend on a balance of prostaglandins which act in opposite ways."

The role of fish lipids in the diet is an exciting one. It can be useful as another supplement to build up the immune system, in stress, P.M.S., Candida, not to mention heart disease and arthritis. This may indeed be the missing link to balance body chemistry.

GERMANIUM

Germanium is a naturally occurring element like gold and silver. It is considered a trace mineral. It is also referred to as a semi-metal or mineral. There is probably no simple differences between a metal and mineral. Many people have become interested and excited about this amazing product.

Dr. Stephen Levine who is the director of The Allergy Research Group, a biochemical development firm located in Berkeley, California is excited about Germanium and the research findings. "I've never seen anything like it. It has three principle benefits, almost instant pain relief, antiviral effects, and anticancer properties. One man I know had kidney cancer, spreading rapidly. He was in terrible pain and losing dangerous amounts of weight. He started taking one gram a day of Ge-132 and within a month his pain was gone and he had gained 40 pounds."

Studies are on going in Japan researching the effects of Germanium-132 or Ge-132 on different forms of cancer and disease. American scientists are also researching this product.

Germanium was first discovered to be very beneficial to health by a Japanese scientist Dr. Kazuhiko Asai. He became interested in it for many reasons. One was that he heard the Russians used it as a rejuvenator. He studied the Germanium in plants. He also found that Germanium enhanced oxygen utilization in plants and animals. He found also that it has an oxygen sparing effect. In studies with mice, he found that less oxygen was required to maintain respiration when those tissues were supplemented with Germanium. Dr. Asai found in his studies that 100-300 milligrams of Germanium a day improved many illnesses such as cancer, AIDS, arthritis, cholesterol, viral infections, and candidiasis. Germanium attaches itself to the oxygen molecules enhancing their function. The body needs oxygen to aid the immune system and rid the body of toxins.

Germanium is found in only small amounts in plants. For this reason it is quite expensive. Germanium is found in sheet fungus, ginseng, sushi, aloe vera, garlic, comfrey, onions, and chlorella.

INTERFERON

Interferon has been touted as a miracle drug for cancer. Drug companies produce interferon artificially.

Interferon is an anti-viral protein produced by the white blood cells. It is an immune substance that counteracts viruses and cancer. It is produced by the body naturally when it is given the proper nutrients. It travels through the blood, casting its protective net over different parts of the body. Interferon, when prompted by one type of virus, can protect cells against other viruses, as well as the original one. Interferon also helps to regulate other immune cells, by increasing the production of fighting T-cells.

The Japanese discovered that a component in LICORICE stimulates the immune system to produce interferon.

The following will stimulate production of INTERFERON—CHLOROPHYLL—ASTRAGALUS — VITAMIN C WITH BIO-FLAVONOIDS—SEA VEGETABLES SUCH AS KELP, DULSE—BLUE-GREEN ALGAE—GINKGO—MILK THISTLE—PAU D'ARCO—SCHIZANDRA—SIBERIAN GINSENG—SUMA—WHEAT GRASS JUICE—DONG QUAI—ECHINACEA—RED RASPBERRY—HO-SHOU-WU—GERMANIUM.

FEVER PRODUCES INTERFERON—We should never suppress a fever unless it is unusually high.

TEA TREE OIL
(Melaleuca alternifolia)

Tea Tree Oil is a gift in a small bottle from New South Wales, Australia. Tea tree oil is the essence produced by the distillation of the leaves of Melaleuca Alternifolia, the medicinal tea tree. There are more than 300 varieties of tea tree but only one is known to produce this valuable medicinal oil. Research shows that pure tea tree oil is an extremely complex substance, containing at least 48 organic compounds. All the compounds work together in synergy to produce the maximum healing power. These compounds consist mainly of terpinenes, cymones, pinenes, terpineols, cineol, sesquiterpenes, and sesquiterpene alcohols. It also contains the organic compound viridiflorence.

Tea tree oil is four to five times stronger than most household disinfectants, yet is gentle to the skin and more versatile and safe to use. Tea tree oil is successfully used around the world for throat and mouth conditions, in gynecological conditions, in dental treatment for pyorrhea, gingivitis, nerve capping and hemorrhages. It is found to be more effective in dirty or pus laden conditions, unlike any other antiseptic, and it also has a remarkable effect on a broad spectrum of skin fungi including candida.

Tea tree oil is an effective bactericide killing a broad spectrum of bacteria and some stubborn fungi such as candida and athletes foot. It is safe for healthy tissue. It is a strong organic solvent and will disperse pus in pimples or infected wounds and neutralize the venom of minor insect bites. It acts as a mild local anaesthetic, soothing to cuts and burns and mouth sores. It kills bacteria to penetrate into skin layers, reaching deep into abscess in gums or beneath fingernails.

TEA TREE OIL USES

ABRASIONS - Use a few drops of the pure tea tree oil.

ACNE & PIMPLES - Use directly on pimples several times a day or mix with water and rinse face, or area of pimples.

ARTHRITIS - Mix about 4 or 5 drops in a small amount of olive oil and massage joints.

ATHLETE'S FOOT - After washing feet thoroughly, apply pure tea tree oil.

BITES - Mosquitoes, stings - dilute 1 part tea tree oil with 3 parts olive oil.

BOILS - Use pure tea tree oil several times a day.

BRUSHING TEETH - Put a few drops on tooth paste to prevent plaque.

BURNS & SCALDS (Minor) - Dilute one part tea tree oil with 10 parts olive oil.

COLD SORES - Apply directly on the sore. Repeat several times a day. It should stop the cold sore before it erupts on the skin.

CONGESTION - Lungs, bronchitis, laryngitis, emphysema - sprinkle a few drops on a cloth and breathe through the mouth, exhaling through the nose.

COUGHS & CROUP - Add pure oil to steam water or vaporizer and inhale. Rub pure oil into chest and back.

CRADLE CAP - Mix with a little olive oil and rub in scalp.

CUTS - Rub pure oil on cuts. It is healing and prevents infections.

DOGS & CATS - Use with shampoo when bathing animals. Kills lice and worms.

FACE CLEANSER - Use a few drops in water and splash on face to prevent infections.

FEET (Smelly) - Add five to ten drops of pure tea tree oil to warm water, let them soak for five or ten minutes.

MOUTH SORES (Sore gums, plague) - Put a few drops in warm water and rinse mouth or dab on sores in mouth.

MUSCLE ACHES - Add a few drops to bath water and soak, or rub pure oil on sore muscles.

NAIL INFECTIONS -Use pure oil under nails.

NASAL ULCERS - Use pure oil on ulcers or mix with water and soak area.

RASHES & RINGWORMS - Apply pure oil to affected area.

SINUS CONGESTION - Use pure oil in boiling water and sniff the vapor.

SPRAINS - Use pure oil directly on sprain.

THROAT (Sore) - Add about 5 drops of pure oil to warm water and gargle.

VAGINAL RINSE (Infections) - 4 parts tea tree oil in 1,000 parts water.

WARTS - Apply directly on warts 2 to 3 times a day.

PHYTOCHEMICALS

Phytochemicals are substances found in fruits and vegetables that appear to play a role in protecting the body against diseases affecting the immune system such as cancer. There are hundreds of different phytochemicals only a few of which have been studied. Many foods contain numerous varieties of these phytochemicals. These compounds interact in complex ways and also overlap in their functions. Many of them are brightly colored and give plants their array of hues.

The difference between phytochemicals and other food components is that they appear to have no actual nutritional value or calories. They don't participate in the normal functions of the body. But they seem to be able to benefit the immune system in fighting disease. New information is appearing rapidly, and it is difficult to keep up with all the data.

"As exciting as scientists find this area of inquiry, they don't pretend to have all the answers yet. 'While there's no doubt that diets rich in fruits and vegetables are cancer-protective, much of what we know about individual phytochemicals is still speculative,' cautioned nutrition researcher Phyllis Bowen, co-director of the University of Illinois' functional foods programs." (Napier, Kristine, M.P.H., R.D., *Harvard Health Letter*, April 1995)

Phytochemicals can be classified by different methods such as chemical name, food sources, and anti-cancer action. The following are some of the phytochemicals listed according to their chemical names.

INDOLES

Indoles are probably the most commonly known phytochemical because of their recent popularity. They seem to increase the activity of enzymes that can detoxify carcinogens and may also change the hormone estrogen into a benign form, reducing the risk of breast cancer as well as other cancers. Scientists think the indoles have the ability to block cancer causing substances before they enter the cells (they are found in cruciferous vegetables).

ALLYL SULFIDES

The allyl sulfides are credited with boosting the production of an enzyme that may actually aid in excreting carcinogens more efficiently. Some have been found to help inhibit the capacity of tumor cells to reproduce (found in onions, leeks, and garlic).

FLAVONOIDS

The flavonoids are often found in vitamin C combinations. They consist of different chemicals commonly found in fruits and vegetables. Flavonoids are considered to be essential in their actions as antioxidants in reducing the risk of cancer. They are able to protect the cells from carcinogens and suppress the malignant changes in cells. Some researchers also believe that they may inhibit the ability of hormones to bind to the cells limiting cancer development (found in fruits and vegetables).

DITHIOLTHIONES

Dithiolthiones help trigger the production of enzymes that may protect the cell's DNA from being damaged by carcinogens (found in cruciferous vegetables).

ISOFLAVONES

These are found in soy beans and soy based products. Studies have found that in countries where soy products are consumed regularly, there is a lower incidence of breast and prostate cancer. This is credited in part to the isoflavones. They act similarly to antioxidants in blocking carcinogens and inhibiting the growth of tumors. (found in soy beans)

LIGNANS

Lignans are found in many foods especially linseed found in flax. They have antioxidant effects in blocking and inhibiting the cancer cell grwoth. Flax is high in omega-3 fatty acids, which are thought to help prevent many different

immune related diseases such as colon cancer and heart disease (found in flax) (See April 1995, *Today's Herbs*).

LIMONENE

The highest concentration of limonene is found in the rind of citrus fruits. It stimulates the production of certain enzymes known to help eliminate carcinogens. It may also reduce the size of mammary tumors (found in citrus fruits).

CAFFEIC ACID

Caffeic acid has been found to make carcinogens easier to secrete from the body by making them more water soluble. It may inhibit the formation of carcinogens and suppress the growth of lung and skin tumors (found in citrus fruit).

SAPONINS

This includes a large group of modified carbohyrates that are found to contain 11 different varieties of saponins. Saponins have been researched and found to contain anti-cancer properties.

INDOLES

Cruciferous vegetables have long been encouraged as part of a healthy diet. In fact, we are often told by the medical and health communities to increase the amount of vegetables in the diet to increase health. But what is the secret ingredient in these cruciferous vegetables that makes them so essential for healing and preventing many ailments including cancer?

The cruciferous vegetables are from the cabbage family which include broccoli, Brussels sprouts, cabbage, cauliflower, collards, kale, radishes, rutabaga, turnips, mustard seed and watercress. These contain a bounty of cancer-fighting substances some of which increase the production of enzymes that are responsible for defusing carcinogens and ridding them from the body. The indoles specifically seem to have a profound effect on the metabolism of estrogen by helping the body to produce benign forms of the hormone, which don't promote some forms of cancer, especially breast cancer.

Different studies have been done researching the effectiveness of indoles. One conducted in 1991 followed 12 individuals for a week as they ate a diet rich in cruciferous vegetables. After the week, there was a 50% increase in good estrogen in the blood levels. An article in the *Ladies' Home Journal*, July, 1994 reported on a study done on one particular indole known as Indole-3 Carbinol. The results seem to indicate that this indole helps change the way in which estrogen breaks down in women's bodies. As this estrogen breaks down it either becomes harmful or benign. This indole helps in preventing estrogen from becoming harmful and increasing the risk of breast cancer. Another Japanese study on mice reported that those exposed to cancer causing agents and given the indole, were much less likely to develop mouth cancer.

Individuals concerned about their health have begun purchasing these cruciferous vegetables in large quantities, and with good reason. there have been over 50 studies conducted in recent years confirming the benefits of this incredible nutrient. These benefits should be taken seriously.

The vegetables eaten raw or lightly steamed seem to have the most benefit. Boiling is known to decrease the nutritional value by half. Supplements are also available containing indoles which make getting an abundance in the diet easier.

AILMENTS

ADDICTIONS ⸻

SYMPTOMS

Anxiety—Depression—Despair—Fatigue—Headaches—Hypoglycemia—Indigestion—Insomnia—Irritability—Skin Problems—Tension—These are the most common. Other ailments arise because of addictions, such as Kidney and Liver Damage—Nervous System Disorders—Immune System Disorders—Malnutrition—

CAUSES

Allergies are one cause of addictions. We usually crave the same foods that cause us physical or mental reactions. Inherited biochemistry weakness occurs when a child is born lacking minerals, vitamins and essential nutrients. The craving for alcohol can be inherited because lack of nutrients causes cravings of all kinds.

Addictive habits can be caused because of chronic fatigue, boredom, to relieve and forget, or from emotional, physical or mental pain. Thyroid disorders are implicated with addictions.

Sugar addiction is the most common and wide spread. It starts when the mother uses sugar when pregnant. It is then supported when sugar water is given in the hospital. Other addictions are tobacco, caffeine, alcohol, heroine, and cocaine. An addiction can result from any substance that causes cravings and prevents eating properly.

NUTRITIONAL THERAPY

Nutritional imbalances are the main cause of addictions. Healthy people have no need for addictions. When cravings are seen as a deficiency of the body, the body can recover with cleansing diets, the proper food and supplements.

Addictive persons have a much higher requirement for extra nutrients than those not addicted. They lack the nutrients even before the addiction starts. This is one of the main causes of craving an addictive substance. Addictions can come from negative emotions, inability to cope with problems and feelings of unworthiness.

Willpower and determination are essential to overcome addictions. A change of diet is essential. Eliminate meat, dairy products, sugar and white flour products.

A liver cleanse is vital to help rid the body of residue of addictive substances. Use an herbal liver formula, milk thistle, along with 1 cup pure water with juices of 1 lemon, 1 lime, 1 T. of fresh grated ginger, and 1 T. of pure olive oil. Take in the morning or before retiring. Use it with a three day cleanse.

Drink fresh carrot, celery and parsley juice because it is rich in iron, calcium, potassium and vitamin A. Fresh juices will help fill nutritional needs rapidly. Herbs that will help strengthen the body to overcome addictions are: Bee Pollen, Ginseng, Ginkgo, Gotu Kola, Burdock, Echinacea, Ho-Shou-Wu, Licorice, Lobelia, Passion Flower, Suma and Valerian.

HERBAL FORMULAS

Herbs are used to clean, restore and maintain health. To detoxify from an addiction, use colon, blood, liver and nervine formulas. Additional formulas are added to treat specific ailments such as allergies, kidney infections, headaches, parasites, hypoglycemia, indigestion, etc.

Blood Cleansers—Colon Cleansers—Digestive System—Energy and Stamina—Glandular System—Immune Builders—Nervous System and Brain—Urinary System—Female or Male Formulas—

VITAMINS, MINERALS AND SUPPLEMENTS

Nutritional support is essential for recovering from an addiction. Clinical studies have found that addicted people tend to eat a lot of sweets and fast foods which are deficient in vital nutrients.

Vitamin C, is essential for the adrenal glands as well as a protection for the immune system. B-complex vitamin deficiency causes cravings for addictive substances. They are necessary for liver detoxification and nervous system function. Vitamin E is an antioxidant which protects the immune system and the adrenal glands. It is essential for the heart, circulatory system and liver. The liver is often damaged by addictive substances.

Calcium and magnesium are essential. Trace minerals and a multivitamin supplement are essential.

Essential Fatty Acids are needed daily. Salmon oil and flaxseed oil are beneficial. Amino acids help restore digestion and assimilation and repair cells and tissues.

Chlorophyll and Blue-Green Algae will help clean the blood and cells.

AGING ──────────

SYMPTOMS

Autoimmune Diseases—Autointoxication— Constipation—Degenerative Diseases—Lack of Exercise—Nutritional Deficiency—

CAUSES

Premature aging can be sped up or slowed down depending on the life style we choose. Hate, anger, resentments and negative thoughts speed up our biological time bomb while love, laughter, and positive thoughts slow down the aging process. A type A personality, who is on the go all the time, and cannot slow down for recreation or relaxation may have an early heart attack and speed up the aging process.

Hearing loss goes along with aging. High fat in the blood can cause hearing problems and some doctors feel that hearing loss is one symptom of future heart disease.

As we reach maturity, at about age 19, there are cells in our body that stop reproducing. They are sensor cells in the intestinal tract, the nervous system, including the brain cells and the myocardiac, and muscles of the ear cells that stop reproducing and gradually lose their functional potential.

Free radicals, when unchecked, disrupt at the cellular level and cause diseases such as cancer, immune disorders, inflammatory conditions and others. Free radicals are similar to an acid burning a cell which creates a chain reaction and causes all kinds of disruptions. These free radicals are caused by many things such as alcohol, tobacco, radiation, nuclear fallout, drugs, over the counter drugs, diet, food additives, stress, air pollution, which contains lead, cadmium and mercury, and even the lack of exercise. Rancid oils also cuase free radical damage.

NUTRITIONAL THERAPY

Exercise is important. Lack of exercise causes the loss of bone and muscle mass and inevitable physical degeneration. Even a little exercise goes a long way. Food assimilates better when one exercises. Good nutrition and exercise protects the cardiovascular system, maintains circulation and oxygen to the cells and tissues. A lack of exercise can speed up the aging process. Exercise is a good investment in your future health.

The following foods contain nucleic acid, which protects against aging. These foods regulate metabolism and cell structure and promote proper enzyme action and hormone balance.

Asparagus, beets, bran, brewer's yeast, buckwheat, chickpeas, honey, kidney beans, lentils, lima beans, millet, navy beans, nuts, especially almonds, sardines, salmon, soy beans, split peas, tuna, vegetables, steamed and fresh (and green leafy), wheat germ, and yogurt, are all beneficial.

Sprouts contain all the essential amino acids. Include in your diet raw fruit and vegetables juices, fresh salads, steamed vegetables, fruit and whole grains, seeds, nuts and beans.

Herbs to help slow the aging process are: Bee Pollen, Cayenne, Echinacea, Ginkgo, Ginseng, Gotu Kola, Hawthorn, Horsetail, Ho-Shou-Wu, Kelp, Pau D'Arco, Saffron and Suma.

HERBAL FORMULAS

As we age, we lose the ability to digest, assimilate and eliminate properly. Herbs contain vitamins, minerals and enzymes to nourish and strengthen the digestive, and eliminative system.

Blood Cleansers—Circulatory System—Colon Cleansers—Digestive System—Energy and Stamina—Immune Builders—Nervous System and Brain—Structural System—Urinary System—Female or Male Formulas—

VITAMINS, MINERALS AND SUPPLEMENTS

The antioxidants are vital for aging. Vitamin A and C are often lacking in the elderly. This can cause a break down in the mucous membranes and cause infections as well as pneumonia. The B-complex vitamins are also lacking and are needed for proper digestion, brain function and stamina, as well as a feeling of well-being.

Minerals are very important for assimilation of nutrients. Calcium and magnesium help in strengthening the bones and muscles. Iron helps nourish the blood. Potassium is essential for the heart muscles. Selenium and zinc help protect the body from free radical damage.

Acidophilus helps in the digestion of food and supplements and provides the friendly bacteria in the colon. Chlorophyll and blue green algae help clean and nourish the blood. They contain properties to help the body produce its own interferon to protect the immune system. CoQ10 and germanium help in providing oxygen to the cells. Lecithin is needed for the nervous system

and brain function. Flaxseed oil and salmon oil are needed to prevent cholesterol from collecting on the artery walls.

AIDS
(Acquired Immune Deficiency Syndrome)

SYMPTOMS

Appetite and Weight Loss—Brain and Neurological Disorders—Candida—Cancer—Fatigue—Fevers—Infections—Intestinal Problems—Immune System Disorders— Skin Diseases—Many more symptoms can develop.

CAUSES

AIDS is caused by a virus that completely breaks down the immune system. Dr. Eva Snead feels that this virus was created in the laboratories. She says that if you have been vaccinated you have the virus. The vaccines were made from the kidney of the green African monkeys. Dr. William Campbell Douglass, M. D., explains in detail in his book, *AIDS The End of Civilization.* When the immune system is weak, germs and viruses can invade the body and cause all kinds of diseases. Sexually transmitted diseases are increasing, and the drugs used in these diseases may be one reason AIDS is growing.

NUTRITIONAL THERAPY

Foods to help heal the body and boost the immune system are raw foods, such as fruit and vegetables, especially those high in vitamins A and C, which are fish liver oils, yellow vegetables and fruits, citrus fruits, strawberries, kale, alfalfa sprouts, papaya, broccoli, parsley and wheatgrass.

Onions, garlic, cabbage, turnips, and winter squash are nourishing. Use kelp and paprika for seasoning along with fresh lemon juice and cold-pressed oils. Use millet or buckwheat and brown rice cooked in a thermos which retain the enzymes for proper digestion. Sprouted grains and beans before cooking will help supply nutrients.

Herbs to help build the immune system are: Garlic, Bee Pollen, Echinacea, Burdock, Ginkgo, Golden Seal, Kelp, Licorice, Pau D'Arco, Psyllium and Suma.

HERBAL FORMULAS

Blood Cleansers—Colds, Flu, Fevers and Allergy Formulas—Colon Cleansers—Digestive System—Energy and Stamina—Immune Builders—Infection Fighters—Nervous System and Brain—Urinary System—Female or Male Formulas—

VITAMINS, MINERALS AND SUPPLEMENTS

The antioxidant vitamins and minerals are needed; vitamin A, C, D, E, and minerals selenium and zinc. The B-complex are needed for digestion and for brain and nervous system health.

A multi-mineral supplement is essential for the proper digestion of vitamins and nutrients. Calcium and magnesium, potassium and chromium are vital for the immune function.

Acidophilus is needed. Candida is common with AIDS. Chlorophyll and Blue-Green Algae have antibiotic properties and are high in vitamins such as K and beta carotene. CoQ10 and Germanium are needed for providing oxygen to the blood. Flax Seed Oil, Lecithin, and Salmon Oil will all strengthen the immune system.

ALCOHOLISM

SYMPTOMS

Arrests for Alcohol related offenses—Blackouts—Cirrhosis—Depression—Delirium—Divorce (seen in 50% alcoholics)—Drugs (illicit)—Emotional Problems—Flushing—Forgetfulness—Heart Palpitation—Hepatitis—Hypertension—Hypoglycemia—Immune Function Disorders—Indigestion—Insomnia—Leg Cramps—Malnutrition—Nicotine Dependence—Numbness in Feet and Hands—Sexual Problems—Ulcers—Urinary Problems—

CAUSES

Little is know about the direct causes, but one half of alcoholics have at least one parent who is an alcoholic. There are certain personality traits typically found, such as low self-esteem, depressive personality, and self-destructive tendencies. Feelings of guilt and frustration are also common.

Children of alcoholics are more likely to use drugs and tranquilizers. Children inherit weakness from their parents, including malnutrition. There is a connection between a genetic factor and a chemical dependency.

Alcohol destroys brain cells and weakens the hypothalamus which controls the appetite. It damages the nervous system. Allergies can be one cause of turning to drinking. Foods such as corn and corn products, milk, wheat, chocolate and sugar, increase hypoglycemia symptoms and causes damage to the body.

Most alcoholics are either hypoglycemic or borderline diabetic. Their digestion is always impaired and hydrochloric acid is usually needed. Licorice root is very helpful for alcoholics. They are usually depleted in minerals and need large amounts to make up for the lack of them in the past. The lack of minerals can be passed on from parent to child. The thyroid has to be dealt with. Kelp is beneficial for the thyroid.

When some alcoholics quit drinking, they often begin eating large amounts of sugar products and drinking strong coffee. Sugar products increases hypoglycemia symptoms. They should be cautioned that it is harmful to the body, and to nourish the system so they aren't dependent on sugar.

NUTRITIONAL THERAPY

Alcohol cravings are associated with poor nutrition. One study of alcoholics placed on a raw food diet showed they began to spontaneously avoid alcohol (and tobacco). In another study a "junk food" diet, when coffee was added, led to increased alcohol consumption. Animal studies showed alcohol was preferred when they were made B vitamin-deficient. (Werbach, M.D. Melvyn R., " Nutritional Influences on Illness.")   A hypoglycemia diet is very beneficial for alcoholics. Meals should be frequent and nourishing. Fresh fruit and vegetables, sprouts, almonds, brown rice, millet, raw fertile eggs, baked potatoes, legumes, whole grains, lentils, soups and salads using lots of vegetables including onions and garlic are excellent. Thermos cooking will provide enzymes to strengthen the stomach. A free-form amino acid supplement would be beneficial.

Herbs to help build up the immune system and cleans the blood are: Bee Pollen, Golden Seal, Burdock, Cayenne, Echinacea, Ginger, Hops, Gotu Kola, Hawthorn, Kelp, Licorice, Milk Thistle, Passion Flower, Pau D'Arco, Psyllium, Saffron, Suma and Valerian.

HERBAL FORMULAS

These formulas listed are to strengthen the immune system, clean the blood and build up the pancreas, liver and brain. Other formulas may be needed for symptoms such as indigestion, headaches, and aches and pains.

Blood Cleansers—Colon Cleansers—Digestive System—Energy and Stamina—Glandular System—Immune System—Nervous System and Brain—Urinary System—Female or Male Formulas—

VITAMINS, MINERALS AND SUPPLEMENTS

All vitamins and minerals are needed to make up for the tremendous loss caused from drinking and from not eating right. Vitamins A and C will help protect the lungs and mucous membranes to prevent infections. The B-complex vitamins help eliminate toxins from the liver and help in digestion. Vitamin E nourishes the veins and the heart.

Calcium, magnesium and potassium are essential for strengthening the bones, flesh and muscles. Selenium and zinc will build up the immune system and are healing.

Acidophilus is needed to protect the body from the bad bacteria. Chlorophyll and Blue-Green Algae are rich in nutrients to help the body produce its own interferon. CoQ10 and Germanium protect the immune system and the veins. Lecithin is needed to protects the nerves and brain.

ALLERGIES ————————

SYMPTOMS

DIGESTIVE—Food Intolerance—Metallic Taste—Dry Mouth—Canker Sores—Stinging Tongue—Heartburn— Indigestion—Nausea— Vomiting—Diarrhea—Constipation— Intestinal Gas—Food Cravings—Pains—Gall Bladder—EAR—Frequent Ear Infections— Hearing Loss—Ears Popping—Imbalance— Itching—Noise Sensitivity—HEADACHES— Can be Allergies— NERVOUS SYSTEM— Confusion—Depression—Anger—Anxiety— Irritability—Hyperactivity—Learning and Memory Problems — Restlessness — MUSCULAR AND SKELETAL— Arthritis— Fatigue—Aches in Neck, Back or Shoulders— Joint Pain—Spasms—RESPIRATORY AND

THROAT—Asthma—Cough—Frequent Colds—Hay Fever—Nose Bleeds—Post Nasal Drip—Wheezing—Shortness of Breath—Chest Tightness—Hoarseness—Dry, Sore or Tickly Throat—SKIN—Acne—Blotches—Dark Circles Under the Eyes—Flushing—Hives— Itching—Psoriasis—Eczema—

CAUSES

Allergies are considered a disorder of the immune system. Approximately 35 million Americans suffer from one type of allergy or another. The causes are due to an internal imbalance and a weakened immune system. An imbalance is created by the food we eat, air we breathe or the chemicals we come in contact with. This causes the mucous membranes to become too thin (runny, drippy nose) or too thick (stuffy nose, congestion in the throat or lungs). Healthy mucous membranes prevent undigested proteins and toxins from entering the bloodstream. Toxins are washed out of the sinuses and down the throat and into the digestive tract, where they are neutralized and eliminated from the body.

Allergies are implicated in hyperactivity, (in adults also), mental illness, arthritis and a host of other seemingly unrelated aliments.

The colon, which is the "intestinal" part of the system, plays a vital function in preventing allergies. Its role is to eliminate waste material. Faulty eating habits, junk food, wrong food combining, heavy meat and sugar diet, and unbalanced diet, plus all the toxins we eat and breathe, cause the colon to become congested or "constipated." The colon harbors all manner of toxins, which when congested, will poison the body when released in the blood stream. This state of autointoxication lowers immune system and sets the stage for allergies.

NUTRITIONAL THERAPY

A cleansing diet using blood purifying herbs. Digestion of food must be complete using is beneficial. Digestive enzymes and hydrochloric acid.

Colon cleansing is essential. Juice fasts, using carrot, celery and raw apple juice can help. When the liver is clogged with fats and accumulated toxins, it cannot produce histaminase, which is the bodies protection against allergies.

The adrenals need to be strengthened. Their job is to provide hormones which render foreign proteins harmless. Healthy mucous membranes do not allow foreign proteins and toxins to enter the bloodstream and cause allergies.

Avoid chemicals that irritate the mucous membranes. A constant contact with chemicals, such as formaldehyde will cause irritation. Formaldehyde is found in wood, carpeting, to treat insulation and in permanent press clothing to prevent wrinkling. Dust mites thrive in household fabrics. They can cause irritation to the mucous membranes.

Try a juice fast for a week. If this is difficult, start with one day, then two, three and so forth. A good liver flush, which can be used every morning while fasting can speed the healing process. Combine 1 teaspoon olive oil, (which cleans the liver and gallbladder), 1/2 teaspoon fresh ginger, (which settles the stomach), 1 teaspoon fenugreek, (which cleans the stomach of mucus), 1 teaspoon of ground dandelion herb, (a nutritive herb, rich in minerals and also cleans the liver), juice of one whole fresh lemon (which neutralizes acids and cleans the liver), and a pinch of cayenne (makes everything work better).

Take 1 cup of boiling distilled water, let the water cool for a few minutes, then add the above ingredients, and add the olive oil , just before drinking.

Herbs to help with allergies are: Bee Pollen, (start with small amounts), Burdock, Cayenne, Echinacea, Ginger, Golden Seal, Kelp Licorice, Lobelia, Pau D'Arco, Saffron, (helps digest oils.)

HERBAL FORMULAS

Blood Cleansers—Colds, Flu, Fever and Allergy — Colon Cleansers — Digestive System — Glandular System — Immune Builders—Infection Fighters—Nervous System and Brain—Urinary System—Female or Male Formulas—

VITAMINS, MINERALS AND SUPPLEMENTS

Vitamin A improves health of mucous membranes. B-Complex is essential for healthy membranes and digestion. Vitamin C is necessary for adrenal function to protect against allergies. Vitamin D works with vitamin A and E which are antioxidants to protect the circulatory system and repair tissues. Multi-mineral formulas help protect against allergies, especially for heavy metal toxins. Calcium and magnesium help protect against toxins and strengthen the mucous membranes. Iron protects against infections. Potassium is good for muscle and nerve impulses.

Acidophilus before meals helps digestion and eliminates undigested proteins. Blue-green algae, cleans blood and nourishes the mucous membranes. Chlorophyll, cleans blood and provides nourishment. CoQ10, germanium and salmon oil protect the circulatory system. Lecithin protects the nerves.

ALZHEIMER'S DISEASE –

SYMPTOMS

Symptoms may be misleading. Many drugs prescribed for the elderly can cause confusion and memory loss.

Some symptoms are Depression—Agitation—Withdrawal—Insomnia—Irritability—Memory Loss—Personality Change—Senility—

There are two types of dementia. One is primary which comes on gradually, without apparent causes. Secondary dementia comes on suddenly from brain injury, operation, drugs or diabetic coma and is usually reversible. Alzheimer's is primary dementia which shows up in the brain as tangled clumps of nerve fibers and patches of disintegrated nerves in the brain.

CAUSES

The cause of Alzheimer's could be a genetic abnormality. When Down's Syndrome victims live to be in their 30's or 40's, some develop Alzheimer's disease. Allergies could play a role because of poor nutrition and improper digestion. Allergies cause swelling in the brain and can cause bizarre behavior.

The brain is sensitive to toxins in the blood stream which are created from autointoxication and constipation. Heavy metals accumulate when minerals are lacking in the body. Minerals help prevent heavy metals from accumulating. Free radicals are seen as one cause of Alzheimer's. Free radicals destroy cells, like acid burning a hole in a cell wall. When stomach acid is lacking and is neutral, it will not break down food, and malnutrition develops. It also causes toxins to accumulate and damage cells.

NUTRITIONAL THERAPY

Most tap water contains aluminum and other heavy metals because of acid rain in our soil that leaks in the water. Purified water is essential to prevent accumulation of toxins. Distilled water works like a magnet, leaching out toxins.

Proper digestion is necessary. A change of diet is needed, with wholesome food that contain vitamins, minerals, and enzymes. Dead food does not contain live enzymes and nutrients are destroyed. Cooking brown rice, millet, and buckwheat in a thermos will assure the that B-complex vitamins are present. Salads, sprouts, and lightly steamed vegetables help.

Fresh fruit and vegetable juices will provide nutrients that are easily digested and assimilated.

Burdock, Butcher's Broom Capsicum, Echinacea, Garlic, Ginger, Ginseng, Ginkgo, Gotu Kola, Ho Shou-Wu, Kelp, Lobelia, Passion Flower, Pau d' Arco, Psyllium, and Suma are useful herbs.

HERBAL FORMULAS

Blood Cleanser—Circulatory System—Colon Cleansers—Digestive System—Energy and

Stamina—Immune Builders—Nervous System and Brain—Structural System—Urinary—Female or Male Formulas—

VITAMINS, MINERALS AND SUPPLEMENTS

Vitamins A, C with bioflavonoids, and E are antioxidants which can prevent free radical damage. Vitamin E helps in brain damage. B-complex vitamins are seen lacking in Alzheimer's victims.

Minerals prevent toxic metals from accumulating. Selenium and zinc are essential. Iron is needed for pure blood. All minerals are necessary for a healthy body.

Blue green algae is rich in vitamins, minerals and amino acids. CoQ10 and germanium provides oxygen to the brain. Lecithin helps clean plaque and nourish the brain. Flaxseed oil and Salmon oil lower cholesterol and prevent blood clotting.

ANEMIA

SYMPTOMS

Anemia is a syndrome, with many disorders. The symptoms can be vague:

Depression—Fainting—Fatigue—Forgetfulness—Headaches—Indigestion—Irritability—Immune Function Disorders causing Colds and Infections—Angina Pectoris—Pallor—Poor Concentration—Weakness—

CAUSES

Excessive bleeding and malnutrition are the two main causes. Ailments such as hemorrhoids or ulcers, diverticular disease, liver damage, infections, thyroid problems, surgery, also heavy menstrual bleeding and repeated pregnancies can also contribute to anemia. Infants and young children on a milk diet, without minerals and essential fatty acids, are prone to anemia.

NUTRITIONAL THERAPY

There are several kinds of anemia. The most common is iron deficiency anemia. There is also folic acid and B12 deficiency anemia. Less common are copper deficiency anemia and Sickle-cell anemia, which is common in African Americans.

The cause should be determined. One of the main causes as we get older is the lack of assimilating iron and other minerals. Scientific experiments have found that in fatal cases of pernicious anemia, a large amount of iron was driven out of the blood (out of circulation), and had settled in the spleen. This revealed that iron was not in short supply. It was not being utilized. The importance of making sure there is enough hydrochloric acid in the body for assimilating minerals is vital.

Foods rich in iron are green leafy vegetables, dried apricots, blackstrap molasses, raw egg yolks, dried bean and peas, soy beans and prune juice. Vitamin C enhances the absorption of iron. Antacids will decrease iron absorption. Aspirin and many other drugs increase bleeding and can cause anemia. Calcium taken at the same time as iron supplements may inhibit its absorption.

Herbs rich in nutrients to help build up the blood are: Alfalfa, Burdock, Dong Quai, Golden Seal, Kelp, Pau D'Arco, Red Raspberry, Slippery Elm.

HERBAL FORMULAS

Blood Cleansers—Colon Cleaners—Digestive System—Immune Builders—Female or Male Formulas—

VITAMINS, MINERALS AND SUPPLEMENTS

B-complex helps in the assimilation of food. Vitamin C with bioflavonoids, helps in iron assimilation. A multi-minerals supplement is essential.

Chlorophyll and blue-green algae are rich in iron and builds the blood, they also contain amino acids, vitamins and minerals.

ANOREXIA NERVOSA —
(Bulimia)

SYMPTOMS

Anorexia and bulimia are obsessive eating disorders associated with ritualistic vomiting and purging. Acidosis—Avid Exercise— Despair—Dehydration—Dizziness—Dry Hair and Scalp—Electrolyte Imbalance—Dental Caries — Blotchy Skin — Coldness — Hypotension—Loss of Menstruation— Restlessness—Heart Problems—Cardiac Arrest—Excessive Vomiting—Weakness— Worthlessness—

CAUSES

Social attitude toward thinness and peer pressure are some of the causes of eating disorders. A deep desire for controlling oneself is another reason. A dread of being fat, unresolved abusive treatment as a child, low self esteem, depression and perfectionism can also be causes. Lack of correct eating habits can increase the symptoms.

NUTRITIONAL THERAPY

An extreme weakness from lack of minerals consist. About one third of those involved die prematurely from starvation, infections, and disorders of the heart or from suicide. The underlying cause must be dealt with. It may take a lot of love and understanding for the one involved. Help may be necessary from someone other than the family.

Nutritional food that builds health is the only answer to permanent weight loss. Vegetables, fruit, whole grains, beans, sprouts, almonds (balance of calcium and magnesium), and avocados, which contain essential fatty acids are good. The nerves need to be nourished so that reasoning with the anorexia or bulimic is possible. Foods high in B-complex vitamins are green leafy vegetables, dried fruits, almonds, whole grains such as millet, buckwheat, oats, barley, wheat, sunflower seeds, pinto and white beans, brown rice, fish and poultry, eggs, and yogurt.

Herbs have nutritional value and will help supply the body with cleansing and healing properties. Bee Pollen, Ginger, Golden Seal, Gotu Kola, Hawthorn Berries, Horsetail, Kelp, Licorice, Lobelia, Passion Flower, Red Raspberry, Saffron, Slippery Elm, Suma and Valerian are all good for their nutritional support.

HERBAL FORMULAS

Blood Cleansers—Circulatory System—Colon Cleansers—Digestive System—Glandular System—Immune Builders—Nervous System and Brain—Structural System—Urinary System—Female or Male Formulas—

VITAMINS, MINERALS AND SUPPLEMENTS

Vitamins A, B-complex, C with bioflavonoids, and E are essential.

Minerals, calcium, magnesium, potassium, mineral formulas, selenium and zinc are beneficial.

Supplements—Acidophilus, blue-green algae, flaxseed oil, CoQ10, germanium, salmon oil, and chlorophyll will nourish the blood.

ANXIETY ATTACKS ——
(Panic Attacks)

SYMPTOMS

Aches and Pains—Fear of Death and Heart Attack—Fatigue—Constipation—Nausea—Diarrhea—Stomach Tightness and Pain—Emotional and Mood Swings—Negative Thoughts—Depression—Headaches—Feeling of going Insane—Feelings of being Outside of Body—Insomnia—Fear of Crowds, Unable to Leave Home—Memory Loss—Mental Confusion—Tightening of Throat with inability to Swallow—Muscle Twitching—Many more symptoms can appear—

CAUSES

Prolonged nutritional deficiency along with extended periods of anxiety without relief can cause this problem. Insecurity as a child and an adult could contribute to anxiety attacks.

Nutritional deficiency prevents the ability to overcome and eliminate panic attacks. The nervous system is depleted. Hypoglycemia has been associated with panic attacks. Dramatic improvements have been seen with dietary changes with additional supplements of B-complex vitamins, calcium and magnesium.

Studies have shown that panic attacks and calcium deficiency tend to go hand in hand. Calcium protects the nerves and prevents toxins from irritating them. Tetany is called the mineral imbalance disease.

NUTRITIONAL THERAPY

Malnutrition has been seen as a caustic factor. Colon cleansing and nutritional supplements are necessary to feed and nourish the nerves. Alcohol, coffee, caffeine drinks, sugar, and drugs are all hard on the body and especially the nervous system. Drugs for panic attacks have been Valium, Xanax, and Prozac. Some physicians have seen rebound anxiety and panic attacks when they are discontinued. Some psychiatrists feel that nutritional therapy along with loving understanding are much more effective.

Dietary change has been beneficial in many people. Using foods that build up the nervous system is recommended. Amino acid supplements are very beneficial. Allergies can give the feeling of a panic attack. Formaldehyde fumes from newly purchased clothes or new carpet give a suffocating feeling and a loss of control which mimics a panic attack. Any allergy could bring on a panic attack.

Herbs can help strengthen the body and protect against panic attacks. Some include: Dong Quai, Ginkgo, Gotu Kola, Ho-Shou-Wu, Kelp, Lady's Slipper, Lobelia, Passion Flower, Slippery Elm, Suma, and Valerian.

HERBAL FORMULAS

Blood Cleansers—Colon Cleansers—Digestive System—Energy and Stamina—Glandular System—Immune System—Nervous System and Brain—Structural System—Urinary System—Female or Male Formulas—

VITAMINS, MINERALS AND SUPPLEMENTS

Vitamins A, and B-complex, build the nervous system, Vitamin C with bioflavonoids and E are also important.

Calcium and magnesium, and a multi-mineral supplement help improve a balance. Potassium helps prevent panic attacks and blackouts from hypoglycemia.

CoQ10, germanium, and lecithin, protect the nerves. Chlorophyll and Blue-green algae nourish the nerves and help in the digestion of nutrients.

ANKYLOSING SPONDYLITIS —
(Rheumatoid spondylitis, Marie-Strumpell disease)

SYMPTOMS

Fatigue—Malaise—Weight Loss—Low Back Pain—Sacroiliac Pain—Back Leg Pain— Stiffness of the Back, especially in the mornings—Stiffness and pain spreading up to and involving the rest of the back—Hips and Shoulder aches and stiff—

CAUSES

This is an autoimmune disorder. The body's immune system attacks the tissues lining the joints. Toxins accumulate in the joints, especially uric acid, which is a by-product of meat. The toxins form crystals and cause inflammation and pain in the joints.

Stress and tension in the body help cause the pain and stiffness. This could be caused by a long-standing bitterness, feelings of being put upon, a problem of loving ones self, or a deep criticism of authority.

Malnutrition could be one main cause. When nutrients are lacking, toxins accumulate in the body. Lack of minerals, especially calcium, magnesium and silicon (helps calcium assimilation) and other essential minerals can promote the disorder.

NUTRITIONAL THERAPY

A cleansing and building diet will help clean the uric acid from the blood and joints and rebuild the cartilage between the joints. A three day fast, using chlorophyll, vegetable juices, green drinks, wheat grass juice and a lower bowel formula and a blood cleanser, containing red clover will help clean the blood and colon and eliminate the toxins from the body.

A change of diet is necessary. Eliminating meat and increasing whole grains, beans, nuts, seeds, sprouts, fruit, vegetables, and vegetable juices is recommended.

Relaxing therapy is essential. The body heals faster when it is relaxed. Use a calcium herbal formula, stress formulas, B-complex vitamins and minerals.

HERBAL FORMULAS

Herbs are rich in minerals and cleansing substances and will supply nutrients to help the body restore immune response.

Blood Cleansers—Colon Cleansers—Digestive System—Energy and Stamina—Glandular System—Immune Builders—Nervous System and Brain—Urinary System—Female or Male Formulas—

VITAMINS, MINERALS AND SUPPLEMENTS

Vitamin C complex is essential to rebuild the cartilage and bones structure along with an herbal calcium formula. The antioxidants, vitamin A, C, E, and minerals selenium and zinc will help strengthen the immune system. B-complex vitamins are necessary for proper digestion, for the nervous system and to prevent toxins from accumulating in the liver.

Essential Fatty Acids are necessary for building the joints. Blue-green algae and Chlorophyll will clean and nourish the blood, help in the digestion of nutrients and supply minerals and vitamins for building the immune system. Amino acids will help build and nourish the cells for healing.

APPENDICITIS

SYMPTOMS

Nausea—Pain or Tenderness in the lower right area of the abdomen—Vomiting—Low—grade fever—Fever in Children can be quite high—The medical profession claims that the appendix serves no useful purpose. No part of the body is without purpose. The appendix is necessary to help clean the cells so the lymphatic system can do its job. The appendix is lymph tissue and protects the body from infections.

CAUSES

Constipation is the main cause of appendicitis. Obstructions in the appendix such as intestinal worms or fecal material prevent proper drainage. Fermentation and digestive disorders from a low fiber diet are the main cause. If the appendix rupture or perforates, the infection spills into the abdominal cavity, causing peritonitis, which can be very serious.

NUTRITIONAL THERAPY

Avoid laxatives and change to a high fiber diet. Fasting and using psyllium combinations to increase bulk will clean the bowels. Cooking whole grains in a thermos will help nourish and provide enzymes and bulk.

Baked potatoes, (eating the skins), whole grains, such as wheat, whole oats, millet, buckwheat, brown rice, beans, nuts, seeds, sprouts and lots of fresh and steamed vegetables are beneficial.

Herbs to help the colon and appendix are Aloe Vera, Burdock, Cayenne, Echinacea, Garlic, Golden Seal, Kelp, Myrrh, Pau D'Arco, Passion Flower, Psyllium, Saffron, Slippery Elm, White Oak Bark, and Valerian.

HERBAL FORMULAS

Blood Cleansers—Colon Cleansers, (worms and parasites)—Digestive System—Glandular System — Infection Fighters — Urinary System—

VITAMINS, MINERALS AND SUPPLEMENTS

Vitamins A, B-complex, vitamin C with bioflavonoids, and E are essential. Mineral supplements, containing calcium, magnesium and potassium will strengthen the body. Iron is needed for rich blood to nourish the organs. Selenium and zinc are healing.

Acidophilus helps in the digestion of nutrients and protects the colon from bad bacteria. Chlorophyll and blue-green algae nourish the blood, help the body produce its own interferon, and help in the digestion of food. CoQ10, and germanium are beneficial.

ARTERIOSCLEROSIS

(Hardening of the Arteries)

SYMPTOMS

Symptoms are hard to detect—Dizziness—Weakness—Heart Palpation—Weakness in the arms or legs—The main symptoms hit suddenly in a heart attack or stroke—Arteriosclerosis develops over a lifetime. Fatty streaks are found in the aortas of babies indicating it starts in the very young and slowly progresses—The brain can "turn to stone" and cause Memory Loss—Headaches—Dimming Eyesight—Senility—

CAUSES

Fatty deposits, called plaque, collect on the smooth inner artery walls. These deposits can thicken and become hard and brittle. This impairs circulation and prevents the blood and nourishment from reaching the organs. Other ailments may arise such as kidney malfunction.

Constipation is the main cause which overburdens the liver. When the liver becomes congested, it dumps excess poisons into the bile. This thickens the bile and clogs the gall bladder. Since the liver is responsible for dealing with cholesterol, it cannot filter properly when overloaded.

The Chinese treat stroke by treating constipation. They are very successful in preventing and treating stroke by cleaning the colon.

NUTRITIONAL THERAPY

To help reduce the risk of arteriosclerosis, use a short juice fast, lower bowel cleansers, and blood purifiers. Add fiber and use whole grains, beans, peas, vegetables, fruit, sprouts, vegetable juices, nuts and seeds.

Controlling stress in life is important. Stress tightens up the organs and prevents them from functioning properly. Relaxation therapy and dealing with inner emotions will help the healing process.

Herbs that help the circulatory system are Alfalfa, Bee Pollen, Burdock, Cayenne, Echinacea, Fenugreek, Garlic, Ginger, Ginseng, Gotu Kola, Hawthorn Berries, Horsetail, Kelp, Pau D'Arco, and Suma.

HERBAL FORMULAS

Circulatory System—Colon Cleansers— Digestive System—Energy and Stamina— Glandular System—Immune Builders— Nervous System and Brain—Structural System—Urinary System—Female or Male Formulas—

VITAMINS, MINERALS AND SUPPLEMENTS

The antioxidant vitamins help protect the veins from free radical damage. Vitamin A, C, E, selenium and zinc should be included in the diet.

The B-complex vitamins help the liver to detoxify and help in digestion. A multi-mineral supplement helps strengthen the body. Iron nourishes the blood. Silicon helps the body assimilate calcium and cleans the veins. Potassium protects the heart.

Acidophilus helps the body assimilate nutrients and aids the colon in preventing the bad bacteria from accumulating. CoQ10 and Germanium provide oxygen in the blood, and Chlorophyll builds blood. Lecithin cleans plaque from veins. Flaxseed Oil and Salmon Oil are essential for healthy veins.

ARTHRITIS

SYMPTOMS

It is estimated that the majority of the United States population over 50 will experience some signs of arthritis. It is considered the number one crippler in the nation. Osteoarthritis is the most common degenerative joint disease. The cartilage in the joints that covers the end of the bones starts to wear away. This involves the tendons, ligaments and muscles. Rheumatoid arthritis attacks the cartilage throughout the body. It is a chronic, inflammatory disorder causing stiffness, deformity, and pain in the joints and muscles. This disease can affect the lungs, blood vessels, the spleen, skin and muscles. Early signs are fatigue, muscular aches and pains, stiffness in the joints and swelling.

This also includes bursitis and gout. Symptoms are pain and inflammation in the joints. This could appear on the neck, back, shoulders, knees, wrist, elbows, fingers, toes, and hips. Stiffness and pain on arising in the mornings is common.

CAUSES

Causes could be autointoxication, constipation, stagnation of blood, and lack of blood supply to the joints, lymphatics and the nervous system. Poor diet and stress can predispose one. It could also be caused from infections, autoimmune disorders, bacterium, rich diet, high in meat, white flour and sugar products. Venereal disease can also be one cause. Allergies to certain foods can increase the symptoms of arthritis such as the nightshade family. Tobacco is from the nightshade family along with tomatoes, potatoes, eggplant and green peppers. They interfere with collagen repair.

Stress causes the destruction of protein which is necessary before ACTH (natural cortisone) can be produced. Arthritis usually means that calcium is out of solution and settles in the joints. The calcium is lost out of the matrix of the bones. Lack of hydrochloride acid is one cause of calcium loss. Another theory of arthritis concerns the role of deep seated repressed emotions, including inflexibility in our lives, resentments, fear, anger, hatred and negative thoughts.

NUTRITIONAL THERAPY

Take care of digestion and the colon. When there are joint problems, there are usually stomach trouble. Sodium herbs and food neutralizes acids. Potassium herbs and broths help drain acids in the body. Hydrochloric acid aids calcium and protein digestion and clears up gastritis. There is a deficiency of minerals found in those with arthritis, especially iron, sulfur, silicon and zinc.

Many people have had success on a vegetarian diet. Use brown rice, millet, buckwheat, fruit, vegetables, seeds, nuts, sprouts, green drinks, and fresh vegetable juices. Avoid citrus juices as they may contribute to swollen joints. Eliminate sugar, refined flour products, salt, alcohol, tea and coffee.

Herbs that will help in arthritis are Alfalfa, Aloe Vera, Burdock, Devil's Claw, Echinacea, Horsetail, Kelp, Pau D'Arco, Saffron, Slippery Elm and Yucca.

HERBAL FORMULAS

Blood Cleansers—Colon Cleansers—Digestive System—Immune Builders—Nervous System and Brain—Structural System—Urinary System—Female or Male Formulas—

VITAMINS, MINERALS AND SUPPLEMENTS

Vitamin A and E help prevent free-radical damage. Vitamin C helps to rebuild cartilage, necessary for the formation of collagen found in the bones, cartilage and connective tissues. Vitamin B-complex and iron are necessary for nerves, digestion and rich blood.

Minerals are essential for joint, muscle and bone repair, especially silicon, calcium, magnesium, selenium and zinc.

Chlorophyll and Blue-green algae are rich in nutrients and help in the assimilation of essential vitamins and minerals.

Lecithin eliminates cholesterol and toxins and helps in repairing the nerves. Salmon oil and flaxseed oil are necessary for joint repair.

ASTHMA

SYMPTOMS

Coughing—Wheezing—Difficult Breathing—Tight Chest. Respiratory distress can come on suddenly with multiple symptoms or gradually and insidiously. Sometimes there is coughing with thick, tenacious sputum that may be clear or yellow. There is a feeling of suffocation.

CAUSES

The flow of air is obstructed in the bronchial tubes. There is swelling of the membranes lining the bronchial tubes and a plugging of the tubes with thick mucus. Catarrh of the bronchi becomes suppressed over the years and hardens and solidifies. These symptoms are the way the body is trying to release this hard catarrh. The main underlying cause is constipation. The lungs are organs of elimination and when the colon is congested, the lungs take over the cleansing process. The lungs are sensitive to these toxins and when irritated can form scar tissue.

Air pollution further irritates the lungs along with food allergies, improper digestion, poor nutrition, free radicals and rancid fats. This results in particles of matter which gradually close the "pores". The lungs then lose their elasticity.

Resolving emotions from suppressed sadness has been shown to help, along with diet. The inability to cry and release these emotions can also be a cause. Smothering love can create the inability to breathe for oneself. The over protection of children can cause asthma in childhood.

NUTRITIONAL THERAPY

When food is held in the colon too long, it becomes putrid and is poisonous. It is capable of producing poisonous toxins, which are absorbed into the circulation with deleterious and harmful results. A colon cleanse is essential when there are lung problems.

Use a vegetarian diet, making sure there is adequate protein, which is abundant in grains, potatoes, seeds, nuts, herbs and vegetables. Avoid sugar, which robs the body of nutrients. White flour products act like glue in the intestines. This includes white pasta products.

Juice fasting will help eliminate toxins and clean the colon and lungs. The best juice to drink is carrot, parsley, celery with a clove of garlic and a piece of onion. Coughing is natures way of expelling toxic material. Health is improved until concentration of toxins are built up again. Changing the diet is essential to eliminate and heal the lungs. Garlic and onion soup will dissolve mucus.

Herbs helpful for asthma are Cascara Sagrada, Ephedra, Fenugreek, Garlic, Ginger, Golden Seal, Licorice, Lobelia, Marshmallow, Mullein, Passion Flower, Pau D'Arco, Psyllium and Valerian.

HERBAL FORMULAS

Blood Cleansers—Circulatory System—Colds, Flu, Fever and Allergy—Colon Cleansers—Glandular System—Immune Builders—Nervous System and Brain—Structural System—Urinary System—Female or Male Formulas—

VITAMINS, MINERALS AND SUPPLEMENTS

Vitamin A, using both the fish oil and beta carotene, heals and protects the mucous membranes in the lungs.

Vitamin E works with vitamin A to prevent destruction of tissue. Vitamin C with bioflavonoids is needed daily for protection and acts as a natural antihistamine, and increases bronchial capacity.

B-complex vitamins are needed for healthy nerves and gastrointestinal tract. B12 injections have helped in wheezing. Low levels of vitamin C are seen in asthmatics.

Minerals are important especially selenium and zinc. They protect the immune system. All minerals are needed. Iron is needed for healthy blood to nourish the lungs. Potassium provides proper acid and alkalinity balance. Calcium and magnesium are needed. Magnesium has bronchiodilating properties.

Acidophilus helps protect from bad bacteria. Flaxseed and salmon oil are important to prevent mucus build-up. They also have anti-inflammatory properties and boost the immune system. Blue-green algae has anti-inflammatory properties, and builds the body. CoQ10 and germanium provide oxygen to the cells and increase the production of interferon to fight diseases. Lecithin protects the cells and is essential for protection to the brain and nerves.

ATHLETIC HEART SYNDROME

SYMPTOMS

It can cause Chest Pounding—Irregular Heart Beat, especially after strenuous exercise. Athletes have dropped dead from this syndrome. X-rays revealed enlarged arteries and irregular heart beat.

CAUSES

Causes can be poor diet, drug use, steroid abuse which is associated with an increased risk of developing circulatory and heart problems, and alcohol abuse.

Lack of electrolytes or an imbalance can cause respiratory failure. Muscular weakness due to lack of minerals can lead to paralysis, and put stress on the heart. Lack of liquids can cause dehydration and increase the risk of heart weakness.

NUTRITIONAL THERAPY

Diets rich in complex carbohydrates, vegetables, fruit, seeds, nuts, salads, and essential fatty acids will build a healthy and strong body. Amino acids will build and nourish the system. Natural food can help build muscle and strength. Avocados have the ability to build muscles naturally.

Dr. Graham Reedy, M.D., emphasis in his practice on sports medicine that "anabolic steroids can cause liver tumors, and testicular or ovarian atrophy", and "once the steroid treatments are stopped all the buildup is lost, and fat tends to infiltrate the tissue. (*Complementary Medicine-Sports Medicine:* An interview with Graham Reedy, March/April 1986, p. 33).

Sugar is not necessary for energy. The body is designed to furnish all the sugar it needs from complex carbohydrates in grains, vegetables and fruit. Sugar leaches out essential minerals from the body; it also increases pain in injuries.

Herbs to build and strengthen the body are Bee Pollen, Burdock, Butchers Broom, Cayenne, Garlic, Ginkgo, Gotu Kola, Suma, Ginseng, Ho-Shou-Wu, and Pau D'Arco.

HERBAL FORMULAS

Blood Cleansers—Circulatory System—Colon Cleansers—Energy and Stamina—Immune Builders—Structural System—Urinary System—Female and Male Formulas—

VITAMINS, MINERALS AND SUPPLEMENTS

Antioxidants vitamins A, C, E, selenium and zinc prevent free-radical cell damage. Vitamin E, improves circulation, and helps prevent blood clots. B-complex vitamins help in mental and physical stress. Vitamin C with bioflavonoids protects against injuries and speeds healing. Vitamin supplements cleanse and nourish the veins and blood.

Calcium and Magnesium protect the heart and strengthen bones, muscles, and ligaments. Potassium is essential for normal heart function. Iron supplements help prevent anemia from heavy sweating. Zinc speeds healing. Mineral supplements contain trace minerals that act as catalysts for enzyme action and is needed for strong bones, muscles and ligaments.

Acidophilus promotes nutrient absorption and utilization. CoQ10 and Germanium enhance immune function and provide oxygen to the blood and cells. Flaxseed Oil and Salmon Oil, protect the heart and veins. Lecithin is vital for breaking down fat and cholesterol. L-carnitine strengthens the heart and dissolves fatty deposits. Chlorophyll nourishes and purifies the blood.

BACKACHE

(Aches, Pains, Sciatica, Scoliosis)

SYMPTOMS

Pain—Fatigue—Breathing Difficulties—Muscle Pain from Tension, lack of exercise, or strain—Emotional Tension can cause muscle pain—Incorrect posture puts a strain on the spine—

CAUSES

Abuse is the main cause of backaches. Overeating, overdrinking, and eating the wrong kinds of food can also contribute. Constipation is a major cause of back problems. A congested colon can put pressure on the back. Lack of exercise and nutrients can also be a cause.

Spinal subluxation can cause back pain. Diseases in the body can cause back pain such as kidney or bladder infections, which are located in the middle of the back.

Scoliosis can be caused from poor posture or discrepancy in leg length. Congenital defects can be caused by a lack of nutrients. Muscle pain or "Charlie horse" can result from a lack of calcium and magnesium.

NUTRITIONAL THERAPY

A recent issue of *Let's Live*, reported a study cited in the British Medical Journal that Chiropractic treatment proved more successful than hospital treatments in every way. Chiropractic reduced pain better and increased mobility, and the worse the back pain, the better the chiropractic results. After two years, those treated with chiropractic maintained their improvement better than those who received hospital (including surgery) treatment.

A change of diet and a healthier live style, need to be followed. Minerals to build strong bones, flesh, cartilage and muscles are important. Food rich in nutrients, whole grains, beans, sprouts, fresh fruit and vegetable juices should be eaten regularly. Vegetable salads, steamed and fresh vegetables are rich in minerals.

Walking and rowing are good for the back. Learn how to bend and avoid using muscles of the back. Use legs and arms and avoid bending at the waist.

Herbs that help clean and nourish the structural system are Alfalfa, Bee Pollen, Burdock, Dandelion, Kelp, Echinacea, Pau D'Arco, Horsetail, Ho-Shou-Wu, Lobelia, Passion Flower, Valerian, White Willow, Slippery Elm, and Cayenne.

HERBAL FORMULAS

Blood Cleansers—Colon Cleansers—Digestive System—Immune Builders—Nervous System and Brain—Structural System—Urinary System—Female or Male Formulas—

VITAMINS, MINERALS AND SUPPLEMENTS

Vitamin A and D are beneficial. D is essential for calcium and phosphorus assimilation. B-complex protect against muscle weakness, pain, depression, fatigue, and helps absorption of all nutrients. Vitamin C with bioflavonoids strengthens bones and muscles. Vitamin E prevents muscular disorders.

All minerals are important for strong bones, muscles and cartilage. Calcium assimilates when silicon is present along with all minerals. Zinc is healing. Lack of iron can cause pain.

Blue-green algae is rich in minerals. Chlorophyll helps purify and nourish the blood for mineral assimilation. Lecithin is good for the nerves. Flaxseed oil and salmon oil help balance body chemistry and ease pain.

BEDWETTING _____

SYMPTOMS

Loss of bladder control at night—It can also be a problem in the day time—

CAUSES

Bedwetting is common in hyperactive children. Dr. Benjamin Feingold works with diets of hyperactive children and says a diet change is often helpful. Milk is high on the list of allergic foods. Next are wheat, chocolate, eggs, and citrus. Allergies can cause the bladder to shrink. It can shrink because the detrusor muscle is in a spasm, a spasm which is often caused by an allergic reaction.

NUTRITIONAL THERAPY

Carbonated drinks, and cola drinks stimulate urine increase. Sugar irritates the kidneys and can cause bedwetting, especially when eaten with milk, as in ice cream. Constipation can put pressure on the bladder, as well as cause autointoxication which creates allergies. Low blood sugar can be a cause as well as allergies.

Children will usually outgrow this problem. Parents need to be patient and understanding. They don't deliberately wet the bed. They should not make a big issue of it. It is hard enough on the child knowing he cannot help the bedwetting. An immature nervous system is one of the problems. Emotional upsets can cause bedwetting as well as infections or extreme tiredness (allergies can cause fatigue).

Drugs are not the answer. One drug called Tofranil is given to children for controlling bedwetting. It could be dangerous. It is a drug also given in aiding cocaine withdrawal; in the management of chronic, severe pain, in relieving symptoms of attention deficit disorder; in preventing panic attacks; and in controlling binge eating and purging in bulimia.

Herbs used to help in bed wetting are Bee Pollen, Black Walnut, Golden Seal, Hydrangea, Kelp and Slippery Elm.

HERBAL FORMULAS

Blood Cleansers—Colon Cleansers—(worms and parasites)-Colds, Flu, Fevers and Allergy—Nervous System and Brain—Urinary System—

VITAMINS, MINERALS AND SUPPLEMENTS

Vitamins A, D, and C with bioflavonoids will strengthen the body and protect against infections. Vitamin E, a natural antioxidant, protects the body. B-complex strengthens the nerves.

Minerals are essential for a strong bladder. Use a powdered beverage drink containing vitamins and minerals to replace soda pop, cool aid and cola drinks. Sodium helps in bladder ailments.

Chlorophyll cleans and nourishes the blood. Blue-green algae is very nourishing. Lecithin builds the nerve sheaths surrounding the nerves. Essential fatty acids are vital for all body functions.

BLADDER AND KIDNEY INFECTIONS _____

(Cystitis, Nephritis)

SYMPTOMS

Inability to Urinate—Blood in Urine— Burning when Urinating—Bags under the Eyes—Infections—Fever—Kidney Stones— Lower Abdominal Pain—

CAUSES

The kidneys are the body's filtering system, and can become plugged like a strainer with toxins. When they are congested with toxins and mucus, irritation to the kidneys can occur and can cause infection. Constipation causes a back-up in the bloodstream which irritates the bladder and causes irritations and infections.

Kidney failure is very serious and can be caused by repeated infections that leave scarring. Painkillers, such as phenacetin can irritate the kidneys. Overuse of aspirin and other pain killers damage the kidneys. Environmental toxins such as heavy metals can cause kidney damage. Anti-hypertensive drugs that reduce circulation can cause kidney damage.

Beer drinking can cause kidney failure or high blood pressure. Kidney failure can cause high blood pressure. Cyclamate, an artificial sweetener like saccharin, was banned by the FDA after it was found to induce cancerous tumors in bladders of rats and mice. Saccharin is widely used and is found in many food products. It is even recommended for diabetics.

NUTRITIONAL THERAPY

Drink plenty of pure water; the bladder collects the body's fluid wastes which contains toxin that can cause cancer. Avoid coffee, alcohol, and artificial drinks.

Use fresh, unsweetened cranberry and apple juice. It helps reduce the built-up calcium that irritates the kidneys and it also inhibits bacterial growth.
Carrot, parsley and celery juice is healing and rich in vitamins A and celery is high in sodium which prevent urine acidity.

Eat more fresh and steamed vegetables, fresh fruit, whole grains, sprouts, beans, seeds and nuts. Almonds and sesame seeds are rich in calcium which nourishes and are assimilated in the body. Use whole grain breads. Millet is rich in calcium and magnesium and is easy to assimilate.

Garlic, Echinacea and Golden Seal contain antibiotic properties. Hydrangea and Juniper are healing, a natural diuretic and cleansing for the kidneys. Parsley and Uva Ursi strengthen and tone the urinary system. Marshmallow is soothing and healing. Burdock and Pau D'Arco clean and nourish the blood.

HERBAL FORMULAS

Blood Cleansers—Colon Cleansers—Digestive System — Immune Builders — Infection Fighters—Urinary System—Female and Male Formulas—

VITAMINS, MINERALS AND SUPPLEMENTS

Vitamins A and C protect against bladder infections and cancer. Vitamin C with bioflavonoids helps prevent the accumulation of toxins in the bladder. B-complex vitamins are needed every day for energy, being essential for the metabolism of carbohydrates, fats, and proteins. They are good for muscle tone in the gastrointestinal tract. Deficiency of choline (found in lecithin), can cause kidney damage. Potassium deficiency can result in renal disorders. Magnesium and B6 can help prevent stones.

Acidophilus helps prevent infections. Chlorophyll cleans and nourishes the kidneys and bladder. Blue -green algae heals infections and cleans the blood. Flaxseed oil, salmon oil along with vitamin E help prevent scarring.

BLOOD POISONING ———
(Gangrene, Infections)

SYMPTOMS

Severe Localized Pain—Swelling—Discoloration—Red Streak from the wound towards the Heart—Sores that do not heal—Deep Frostbite produces Pain, Skin Blisters, Gangrene—When a sore, cut or abrasion becomes red and infected it could turn into blood poisoning—

CAUSES

Faulty diet and hard water causes the walls of the arteries, veins and capillaries to become coated with inorganic waste material and become hard and brittle. This can cause problems when injury occurs.

Impaired circulation can cause gangrene when the arteries become clogged. This impedes the flow of blood which can become deprived of nutrients and oxygen. Dry gangrene is caused by decreased blood flow, oxygen and nutrients to the area, as in hardening of the arteries, diabetes, and poor circulation.

Wet gangrene is caused by a wound or injury that becomes infected from toxic blood.

Weakened and injured areas of the body accumulate toxin and poisons because vitality is lacking in these areas and nutrients are deficient.

NUTRITIONAL THERAPY

Use juice fasting with fresh vegetable juices made with parsley, carrots and celery. Citrus juices will clean and eliminate toxins: orange, grapefruit, lemons and limes. Wheatgrass juice is purifying to the blood. A change of diet is indicated when blood poisoning is present. Blood purification and colon cleansing is beneficial to eliminate toxin accumulation in the body. Use herbs that purify the blood such as Red Clover formulas, Burdock, Echinacea, Golden Seal, and Garlic. Teas and extracts will enter the blood stream faster.

External: Plantain Poultice, Clay Packs, Charcoal Poultice, Echinacea, Comfrey Powders with Aloe Vera Juice all will help when applied to the wound.

Aloe vera, repairs tissues and aids in the treatment of frostbite. Black Walnut, contains iodine which is healing and an antiseptic. Burdock, Cayenne, Echinacea, Ginger, Golden Seal, Horsetail, Kelp, Lobelia, Myrrh, Pau D'Arco, Slippery Elm and Suma are all useful herbs.

HERBAL FORMULAS

Blood Cleansers—Circulatory System—Colon Cleansers—Immune Builders—Infection Fighters—Urinary System—

VITAMINS, MINERALS AND SUPPLEMENTS

Vitamins A and C are healing. Vitamin B-complex helps fight infections. Vitamin E increases immunity.

Calcium and Magnesium strengthen the nerves and the immune system. Iron builds and nourishes the blood. All minerals are essential for healing especially selenium and zinc. A multi-mineral supplement is essential.

Essential fatty acids found in flaxseed oil and salmon oil increase immunity. Acidophilus, protects against bad bacteria. Chlorophyll cleans the blood. Blue-green algae is healing and nourishing. CoQ10 and Germanium provide oxygen to the cells. Lecithin is needed for all cells and prevents infections.

BRONCHITIS _____

SYMPTOMS

Inflammation of the Bronchi Causes Frequent Coughing—Pain—Back and Chest Pain—Sore Throat— Tight feeling in the Chest—Chills—Fatigue—Fever—

CAUSES

Nutrient deficiency is seen in case of bronchitis, wheezing and other chronic respiratory disorders. An imbalance is seen in high sodium levels compared to potassium and low levels of vitamin C and niacin.

Chronic bronchitis is caused by constant irritation of the lungs, such as smoking, air pollution, breathing toxic chemicals or autointoxication. The lungs become irritated when the kidneys and colon are congested. The lungs attempt to eliminate toxins, and this is very irritating to the lungs and causes congestion. Dairy products cause excess mucus and toxins. Low fiber diet cause a build-up of toxins.

Grief is the emotion that is associated with the colon and lungs. When grief is repressed for long periods, it can cause contraction in the lungs, and they become congested.

Air pollution causes serious health problems. Respiratory problems including asthma, emphysema, chronic bronchitis, coughing and chest pain are caused and aggravated by air pollutants. Some pollutants are lead, cadmium, aluminum, carbon monoxide, nitrogen oxides, sulfur oxides and fine particulates (PM10).

NUTRITIONAL THERAPY

A change of diet will help to eliminate the toxins in the respiratory system. Dairy products, starchy foods, salt, sugar, meat, chocolate, pastries, white flour products, and fried food are all irritating for the lungs. Eliminate all refined foods. Fumes from household cleansers and paint can cause lung irritation.

The particulates, found in the air, can lodge in the lungs and cause irritations and infections. When irritations are present using herbs, citrus juices, herbal teas and extracts will help nature heal faster and prevent chronic bronchitis. Herbs can be used every half hour at the onset of an infection. Cayenne and lobelia extracts will break up the congestion. Fasting will speed the healing. Specific herbs can be used to treat the symptoms.

Burdock cleans the blood, Echinacea acts like an antibiotic. Ephedra is a natural dilator and Eucalyptus soothes the lungs when inhaled.

Garlic, Ginger and Licorice act as expectorants. Marshmallow is soothing and healing.

HERBAL FORMULAS

Blood Cleansers—Colds, Flu, Fever and Allergy Formulas—Colon Cleansers—Digestive System—Immune Builders—Infection Fighters—Nervous System and Brain—Urinary System—

VITAMINS, MINERALS AND SUPPLEMENTS

Vitamin A and beta carotene work with zinc and other essential minerals to heal. Vitamin B-complex strengthens immune function and the nerves. Vitamin C with bioflavonoids heals infections and builds the immune system. Vitamin and mineral supplements help nourish and strengthen the body. Vitamin E is essential and works best with vitamin C, B vitamins and lecithin.

Minerals work with vitamins for preventing and healing the body. Calcium and magnesium protect the immune system and nerves. Potassium protects the heart. Iron is needed to nourish the blood. Selenium and zinc heals infections.

Blue-green algae and chlorophyll heal infections and increases assimilation of nutrients. Flaxseed oil and salmon oil protect the veins for a healthy blood supply.

BRUISING

SYMPTOMS

Most bruises are not serious. You can fall or bump yourself and a bruise is the result. The fragile capillaries under the skin's surface rupture, bringing blood to the surrounding bump. This creates black and blue patches.

CAUSES

In rare cases, a bruise is a sign of problems elsewhere in the body. It could be kidney and liver disorders. Anemia can cause bruising as well as blood disorders and allergies. Purplish bumps under the ski that do no heal and look like bruises could be a symptom of AIDS.

Lack of proper nutrition, vitamins and minerals can be a factor. Drugs such as aspirin can cause bruising. Anti-clotting drugs can cause bruising. They can also be a sign of cancer.

NUTRITIONAL THERAPY

Strengthen the blood and vessels. Dark green leafy vegetables in salads, steamed and raw vegetables, juices containing carrot, celery, parsley, wheatgrass, and chlorophyll will build and purify the blood. Eliminating acid foods and adding alkaline foods will clean the blood.

Herbs to help in bruising are Alfalfa, Bee Pollen, Black Walnut, Burdock, Aloe Vera, Cayenne, Horsetail, Kelp, Pau D'Arco, and White Oak Bark.

HERBAL FORMULAS

Blood Cleansers—Circulatory System—Colon Cleansers—Digestive System—Immune Builders—Urinary System—Female or Male Formulas—

VITAMINS, MINERALS AND SUPPLEMENTS

Vitamin A and D are healing. B complex with extra B12 and folic acid can help. Vitamin C with bioflavonoids strengthens the vessels to prevent and heal bruises. Lack of vitamin K can cause bruises. Iron supplements are beneficial; those containing yellow dock assimilate easier. Zinc is very healing. Calcium and magnesium are beneficial. Mineral supplements are essential.

Blue-green algae and chlorophyll nourish and clean the blood. Lecithin is essential for healthy veins. Essential fatty acids play an important role in healthy blood found in flaxseed oil and salmon oil.

BURNS

SYMPTOMS

First degree burns will cause redness, mild swelling and pain. Second degree burns will cause redness and blisters and third degree burns cause destruction of the skin and underlying muscles. Little pain is noticed with third degree because the nerve endings have been destroyed.

CAUSES

Burns range from mild to charring with destruction of all layers of the skin. Sunburns can be serious. Sun exposure should be a gradual process, and sun screen is advised. Steam, fire and chemical burns can all cause serious damage. Children need to be supervised at all times to avoid serious accidents. A small child can accidentally turn on the hot water if left alone or pull a hot pan from the stove and cause hot liquids to spill on them.

First degree burns usually result from the sun or hot water.

Second degree usually result from hot metal

objects, flame-contact burns and severe sunburns.

Third degree are usually from high flame-contact, hot fluid burns, steam from a pressure cooker, X-rays, and electrical burns which can cause death.

Fourth degree burns can cause total destruction of the skin but can also destroy organic bodily function and can be fatal.

NUTRITIONAL THERAPY

Cold water should be applied until the pain has subsided. Cold water will help prevent blistering and reddening of the skin. Clothes that cover the burn should be soaked to prevent the hot cloth from causing a deeper burn. Blisters should not be broken. They protect the burn and help prevent infections.

Aloe Vera plant or lotion is very beneficial. It will help prevent pain and prevent scarring. A paste made with pure honey, wheat germ oil, comfrey leaves, slippery elm and golden seal, with mineral water will heal and prevent infections. Honey has antibiotic properties. ("Honey for superficial wounds and ulcers," *Lancet* Jan. 9, 1993 p. 341.) Comfrey helps in new cell growth, Slippery Elm is healing and draws out impurities. Golden Seal is an antibiotic. Herbs will tend to heal the skin, help replace body cells and rebuild tissue from the inside out to such a point that scar tissue is minimal. (Malstrom, Stan, N.D., M.T., *The Tree of Knowledge*, Burns, p. 13.)

Drink a lot of pure water. High amounts of vitamin C will help prevent infections. Fresh fruits are cleansers, especially citrus juices. Vegetables are rich in minerals; juices will supply large amounts of nutrients. Green drinks are healing, add fresh Ginger, Garlic and Cayenne.

Herbs useful for burns are Aloe Vera, speeds healing, Bee Pollen, internally 1/2 teaspoonful twice daily, Horsetail, Kelp, Passion Flower, relaxing, and Slippery Elm, healing and builds new cells. Externally, apply a Comfrey salve. Salves containing Golden Seal or Cayenne may be applied to the burn with a sterile cloth and will aid in reducing the danger of staph or septic infection.

HERBAL FORMULAS

Blood Cleansers—Colon Cleansers, to prevent infections—Immune Builders—Infection Fighters—Nervous System and Brain—Structural Formulas—Urinary Formulas—

VITAMINS, MINERALS AND SUPPLEMENTS

Take 100,000 units of vitamin A and beta carotene for a while to speed healing. Take B-complex in twice the recommended dosage. Vitamin C, with bioflavonoids is healing and prevents infection. Potassium will help maintain fluid and electrolyte balance. Vitamin E used externally and internally is recommended.
A multi-minerals supplement will help speed healing.

Flaxseed oil and salmon oil help the immune system. Blue green algae and chlorophyll will purify the blood and heal. Lecithin helps fight infections. CoQ10 and germanium help the immune system and veins.

CANCER

SYMPTOMS

A sore that does not heal—Unusual bleeding or discharge—Change in bowel or bladder habits—Lump or thickening in breast or any where on body—Hoarseness or nagging cough—Difficulty in swallowing or prolonged indigestion—A wart or mole that changes or bleeds—Fatigue—Appetite loss—

CAUSES

The main cause of cancer is the presence of poisons or toxins in the bloodstream. The cancer growth acts as a dumping encasement for the poisons. The cancer indicates that the blood is overloaded and is unable to eliminate in the normal way because of constipation and autointoxication.

We have been made to believe that a cancer or tumor is localized, and when it is cut out or destroyed by chemotherapy, the cancer is eliminated. Cancer is more common today because there are more toxins in our food, water and air. The body was designed to eliminate a certain amount of poisons, but when junk food is eaten along with bad living habits, it accumulates.

Cancerous growths require sugar to grow. Rancid oils and fats are dangerous, for they decrease oxygenation, inhibiting the function of every cell. Rancid oils and heavy protein diets cause the blood to become heavy and thickened and limits its transport ability. When the blood is too thick, the elimination organs have a difficult time doing their job. They are the liver, kidneys, bowels and skin. Researchers in Sweden estimate that 30 to 40% of cancer in males and 60% of cancer in females is caused by dietary deficiencies

and toxins.

Diseases are due to substances the body needs and is not getting and to the presence of substances which the body ingests and does not need."

NUTRITIONAL THERAPY

Good nutrition and detoxification will speed the elimination of toxins which destroy the organs that build and clean the blood. Dietary indoles reduce the risk of breast, cervical and colon cancers. Fresh juice fasting and wheatgrass juice inhibit and destroy cancer cells. Sprouts, and seeds are beneficial. Sprouted grains are rich in vitamins and minerals. Cruciferous vegetables protect against cancer (cabbage, broccoli, brussels sprouts, cauliflower), and encourage indole formation in the intestines that prevent the formation of cancer.

Cancer is the second most common killer in the United States and is increasing. Thirty years ago, one in twenty contacted cancer. Today it is one in three. The type of food we eat can gradually create a toxic condition in the body that invites cancer cells to grow. Cancer has a long incubation period which can last many years. Building up the immune system is necessary so the body can heal itself.

Avoid meat because it is dead matter and is low in minerals and produces uric acid which is harmful to the blood. Eliminate fats, salt-cure, salt pickled and smoked foods such as bacon, ham, sausage, smoked fish, bologna and hot dogs. Prevent constipation, which is the main cause of all disease.

Alfalfa, contains anticancer properties. Aloe Vera, Bee Pollen, Black Walnut, Burdock, Echinacea, Golden Seal, Horsetail, Kelp, Pau D'Arco and Suma are all immune builders.

276

HERBAL FORMULAS

Blood Cleansers—Circulatory System—Colon Cleansers—Digestive System—Immune Builders—Nervous System and Brain—Urinary System—Female or Male Formulas—

VITAMINS, MINERALS AND SUPPLEMENTS

Antioxidants vitamins A, C, and E, with minerals selenium and zinc protect against cancer. B-complex vitamins protect the immune system against cancer. Calcium and magnesium supplements may help prevent colon cancer. Natural iron supplements help prevent thyroid cancer. Minerals are essential for protecting the body.

Acidophilus protects against bad bacteria. Blue-green algae and chlorophyll clean and protect the blood. CoQ10 and germanium provide oxygen to the cells and boost the immune system.

CANDIDA _____
(Candidiasis, Thrush, Yeast Infection)

SYMPTOMS

The symptoms are many depending on where it is in the body. They can range from anxiety to chemical sensitivity.

Bad Breath — Constipation — Chronic Infections—Depression—Fatigue—Food Cravings—Gas—Headaches—Adrenal and Thyroid Problems — Hiatal Hernia—Indigestion—Insomnia—Mental Confusion—Odors that cause Discomfort — Panic Attacks— Menstrual Problems—

CAUSES

The overuse of antibiotics is one of the main causes of candida. Antibiotics are also found in beef, chicken, and dairy products. A high sugar diet encourages the candida growth. Repeated pregnancies without time for the body to replenish nutritionally can also be a problem. Nutritional deficiencies, birth control pills, steroid hormones, and many drugs weaken the immune system and set the stage for candida growth.

NUTRITIONAL THERAPY

Yeast multiplies rapidly when starches and sugars are consumed. Eliminate sugar, white flour products, yeasts breads, wine, beer, fruit juices, cheeses, mushrooms, vinegar products, and limit fruit to small amounts. Hydrochloric acid and pancreatic enzymes help to prevent yeast overgrowth.

The liver is responsible for filtering the blood. When overloaded, it is difficult for it to eliminate the yeast growth. Clean the liver and bowels, purify the blood, and stick to a diet rich in vegetables, whole grains, millet, brown rice, buckwheat and other whole grains. Beans are high in protein. Nuts such as almonds are high in nutrients and protein. Avoid peanuts, they carry a cancer causing mold called aflatoxin. Garlic has antifungal properties. A great juice drink is carrots, celery, parsley, 1 clove garlic and ginger.

Herbs to help balance body chemistry and prevent candida are Bee Pollen, Burdock, Echinacea, Ginger, Golden Seal, Kelp, Lobelia, Passion Flower, Pau D'Arco, Psyllium, Slippery Elm, Ginkgo and Suma.

HERBAL FORMULAS

Blood Cleansers—Colon Cleansers—Digestive System—Immune Builders—Infection Fighters—Urinary System-Female or Male Formulas—

VITAMINS, MINERALS AND SUPPLEMENTS

Vitamin A is essential for healthy mucous membranes. Vitamin C with bioflavonoids encourages healing and prevents infections. B-complex (yeast free) are necessary for proper digestion and they also help the liver to eliminate toxins. Extra biotin, B6 and B12 are needed. Vitamin E is an antioxidant for healthy veins and immune function.

A multi-vitamin supplement will build up the immune system. Iron is important for a healthy immune system and energy. Multi-minerals are necessary for proper function and utilization of vitamins.

Acidophilus is important for increasing friendly bacteria and digestion. It is best taken first thing in the morning or just before going to bed so it can reach the colon. Hydrochloric acid can destroy the effects of acidophilus. Chlorophyll and blue-green algae will purify the blood and provide nutrients. They also help the body produce its own interferon. Flaxseed oil and salmon oil help strengthen the immune system. Germanium and CoQ10 improve oxygen supply to the arteries. Lecithin protects the nervous system and brain and also helps prevent fatigue.

CARDIOVASCULAR DISORDERS _____

(Angina Pectoris, Heart disorders, Strokes)

SYMPTOMS

Angina pectoris causes pain or pressure in the chest lasting more than five minutes—Recurrent chest pain—Irregular Heart beat like skipping or twitching feelings—Coughing up blood—Struggling to breath especially when climbing stairs—Heart attacks and strokes can happen without warning. A low fiber diet is a contributing factor to the veins collecting material and causing blockage.

CAUSES

Cardiovascular problems arise when the heart's blood vessels narrow and limit oxygen to the heart. Constipation is the main cause. The bowels back up and the liver cannot eliminate fatty material and toxic deposits that accumulate in the blood and arteries. Recently Chinese statistics have shown that constipation is one of the most common symptoms in ischemic stroke. So when they treat stroke or prevent it, they treat constipation. (C. Keji and S. Jun, "Progress of research on ischemic stroke treated with Chinese medicine," *Journal of Traditional Chinese Medicine 12* (1992): 204-10.

Treating constipation, which causes auto-intoxication, is how doctors before World War II, used to approach their patients with heart problems. (Kellogg, M.D, John Harvey, *"Colon Hygiene"*)

NUTRITIONAL THERAPY

A change of diet is necessary. A high fiber diet using whole grains, brown rice, beans and fresh fruit and vegetables is recommended.

Exercise is beneficial to help provide oxygen to the cells. It also strengthens the lungs and heart.

Bee pollen provides nutrients, Burdock cleans the blood, Cayenne cleans and strengthens the veins. Hawthorn berries feed and build the heart. Kelp cleans the veins. Psyllium cleans the colon. Gingko and Suma help to eliminate blood cholesterol.

HERBAL FORMULAS

Blood Cleansers—Circulatory System—Colon Cleansers—Digestive System—Energy and Stamina—Glandular System—Immune Builders—Nervous System and Brain—Urinary System—Female and Male Formulas—

VITAMINS, MINERALS AND SUPPLEMENTS

Vitamin A strengthens the veins. B-complex vitamins strengthen the heart muscles. Vitamin C with bioflavonoids strengthens the heart muscles and protects the immune system. Vitamin E with lecithin strengthens the heart and veins.

Calcium and magnesium protect the heart, veins and nervous system. Potassium strengthens the heart. Iron is necessary for healthy blood. A multi-mineral supplement keeps the heart healthy.

Acidophilus provides friendly bacteria and is needed for protection. Blue-green algae and chlorophyll helps build rich, healthy blood.

Flaxseed oil and salmon oil contain Omega-3 fatty acids. New evidence links their daily intake with reduced risk of coronary heart and cardiovascular diseases. L-carnitine help dissolve fat around the heart. Lecithin helps dissolve cholesterol deposits. CoQ10 and germanium strengthen veins and provide oxygen to the blood and cells.

CARPAL TUNNEL SYNDROME

SYMPTOMS

Pain is the main symptom which seems to come on at night—when severe, it prevents sleep—Numbness—Burning Sensation—Tingling—Weakness in the hand muscles—

CAUSES

Carpal Tunnel is the most common nerve entrapment syndrome. It results from compression of the median nerve at the wrist. It is seen in computer workers, assembly-line workers, and persons who repeatedly use their wrist. It is most often seen in women between ages 30 to 60.

There are conditions that can cause the structure of the carpal tunnel to swell and press the median nerve against the transverse carpal ligament. Some conditions are: pregnancy, rheumatoid arthritis, renal failure, menopause, diabetes mellitus, hypothyroidism, benign tumors, Raynaud's disease, tuberculosis and an injury. The main causes is nutritional deficiency and fatty deposits in the wrist.

NUTRITIONAL THERAPY

A change in diet is important, using more whole grains, fruit and vegetables. Pure water is vital. Hard water deposits can accumulate in the joints and tap water should not be used. High fiber diets will help eliminate fatty deposits. A low animal protein diet may help since uric acid may accumulate in the joints. A low fat diet will help the liver filter out built-up deposits. An arthritis formula will help clean joints and ease pain.

Sugar can also cause accumulation in the veins because it turns to fat in the liver. A low sugar diet may help since sugar causes calcium, minerals and B vitamins to be eliminated from the body.

Herbs that will help in carpal tunnel are Alfalfa, Bee Pollen, Burdock, Cayenne, Devil's Claw, Echinacea, Ginseng, Horsetail, Kelp, Pau D'Arco, Saffron, and Valerian Root.

HERBAL FORMULAS

Blood Cleansers—Circulatory System—Colon Cleansers-Digestive System—Immune Builders—Nervous System and Brain—Structural System—Urinary System—Female or Male Formulas.

VITAMINS, MINERALS AND SUPPLEMENTS

Vitamin A is essential for healthy cartilage and bones. B-complex is essential with extra B6. A deficiency has been seen in patients with carpal tunnel syndrome. Lack of vitamin C with bioflavonoids can cause weak capillaries, bones and joints. It is essential in the assimilation of calcium. Calcium and magnesium are vital for healthy joints. Potassium helps prevent kidney failure, and is involved with muscle contraction. All minerals are involved in joint and ligament health.

Acidophilus helps in vitamin and mineral assimilation. Flaxseed oil and salmon oil are essential fats the body needs to protect the immune system. CoQ10 and Germanium helps prevent cell damage. L-carnitine helps in dissolving fatty deposits. Lecithin dissolves cholesterol deposits.

CATARRH

(Mucus accumulation)

SYMPTOMS

Runny Nose—Coughing—Bronchitis—Croup—Enlarged Tonsils—Dull Frontal Headache—are all symptoms of catarrh in the head. It depends where the catarrh settles, what the symptoms are. Catarrh of the stomach is called gastritis—The bronchi is called bronchitis—The eyes, conjunctivitis—Ears otitis—The brain, meningitis—Small intestines, enteritis. If it is found in the appendix, its appendicitis—In the kidneys, nephritis—In the joints, arthritis, veins, phlebitis, or in the bladder, cystitis.

CAUSES

The main cause of catarrhal conditions is a diet high in mucus forming and overcooked food. The congestion collects in many areas of the body, usually the weakest part. Pasteurized milk, a high meat diet, white flour and sugar products, cooked oils, and not enough live food will cause congestion in the body.

A common example is indigestion, which indicates too much catarrh in the stomach and constipation which is catarrh in the colon. The immune system is weakened by too much cooked food and lacks raw food to balance the body chemistry.

When cooked food is eaten, white blood cells (which is part of the immune system) increase in the intestines, where cooked food is treated as a poison. Eating raw vegetables before a cooked meal prevents the white cells from coming to the rescue.

NUTRITIONAL THERAPY

Use a high fiber diet using raw food, thermos cooking, sprouts, nuts, seeds, raw fruit and vegetable juices. Whole grains such as millet, buckwheat, brown rice, and beans are recommended. Steamed vegetables and raw salads should be eaten. Catarrh is formed to protect the lining of the stomach and intestines, but when too much is produced and toxins are accumulated, it becomes hard in the colon and causes constipation and autointoxication. A psyllium and herbal formula will help prevent and eliminate toxins in the colon.

Herbs will help clean the colon clean such as Alfalfa, Aloe Vera, Black Walnut, Burdock, Cascara Sagrada, Ginger, Golden Seal, Kelp, Lobelia, Pau D'Arco, Psyllium and Slippery Elm.

HERBAL FORMULAS

Blood Cleansers—Colds, Flu, Fever, and Allergy—Colon Cleansers—Digestive System—Glandular System—Nervous System and Brain—Urinary System—

VITAMINS, MINERALS AND SUPPLEMENTS

Vitamin A, D and C heal the mucous membranes. B-complex helps in eliminating catarrh. Vitamin E, an antioxidant, helps protect the mucous membranes. Calcium and magnesium work together to improve nerve and muscle function. Potassium is good for a healthy stomach and colon and can also prevent acidity and autointoxication.

Mineral supplements are all needed to prevent catarrh accumulation.

Acidophilus helps in assimilation of nutrients.

Blue-green algae and chlorophyll cleans the blood.

CELLULITE

SYMPTOMS

Cellulite is the excess fat that looks like lumps, bumps or dimple deposits on the hips, thighs and buttocks. Cellulite is most often found in women.

CAUSES

The causes of cellulite are lack of exercise, too much starches and sweets, and the wrong kind of fats. This is most often found in women, who produce extra estrogen. When the liver cannot excrete the estrogen properly, it encourages fat accumulation in the wrong places.

Fatty buildup in the fatty tissues results from an underactive bowel created by poor nutrition and elimination which is incomplete removal of wastes from the colon, whether or not you have one or two bowel movements a day. Lack of exercise and poor circulation are also causes.

Poor lymphatic drainage can be a problem and exercise will help. This bad fat is trapped between the cells where they are held by hardened connective tissue and where they collect pockets of water, toxins and fat that give the skin the orange color appearance.

NUTRITIONAL THERAPY

A lasting approach to eliminating cellulite consists of a matter of changing lifestyle, keeping the colon functioning properly and eating lots of raw fruits and vegetables. Cellulite is ugly, unwanted fat and is very hard to eliminate, but with desire and determination, it can be done.

Skin brushing will also speed up the elimination of cellulite. Skin brushing is a well known and proven method for encouraging better lymphatic circulation. Brushing with a long-handled, natural bristle or a loofa "sponge" creates surface friction which promotes circulation and brings nourishment to the skin.

Herbs to help are Alfalfa, Dandelion, Cornsilk, Parsley, Uva Ursi, Bee Pollen, Burdock, Cascara Sagrada, Ginseng, Golden Seal, Hydrangea, Kelp, Psyllium and Saffron.

HERBAL FORMULAS

Blood Cleansers—Circulatory System—Colon Cleansers—Digestive System—Structural System—Female or Male Formulas—

VITAMINS, MINERALS AND SUPPLEMENTS

B-complex vitamins help to eradicate cellulite, especially B3 and niacin, which improve circulation and help lower blood fats. Vitamin E and lecithin are also beneficial for circulation. Lecithin helps eliminate cholesterol. Vitamin C, potassium and B6 will speed up the elimination of cellulite.

Acidophilus helps utilize nutrients. Blue-green algae and chlorophyll help clean blood and nourish the skin. Flaxseed oil and salmon oil, help in burning bad fat in cells. CoQ10 and germanium help supply oxygen to the cells. Lecithin helps utilize oils, and eliminates cholesterol.

CELIAC DISEASE
(Celiac-Sprue, Gluten Intolerance)

SYMPTOMS

Diarrhea—Large and Frequently Foul Smelling Stools—Anemia—Skin Rashes— Nausea — Abdominal Distention — Flatulence—Stomach Cramps—Weakness— Weight Loss—

CAUSES

Celiac is a rare disease found mostly in children but can occur in adults. It is caused when the villain, the small intestines, are damaged by gluten, the protein part of wheat or other grains.

281

Breast fed babies rarely get celiac disease. Usually the first solid foods introduced to babies are cereals. Babies cannot digest cereals, because the enzyme to digest grains is found in the saliva, and chewing is necessary. This can irritate the delicate lining of the small intestine. The lining becomes damaged and loses the ability to absorb essential nutrients.

A tendency toward this disease seems to be inherited. This is probably due to the diet of the parents. Intestinal damage can bring on celiac disease. It can be caused by emotional stress, laxative abuse, intestinal infections, parasites, and excessive coffee intake.

NUTRITIONAL THERAPY

Celiac-Sprue is the name given for the disease in both adults and children. It is caused by the gluten found in wheat, barley and rye grains. Gluten is a gray, sticky, insoluble, nutritious protein. Corn, rice, millet, oats, soybeans, buckwheat, quinoa and amaranth do not contain gluten. Good health can be maintained by eliminating gluten products. Read labels to make sure they do not contain gluten products.

Chinese doctors believe that the inability to digest any healthful food is due to a weakened spleen-pancreas, which is severely lacking in energy and/ or digestive fire.

Malnutrition is seen because of the inability to digest Vitamins A, D and K. Bone pain and lower back rib cage pain may exist because vitamin D is necessary for absorbing calcium. Avoid an over consumption of sugar and white flour products. Anemia is common due to poor absorption of folic acid, iron, vitamin B12 and K.

Herbs to help in celiac disease are Alfalfa and Kelp which contain vitamin K. Aloe Vera helps heal scar tissues. Bee Pollen is nourishing, Burdock, Cascara Sagrada, Golden Seal, Gentian, Pau D'Arco, Psyllium, Saffron, Slippery Elm, and Suma are also useful herbs.

HERBAL FORMULAS

Blood Cleansers—Circulatory System—Colon Cleansers—Digestive System—Glandular System — Immune Builders — Infection Fighters—Nervous System and Brain—Urinary System—

VITAMINS, MINERALS AND SUPPLEMENTS

Supplements are essential since the diagnosis for Celiac-Sprue can take years. Vitamins A, D and K are probably lacking and supplements, are essential. B-complex vitamins are beneficial and needed for many functions of the body. Calcium, magnesium, and potassium are essential to build bones, muscles and protect the heart.

Vitamin C is essential for a healthy immune system. Iron is very essential because anemia is usually present. Minerals are necessary and selenium and zinc are essential.

Acidophilus helps in digestion. Blue-green algae and chlorophyll contain vitamin K and other essential minerals. They also helps in the digestion of nutrients. Flaxseed oil and salmon oil build blood and the immune system. Germanium and CoQ10 provide oxygen to the cells. Lecithin breaks up fat deposits and lowers cholesterol.

CHEMICAL IMBALANCE

SYMPTOMS

Emotional Disturbance—Anorexia and Bulimia can create a Chemical Imbalance—Confusion—Forgetfulness—Irritability—Inability to make Quick Decisions—

CAUSES

What is "Chemical Imbalance?" Dr. William J. Goldwag, M.D, said in *Bestways*, April 1984, that "Chemical Imbalance," is not a specific disease. Instead, it refers to any condition or set of circumstances which change the normal pattern of chemical reactions in the body. This can occur in any disease or especially prior to the development of an illness."

The brain has a set of chemicals called neurotransmitters which may become unbalanced when the rest of the body seems healthy. The brain is extremely sensitive and when not nourished properly, can cause problems. In autointoxication, the brain suffers toxic effects which will alter brain function and cause emotional problems.

Alfalfa, Bee Pollen, and Kelp provide nutrients. Burdock, Echinacea, and Pau D' Arco clean the blood. Horsetail aids in the assimilation of calcium and other minerals. Gotu Kola, Ginkgo and Suma nourish and stimulate brain function.

NUTRITIONAL THERAPY

When it comes to chemical imbalance in the brain, there is only one natural source to correct it: Food (including vitamins, minerals and herbs). The brain is the seat of our emotions and is another organ in the body. It needs to be fed and nourished and looked after as much as the heart, lungs, liver or any other part of the body.

Research has found that what we lack in our diet causes an imbalance of the brain neurotransmitters. A toxic colon and congested liver need to be cleaned. People with emotional problems need more nutrients than the normal dosage.

A diet rich in fresh fruit and vegetables is essential. Fresh vegetable juices help to nourish and clean the body and are easy to assimilate in a weakened state. Whole grains, especially millet, brown rice, whole oats, yellow corn meal, and buckwheat are beneficial. Use almonds, sesame seeds and pine nuts. Green drinks help nourish and clean the blood.

HERBAL FORMULAS

Blood Cleansers—Circulatory System—Colon Cleansers—Digestive System—Energy and Stamina—Glandular System—Immune Builders—Nervous System and Brain—Urinary System — Female and Male Formulas—

VITAMINS, MINERALS AND SUPPLEMENTS

Vitamins A, C, E and the minerals selenium and zinc are antioxidants and will protect against cell damage and disease. B-complex vitamins help to boost brain function, and choline stimulates acetylcholine levels in the brain. Serotonin levels in the brain can be increased by sunlight. Passion flower will boost serotonin levels. B6 helps in depression.

Calcium, magnesium and potassium are needed for proper brain function. Iron will strengthen the blood. Minerals are necessary for vitamins to work properly. Acidophilus protects against bad bacteria in the colon. Blue-green algae and chlorophyll will build the blood, speed the assimilation of nutrients and increase health.

Flaxseed oil and salmon oil are essential nutrients for health. COQ10 and germanium provide oxygen to the blood and cells. Lecithin is needed for healthy brain function.

CHEMICAL POISONING —

SYMPTOMS

Neurological symptoms are: Mental Confusion—Mental Illness—Nervous System Disorders—A Low Immune System will cause Autoimmune Diseases—When it settles in the bones it can cause Anemia—Leukemia—Sarcoma of the Bones— Hodgkins Disease and Immune System Disorders—

CAUSES

There are all kinds of chemical additives and environmental toxins. They are present in the air, water and in our food. Plutonium is created from nuclear plants and there are tons of nuclear waste sites in the United States which are leaking into our water supplies. Radioactive isotopes are invisible, odorless and tasteless. Radiation of any kind is cumulative.

Strontium 90 is very prevalent. Scientists say that everyone has potentially dangerous amounts of radioactive strontium in their bones. Our one defense and protection is to strengthen and protect the immune system.

NUTRITIONAL THERAPY

Pectin protects against strontium 90 and prevents absorption in the bones. Foods rich in pectin are grapefruit, soybeans, oranges, carrots, bananas, beets, potatoes, apples, brussels sprouts and beans.

Sulfur foods can also protect against chemical poisoning. Foods that contain sulfur are kale, watercress, brussels sprouts, horseradish, cabbage, cranberries, turnips, cauliflower, savoy cabbage, garlic, onions, almonds, parsnips, leeks, okra, and chard.

Whole grains help eliminate toxins such as millet, brown rice, whole oats, and buckwheat.

Herbs that help protect against the effects of chemical pollutants are Alfalfa, Aloe Vera, Bee Pollen, Burdock, Cascara Sagrada, Echinacea, Ginseng, Golden Seal, Gotu Kola, Kelp, Pau D'Arco, Psyllium, Ginkgo and Suma.

HERBAL FORMULAS

Blood Cleansers—Circulatory System—Colon Cleansers—Digestive System—Immune Builders—Nervous System and Brain—Structural System—Urinary System—Female and Male Formulas—

VITAMINS, MINERALS AND SUPPLEMENTS

Antioxidants vitamins A, C, and E and the minerals selenium and zinc protect against toxins. Vitamin C with bioflavonoids counteracts radiation and chemical toxins. B-complex vitamins protect against toxins and chemical poisoning. Calcium, magnesium and potassium protects against lead poisoning and radioisotopes. Iron builds red blood cells. Radiation in the air increases the need for iron. Mineral supplements protect against chemical poisoning. Amino acids high in sulfur are Cysteine and Methionine.

Acidophilus protects the immune system. Blue-green algae contains nucleic acids to protect against radiation. Chlorophyll can decrease toxins from radiation. Lecithin contains choline and inositol to help counteract the effects of chemical poisoning. It regulates blood cholesterol and prevents hardening of the arteries. It protects the liver, kidneys and heart, and protects against strontium 90, X-rays, radiation, and fine particles in the air.

CoQ10 and germanium protect against toxins from metals mercury and cadmium. Flaxseed oil and salmon oil strengthen and protect the body.

CHILDHOOD DISEASES

SYMPTOMS

Fevers, in varying degrees—Rashes—Coughs—Sore Throat—Weakness—Loss of Appetite—The childhood diseases are Chicken Pox—Measles—Mumps—Rubella—(German Measles)—Rheumatic Fever—Scarlet Fever—Whooping Cough. Mumps can be serious in teenagers and can spread to the ovaries, pancreas, testicles and the nervous system.

CAUSES

Childhood diseases serve to cleanse the system from inherited or acquired weaknesses in the body. Germs are nature's scavengers and can live only on toxins and excess mucus in the body. Sugar and white flour products weaken the body, especially in small children, who consume junk food and leave little room for nourishing food.

NUTRITIONAL THERAPY

To protect against childhood diseases, keep the bowels moving and protect with herbal formulas. These diseases can be treated at the first sign of symptoms. Treat the kidneys and bowels. Sweating therapy can be used to bring out toxins through the skin. Herbal garlic extract formulas will help treat as well as prevent serious complications. Drinking juices such as orange, lemon, lime and grapefruit will speed the cleansing. They can be used with an herbal tea bowel formula which will clean the kidneys and bowels. Herbs can be given every 30 minutes to ease the symptoms. Diaphoretic herbs to produce perspiration are Angelica, Blue Vervain, Boneset, Catnip, Cayenne, Chamomile, Elder Flowers, and Linden Flowers.

Alfalfa can be made into a tea. Aloe Vera in small amounts cleans the colon. Black Walnut, Burdock, Echinacea, Ginger, Golden Seal, Kelp, Licorice, Lobelia, Passion Flower, Psyllium, and Slippery Elm are useful herbs.

HERBAL FORMULAS

Blood Cleansers—Colds, Flu, Fever and Allergy — Colon Cleansers — Immune Builders—Infection Fighters—Nervous System and Brain—

VITAMINS, MINERALS AND SUPPLEMENTS

Vitamin A and C with bioflavonoids help with healing in childhood diseases. A multi-mineral supplement and potassium are good for colds and fevers. Blue-green algae heals and strengthens the lungs and throat. Chlorophyll helps clean toxins from the blood. Acidophilus helps protect the body and improve digestion.

COLDS, FLU, AND FEVERS

SYMPTOMS

Runny Nose—Watery Eyes—Sneezing—Coughs—Sore Throat—Nausea—Diarrhea—Swollen Glands. With the flu there can be Chills—Headache—Backache—Aches All Over—and Nausea—

CAUSES

Colds, flu and fevers are acute diseases which are nature's natural cleansing of the body. Germs and viruses are a result of toxins in the body. They will not invade a body that is clean with a strong immune and nervous system.

Poor eating habits and stress can cause toxins to accumulate and germs and viruses to invade. Constipation causes an accumulation of toxins in the bloodstream and settles in different parts of the body. When toxins in the body increase and elimination is decreased, nature causes an acute disease. Acute diseases are nature's way of protecting the body. When acute diseases are treated naturally, it will prevent chronic diseases from accumulating.

NUTRITIONAL THERAPY

Natural treatment is to stop eating and use citrus juices. Oranges, grapefruit, lemons and limes help clean the blood, stimulate liver function and eliminate toxins and mucus from the body. Use herbal teas and specific herbs to fit the symptoms. When vomiting occurs, use peppermint tea to settle the stomach.

Herbal laxatives will speed the cleansing process. Enemas will help bring down a fever and clean the colon. Hot herbal teas will increase sweating and reduce fevers and boost elimination of toxins through the skin. Rest will help the body heal faster. When you eat large amounts of food with an acute disease, it stops the cleansing process and the toxins deposit in different parts of the body. It could be the lungs, stomach, head, or any organ of the body.

Using drugs will also stop the cleansing process. Aspirin causes the stomach to bleed. Cold medication can also stop the cleansing process. Using natural remedies will make you feel better while acute diseases run their course. Use pure water to help eliminate toxins.

Single herbs that help in acute diseases are Burdock, Echinacea, Elder Flower, Ginger, Golden Seal, Kelp, Licorice, Lobelia, Passion Flower, Pau D'Arco, Psyllium and Slippery Elm.

HERBAL FORMULAS

Blood Cleansers—Colds, Flu, Fever and Allergy — Colon Cleansers — Infection Fighters—Nervous System and Brain—Urinary System—

VITAMINS, MINERALS AND SUPPLEMENTS

Vitamin A and beta-carotene protect the mucous membranes. Vitamin C with bioflavonoids has been shown to shorten the course of colds and also has antiviral properties. Zinc has antiviral activity and speeds healing. Minerals, especially selenium are healing. Calcium and magnesium, balance, build the blood and sustain the nerves.

Blue-green algae and chlorophyll will help clean toxins from the blood.

COLITIS

SYMPTOMS

Diarrhea—Stomach Cramps—Blood in Stools—Incomplete elimination of the Bowels—Alternate Constipation and Diarrhea — Weakness — Weight Loss — Headaches—Indigestion—Fatigue—It is also called spastic colon. If bleeding occurs anemia could result—

CAUSES

Colitis is a disease of the large intestine. A soft diet using refined food can be harmful. This type of diet results in constipation and causes colitis in the first place. Some causes could be the overuse of over-the-counter laxatives, cooking in aluminum utensils, food allergy, over-consumption of refined carbohydrates, and eating too much sugar.

Colitis is a chronic infection in the lower colon. It is caused by infection of the mucous membranes as a result of prolonged irritation of toxic fecal matters which accumulates and is retained day after day. Toxic bacteria multiplies quickly when retained in the lower bowel too long. Low fiber food and wrong combinations of food causes accumulation of toxic waste in the colon.

Stress can add to the problem. The colon tightens up under stress. Stress and emotions need to be dealt with. The nervous system needs to be strengthened and nourished so the body can handle stress.

NUTRITIONAL THERAPY

Chewing food well is essential for proper digestion. Eliminate milk products, because they are irritating to the colon. Wheat products could be irritating to the colon, and can also cause an allergic reaction. Include mineral drinks to prevent electrolyte imbalance.

Use juice drinks containing cabbage, carrots, celery and parsley to help heal colitis. Brown rice and millet are beneficial for colitis, and are easy to digest. Cook grains in a thermos overnight to obtain enzymes which will help heal the colon. Eat boiled potatoes, sweet potatoes, cooked carrots, squash, avocados, and bananas which will provide protein, fat and carbohydrate, vitamins and minerals.

Slippery elm is very healing and soothing and provides protein. Make a gruel with one teaspoon of powdered slippery elm to one pint of pure boiling water and blend well. Add cinnamon, nutmeg or cardamon for flavor. Drink slowly on an empty stomach to coat the lower colon.

Aloe Vera is healing. Alfalfa contains minerals. Garlic and Echinacea are healing and act like antibiotics. Hops, Kelp, Lobelia, Marshmallow, Myrrh, Papaya, Pau D'Arco, Psyllium, and Slippery Elm are useful for colitis.

HERBAL FORMULAS

Blood Cleansers—Circulation System—Colds, Flu, Fever and Allergy—Colon Cleansers—Digestive System—Immune Builders—Infection Fighters—Nervous System and Brain—Urinary System—Female and Male Formulas—

VITAMIN, MINERALS AND SUPPLEMENTS

Vitamins A and E repair tissue. B-complex vitamins help in healing and in stress. Vitamin C with bioflavonoids is healing and helps prevent infections. Calcium, magnesium and potassium help prevent colon cancer and relax muscles of the colon. Iron, in a natural form, helps to prevent anemia and increase stamina. Trace minerals in extract form are essential for healing, assimilation and digestion.

Acidophilus is essential for healing the colon and provides friendly bacteria. It also helps in the digestion of food, vitamins and minerals. Blue green algae and chlorophyll are very healing and contain vitamin K, which has been linked with colitis.

CONSTIPATION ——————

SYMPTOMS

Hard, dry stools—Straining at the Stool—Bad Breath—Heartburn—Delays in Elimination, Days or Weeks—Gas—Autointoxication—Headaches—Bloated Feeling—Lack of Energy— Feeling of not Completely Eliminating—

CAUSES

Constipation can be caused by bad eating habits, lack of fiber and nutrients, eating white flour products, (glue foods), overeating, bad food combining, stress (tightening of the anus), lack of exercise, bad drinking habits, poor living habits, (drinking, smoking, drugs, lack of proper rest).

Constipation can cause numerous problems if left untreated. Every system of the body can be effected through autointoxication caused by constipation. The following can cause constipation: aspirin, atropine used to prevent motion sickness, Pepto-Bismol®, pepcid and Tagamet®, aluminum products, and many other drugs.

NUTRITIONAL THERAPY

A change of diet is essential for the bowels to be healthy and regular. A high fiber diet will help to clean and completely eliminate the colon of waste products soon after eating. Eat whole grains, whole wheat, brown rice, yellow corn meal, whole oats, millet, buckwheat, amaranth, and quinoa. They contain bran and are rich in fiber, vitamins and minerals as well as complex carbohydrates and protein.

Use fresh steamed vegetables and fresh fruit of all kinds. Juices that are good for constipation are: prune, apple and peach, which have a laxative effect. Beet greens, cabbage, parsley and carrots are also beneficial.

Eliminate constipating foods such as: fried foods, sugar, white flour, beef, cheese, junk food, coffee, carbonated drinks, wine, pastries and fast foods.

Exercise and drinking plenty of pure water are necessary to prevent constipation. A gradual change in diet helps the body and mind adjust to a new way of eating.

Start with a lower bowel cleanser, which will clean deep while rebuilding the colon. If constipation is stubborn, you can add Cascara Sagrada. Start slowly and increase amounts as needed. A Psyllium hull herbal combination can be added.

Aloe Vera is a natural laxative. Black Walnut eliminates worms. Burdock neutralizes toxins and cleans blood. Cascara Sagrada is a natural laxative. Ginger soothes and helps to prevent cramps. Golden Seal kills parasites and heals the colon. Lobelia relaxes the colon. Psyllium creates bulk and loosens material from the colon. Slippery Elm heals the colon.

HERBAL FORMULAS

Blood Cleansers—Circulatory System—Colon Cleansers—Digestive System—Immune Builders—Urinary System—

VITAMINS, MINERALS AND SUPPLEMENTS

Vitamins A and E protect the mucous membranes. B-complex vitamins help regularity, protect the intestine and improve digestion. They also help to eliminate toxins from the liver. Vitamin C destroys toxins in the colon.

Calcium and magnesium help relax the bowels. Potassium is healing for the stomach and colon. Iron helps liver to detoxify. Minerals are essential for a healthy colon.

Acidophilus restores health to the colon. Chlorophyll is a blood cleanser and helps in digestion. Blue-green algae heals and nourishes the colon. Lecithin is beneficial to the colon and kidneys.

COUGHS ─────────────

SYMPTOMS

Croupy—Hard, Unproductive—Feverish—Catarrhal—(Phlegm)—Watery—Chronic—Flu—(Congestion in the Chest)—Allergies—Bronchitis—

CAUSES

Coughs are nature's reflex action to try to clear the airways of mucus, phlegm, foreign bodies, or an irritant or blockage. These could be dust, smoke or mucus dripping from the sinuses.

Coughs can be caused by allergies, acute diseases, air pollution, colds developing into bronchitis, pneumonia, asthma, tuberculosis, and cancer of the lungs.

Croupy coughs usually comes on suddenly with a loud rasping sound. The phlegm is difficult to cough up. When a croupy cough starts, using a few drops of Lobelia under the tongue every few minutes will sometimes loosen the mucous.

A bronchial cough is tight and painful. A feverish and catarrhal cough usually accompanies infections. A sinus infection or allergy will cause drainage down the throat that produces a cough.

Acute coughs are nature's way of eliminating toxins in the form of mucus. Chronic coughs can be a sign of a serious disease.

Damage to the lung tissues caused by pneumonia, asthma, or tuberculosis can cause a cough. Lung cancer or tumors can cause a mild cough at first, then becomes more severe and may accompany blood-stained phlegm.

An inhaled foreign object, such as a popcorn kernel, can lodge in the larynx and cause a violent cough to relieve choking. It can travel down further and block a bronchus, which can lead to a persistent cough.

Smoker's cough is seen as a recurrent one and is common. The sufferer becomes accustomed to it and regards it as normal.

NUTRITIONAL THERAPY

An acute cough in the form of a cold or flu should be treated naturally. Stop eating and use only citrus juices and herbal teas to drink. Use herbs to help congestion, relax, and help eliminate built-up toxins. Air pollution puts an extra burden on the lungs and lowers resistance. Vitamins A and C are essential for healthy lungs. The stomach needs to eliminate the mucus and toxins to repair and heal the body. Avoid cough medicines, antibiotics and all drugs which only suppress the cough and drainage.

Single herbs to help prevent as well as heal coughs are: Burdock, Blue Vervain, Echinacea, Kelp, Licorice Root, Lobelia, Passion Flower, Pau D'Arco, Psyllium, Red Raspberry, Slippery Elm and Valerian.

HERBAL FORMULAS

Blood Cleansers—Colds, Flu, Fevers and Allergy — Colon Cleansers — Digestive System — Immune Builders — Infection Fighters—Nervous System and Brain—Urinary System—

VITAMINS, MINERALS AND SUPPLEMENTS

Vitamins A and C are important in coughs. They help heal as well as protect against infections. Vitamin E builds the immune system. B-Complex, builds blood.

Calcium and magnesium are relaxing, and help in infections. Iron helps in colds, sore throats, and builds blood. Potassium calms nerves and is healing. Selenium and Zinc build the immune system and heal. A multi-mineral supplement helps provide nutrients for healing.

Acidophilus protects and heals. Blue-green algae is good for infections. CoQ10 and germanium build the immune system. Lecithin fights infection and builds resistance to disease. Flaxseed oil and salmon oil help protect against disease and help balance body chemistry.

CHRONIC BRAIN SYNDROME

SYMPTOMS

Lack of Reasoning—Errors in Judgement—Neglect of Personal Hygiene—Short Term Memory Loss—Disorientation—Poor Intellectual Function—Severe Symptom: Hallucinations—Incoherent Speech—Restlessness—Agitation—

CAUSES

Adrenal or Thyroid Dysfunction—Pulmonary Insufficiency—Wilson's Disease—Vitamin B Deficiencies—Hemorrhage—Vascular Disorder — Brain Abscess — Parasite Infections—Injury—Brain Tumor—Venereal Disease—Chemical Poisoning—(lead, mercury, or organic solvents)—

NUTRITIONAL THERAPY

Subclinical malnutrition can bring on the symptoms of senility. Cooking robs the food of enzymes, some vitamins especially vitamins B, and C. Fresh fruit and vegetables, whole grains, brown rice, beans, sprouts, raw vegetables, fruit juices and natural supplements are beneficial.

Because of poor nutrition and lack of fiber, the colon becomes congested and the tiny capillaries become narrowed and reduce the supply of oxygen and nutrients available to the brain and tissues. This results in memory loss, confusion, disorientation and agitation. Agitation is from not realizing what is going on. Much of what is considered "senility," is the result of deficiency. A change of eating habits will do much to improve brain function.

Herbs that can help in brain disorders are Burdock, Butcher's Broom, Capsicum, Echinacea, Garlic, Ginseng, Ginkgo, Gotu Kola, Psyllium, and Suma.

HERBAL FORMULAS

Blood Cleansers—Circulatory System—Colon Cleansers—Digestive System—Energy and Stamina—Immune Builder—Nervous System and Brain—Structural System—Urinary System—Female and Male Formulas—

VITAMINS, MINERALS AND SUPPLEMENTS

Decreased amounts of vitamins A, C, and B-complex are seen in senility, especially B12 and B3. Vitamins A, C with bioflavonoids, E with minerals selenium and zinc are antioxidants to prevent free radical damage. Vitamin E repairs brain damage. B-complex are essential. Cooked food destroys vitamin C and B vitamins. Minerals prevent toxic metals from accumulating in the brain. Iron is needed for clean blood. All minerals are essential for a healthy brain. Manganese improves memory. Sulphur helps clean the brain tissues. Silicon is essential for strong nerves. The brain needs calcium, magnesium and phosphorus to think clearly. Blue-green algae and chlorophyll will help dissolve hard deposits and nourish the brain. CoQ10 and germanium provide oxygen to the brain. Lecithin helps clean plaque and nourishes the brain. Flaxseed oil and salmon oil lower cholesterol and prevent blood clotting.

CROHN'S DISEASE

SYMPTOMS

At first symptoms can be mild—Acute inflammatory symptoms mimic appendicitis and include lower right pain—Cramping—Tenderness, Flatulence—Nausea— fever—Diarrhea—Bleeding may occur—Chronic Symptoms—Diarrhea (four to six stools a day) Lower right pain—Weight loss—Weakness—(loss of potassium and other minerals)—Abscesses—Fistulas—

CAUSES

Crohn's disease, which most often affects the small intestine is seen as a bacterial or viral infection. The ileum is its most common site but can affect the small and large intestine.

The most common cause of symptoms is due to the inflammation of the walls which prevent absorption of essential nutrients. It is felt that Crohn's disease is an "autoimmune" disorder. I feel that the gastrointestinal tract becomes so toxic from many years of toxin buildup from poor eating habits, medications, etc., that the immune system becomes confused. It then attacks the toxic tissues, and begins to destroy them thinking they are a foreign organism. Autointoxication and parasites are two of the main causes.

NUTRITIONAL THERAPY

A diet free of meat has helped Crohn's patients. (meat can cause constipation and parasite infestation). Eliminating white sugar and white flour products has been effective. A high fiber diet is beneficial. Eat a lot of fresh fruit and vegetable juices, salads, and steamed vegetables. A program of healing, cleaning and building will provide nutrients that have been lacking. The small intestine assimilates nutrients and can be lacking because of Crohn's disease.

Herbs that will help heal are Alfalfa, Aloe Vera, Bee Pollen, Black Walnut, Burdock, Cascara Sagrada, Fenugreek, Golden Seal, Kelp, Passion Flower, Pau D'Arco, Psyllium, Saffron, Slippery Elm and White Oak Bark.

HERBAL FORMULAS

Blood Cleansers—Colon Cleansers—Digestive System — Immune Builders — Infection Fighters—Nervous System and Brain— Urinary System—

VITAMINS, MINERALS AND SUPPLEMENTS

Supplements are very important because of the depletion from poor absorption and diarrhea. Vitamin A and E repair tissue. B-complex vitamins help in healing and in stress. Vitamin C with bioflavonoids is healing. Calcium, magnesium and potassium prevent colon cancer and strengthen muscles of the colon. Iron is important to prevent anemia and increase energy.

Trace minerals in extract form are essential for healing. Acidophilus is essential to heal the colon and provide friendly bacteria. Blue-green algae is very healing and rich in vitamins and minerals especially vitamin K. Deficiencies have been linked with Crohn's disease. Liquid chlorophyll is rich in nutrients and is healing.

CYSTIC FIBROSIS

SYMPTOMS

Abdominal Distention — Vomiting — Constipation—Dehydration—Electrolyte Imbalance—Sweat Gland Dysfunction— Recurrent Bronchitis and Pneumonia—

CAUSES

This disease is a hereditary disorder caused by a recessive genetic trait carried by both parents. Cystic fibrosis creates a lot of mucus in the body which contains toxins and are irritating to the colon. The child inherited the mucus and toxins from their parents. There is a weakness in the exocrine glands, those secreting mucus, which are the pancreas and sweat glands. This is a weakness which comes from the parents.

A lack of digestive enzymes, exists and minerals and vitamins are poorly absorbed and may cause malnutrition. The mucus membranes in the lungs accumulate mucus and attract virus and germs which creates constant infections.

NUTRITIONAL THERAPY

Many nutritionist see CF as a defect in the ability to absorp selenium, zinc, essential fatty acids and other mega and trace elements as a result of subclinical celiac disease. If the disease progresses unmanaged, it will spread through the intestines resulting in malabsorption of protein, minerals and essential fatty acids and lung infections.

Diet change has improved CF patients. Learning what foods are irritating to the intestines and eliminating or reducing them through rotation diet can help. This gives the small intestine time to heal and repair while improving absorption of nutrients. The most common irritating foods are wheat and dairy products.

The diet should include raw fruits and vegetables, steamed vegetables, fruit and vegetable juices, (carrot juice is a source of calcium and carotene, which converts into vitamin A in the liver. Parsley, green peppers, garlic are a source of magnesium, selenium and zinc.) Raw oils, nuts, seeds, honey, sprouts, baked potatoes, squash and yams are beneficial.

Cleanse the colon. A congested colon can balloon and cause a dysfunction of the Ileocecal Valve which causes toxic poisons to enter the small intestine and cause irritations. These poisons are 20% more toxic then when toxins come from the large colon.

Take Alfalfa, which is rich in vitamin K and is usually lacking. Aloe Vera heals tissues and adhesions. Black Walnut kills parasites and worms. Burdock cleans blood. Cascara Sagrada is a colon cleanser. Golden Seal heals and kills parasites. Kelp supplies minerals and cleans. Passion Flower relaxes nerves for proper healing. Pau D'Arco cleans blood and liver. Psyllium cleans colon. Saffron helps digest oils. Slippery Elm is healing and nourishing. White Oak eliminates catarrh and heals.

HERBAL FORMULAS

Blood Cleansers—Colon Cleansers—Digestive System—Immune Builders—Infection Fighters—Nervous System and Brain—Urinary System—

VITAMINS, MINERALS AND SUPPLEMENTS

The fat-soluble nutrients are deficient in CF individuals because pancreatic obstruction prevents release of the enzymes needed for their absorption. These nutrients are vitamins A, E, D, K and essential fatty acids.

Vitamin A is needed to protect the mucous membranes and prevent infections. Beta carotene would absorb better and not endanger the liver. Vitamin A derived from carrot powder would also supply calcium. Vitamin E is difficult to absorb, and CF patients test low in this vitamin. The exocrine glands show signs of oxygen starvation. Lack of vitamin E causes blood cells to die prematurely without being replaced quickly and lowers resistance to infections. Anemia can also develop. Water soluble vitamin E would be absorbed better. Vitamin C with bioflavonoids is essential to those with CF who are plagued with frequent infections. Vitamin C helps remove waste out of the body. Small frequent doses are better tolerated and some feel that buffered vitamin C is absorbed better. B-complex vitamins are important and keep all cells healthy. Using this with pancreatic enzymes has been beneficial to some with CF. Pancreatic digestive enzymes can benefit CF sufferers. They usually lack nutrient absorption and have poor pancreatic function which causes certain allergy-like responses, mucus build-up(where germs breed), and poor colon function. Free-form amino acids can be used until the small colon is healed. Acidophilus is needed because of all the antibiotics given to prevent infections as well as during infections. Since antibiotics destroy intestinal flora, this inhibits the absorption of B-complex vitamins. This also leads to Candida which lowers the immune system.

Chlorophyll and blue-green algae will heal and nourish the colon.

CYSTS, POLYPS, AND TUMORS

SYMPTOMS

Growths on body—Cysts contains fluid, Semifluid or Solid Material—Tumors—Abnormal Growths of Tissue—could be Cancerous—

CAUSES

Cysts and Tumors collect in the body when toxins are allowed to accumulate creating mucus from a bad diet or living habits. They can harden in the body over a time period. They accumulate when the body does not eliminate naturally through normal channels such as the kidneys, colon, and skin.

Using drugs and rich food with acute diseases suppresses the mucus and toxins and solidifies in the body.

NUTRITIONAL THERAPY

A complete change of diet is necessary in order dissolve cysts and tumors. The harder they are the longer it will take to eliminate. One cause of growth of cysts and tumors is the lack of potassium food, such as almonds, apples, dried apricots, bananas, beans, beets, broccoli, carrots, dulse, figs, goat milk, grapes, kale, olives, parsley, pecans, rice bran, sunflower seeds, watercress and wheat bran and germ. These foods are very beneficial to help eliminate cysts and tumors.

Herbs to help this condition include Alfalfa, which supplies minerals and is healing, Burdock which cleans the blood, Cayenne which stimulates and heal, Echinacea also cleans the blood and has antibiotic properties, Golden Seal which also has antibiotic properties and eliminates toxins, Horsetail which supplies silicon for assimilation of minerals, Kelp which is rich in minerals, Pau D'Arco which is a blood cleanser, Suma which increases circulation, and Garlic which has been shown in studies to have tumor reducing abilities.

HERBAL FORMULAS

Blood Cleansers—Colon Cleansers—Digestive System — Immune Builders — Urinary System—

VITAMINS, MINERALS AND SUPPLEMENTS

Vitamin A and E are powerful antioxidants and immunostimulants essential for preventing stagnation in the body. Vitamin C with bioflavonoids cleans the veins, promotes a healthy immune system and helps prevent cysts and tumors. B-complex vitamins repair cells. Calcium, magnesium, potassium, selenium and zinc protect the immune system.

CoQ10 and germanium promote immune function and carry oxygen to the cells and increase circulation in the blood. Digestive Enzymes aid in the breakdown of undigested foods in the system to help prevent stagnation. Chlorophyll and blue-green algae clean and nourish the blood. Lecithin helps to regulate metabolism and break down fat and cholesterol and prevent cysts and tumors.

DEPRESSION ——————

SYMPTOMS

Depression has been defined as "A state of excessive sadness or hopelessness, often with physical symptoms." Insomnia—Sleeping too much—Loss of Appetite—Negative Attitude—Dissatisfaction with Life—Fatigue—Anger—Anxiety—Worthlessness—Manic Depression have periods of high elation—Working sprees—Spending Sprees—Constant Moving—Followed by Deep Depression

CAUSES

An imbalance in body chemistry can trigger depression, which can result from a lack of nutrients. Events connected with extreme loss such as death, divorce, losing a job, along with a bad diet can lead to depression. Allergies to certain foods and chemicals and hormonal changes in women can precipitate depression. Epstein, candida, hypoglycemia, poor diet, and poor digestion along with poor absorption and elimination also contribute. Lingering illness and mind altering drugs can cause depression. The main cause is autointoxication.

NUTRITIONAL THERAPY

The mind is very sensitive to toxins, constipation and autointoxication can cause bad estrogen in women to accumulate, especially when the liver is congested from constipation. Toxins can travel in the blood and into the brain and cause an imbalance in our rational thinking.

Studies have been conducted on mentally disturbed patients participating in a diet change by eliminating meat, sugar, processed foods and synthetic foods and additives. Included in their diets were whole grains, brown rice, beans, fresh vegetables and fruit. A noticeable change was seen in the reduction of agitation and psychosis among the patients.

Blood and colon cleansing are necessary to eliminate toxins in the body. A wholesome diet will strengthen the nerves and brain.

Some herbs that are beneficial for depression are Ginseng, Gotu Kola, Ginkgo, and Suma. Bee Pollen is very beneficial for nourishing the brain.

HERBAL FORMULAS

Blood Cleansers—Circulatory System—Colon Cleansers—Digestive System—Energy and Stamina—Immune Builders—Nervous System and Brain—Structural—Urinary System—Female or Male Formulas—

VITAMINS, MINERALS AND SUPPLEMENTS

Vitamin A benefits tissues of the glands which maintain hormonal balance. A deficiency of the B vitamins slows the liver's ability to eliminate the excess estrogen that most women have. Vitamins C and E are known to help the liver deal with toxins and eliminate them. Vitamin E has been called the "anti-estrogenic vitamin."

Magnesium, calcium, selenium and zinc are important for preventing depression. The brain needs minerals, and a lack can cause depression and create a chemical imbalance. Chromium is needed for utilizing fats in the body. Potassium helps in maintaining normal heart beat. Silicon, found in horsetail, helps in the assimilation of calcium and other minerals.

Germanium and CoQ10 prevent free radical damage and act as antioxidants and provide oxygen to the brain cells. Chlorophyll and blue-green algae clean and nourish the blood, liver and brain. Lecithin is needed in the brain and contains choline and inositol, which eliminate toxins in the brain as well as nourish it.

DIABETES

SYMPTOMS

The symptoms of Type l called insulin-dependent or juvenile diabetes—Excessive Thirst and Urination—Excessive Hunger—Depression—Weakness—Dry Mouth—Blurred Vision-Nausea—Vomiting—Type II Diabetes (Maturity-Onset Diabetes) Symptom are Frequent Urination—Unusual Thirst—Obesity—General Weakness—Skin Disorders—Boils—Blurred Vision—Impotence—Dry Mouth—
Complications of diabetes may include Blindness—Heart Disease—Kidney Problems—Circulatory problems in the extremities—

CAUSES

One thing Dr. John Harvey Kellogg observed when he X-rayed diabetic patients was that their ileocecal valve was usually incompetent. The ileocecal valve protects the small intestine from infection. The regurgitation of the colon contents into the small intestine is estimated to be 20 times faster than in the large colon. Alloxan, a toxin produced in the colon, was injected into animals and found that it destroyed the Islets of Langerhans in their pancreas. This poison is produced by the action of any oxidizing agent on a factor of the vitamin E complex. These poisons are found in chlorine in the municipal drinking water and in the bleach used in commercial flour products.

Other causes of diabetes include obesity, stress, pregnancy and oral contraceptives: increased levels of estrogen and placental hormones which antagonize insulin. Other medications that are known insulin antagonists are: Thiazide diuretics, adrenal corticosteroids, and phenytoin. A diet high in sugar and white flour products can put extra burden on the pancreas. Parasites are also implicated in diabetes, especially childhood onset diabetes. This seem very logical because parasites are known to harbor in the cecum, below the ileocecal valve, and when it is incompetent, the parasites are dumped into the pancreas or other organs.

NUTRITIONAL THERAPY

Eliminate sugar, white flour products, fruit juices, greasy and fatty foods, (meat, eggs, cheese, excess oil, rancid nuts and seeds), high fat (which encourages diabetes and also causes damage to the liver, which causes an imbalance in the spleen and pancreas causing pancreatic secretions such as insulin less effective). Eat small, frequent meals, (avoid big heavy meals) which help stimulate insulin production. Avoid eating late at night.

A high carbohydrate and high fiber diet reduces the need for insulin and lower the fat levels in the blood. Proper chewing, particularly with complex carbohydrates where digestion begins with saliva, is essential for adequate minerals and nutrients to be absorbed. Exercise improves circulation which tends to be poor in diabetics. It also lowers blood sugar levels.

Vegetable broths are rich in mineral and very healing for the pancreas. Fresh fruit contains natural sugar called fructose which is not hard on the pancreas. Short fasts will help speed up the elimination of excess sugar in the cells. Golden Seal helps to regulate blood sugar and Cedar Berries help to heal the pancreas. Black Walnut kills parasites and worms. Echinacea and Burdock clean the blood. Hydrangea cleans the kidneys and Ginkgo, Gotu Kola and Suma help strengthen the immune system.

HERBAL FORMULAS

Blood Cleansers—Circulatory System—Colon Cleansers—Digestion System—Energy and Stamina—Glandular System—Immune Builders—Nervous System and Brain—Urinary System—

VITAMINS, MINERALS AND SUPPLEMENTS

Vitamin A heals tissue. A vitamin and mineral supplement is needed every day. B-complex is needed for utilization of nutrients. Vitamin C with bioflavonoids speeds healing and prevents gangrene. Vitamin E protects the heart and helps in circulatory problems.

Calcium and magnesium are natural tranquilizers. Potassium protects the heart and kidneys. Mineral supplements are necessary for digestion and utilization of all nutrients. Chromium is lacking in diabetes. It is found in whole grains. Manganese and zinc are needed.

Flaxseed oil and salmon oil will enable insulin to be more effective. L-Carnitine burns fat. Acidophilus is used to restore friendly bacteria. Lecithin is needed for the myelin sheath around the nerves.

Chlorophyll and blue-green algae are considered catalysts to increase the utilization of all nutrients. They will also help in rebuilding a damaged pancreas.

DIARRHEA AND DYSENTERY

SYMPTOMS

Frequent Runny Bowel Movements— Cramping—Intestinal Upset—Vomiting— Extreme Thirst—Sudden Need to Eliminate— Severe Diarrhea causes Loss of Essential Electrolytes such as Potassium—Diarrhea in Infants is serious—Can cause Listlessness, Pale Pallor—Dark Circles around Eyes—A doctor should be contacted.

CAUSES

Most acute diarrhea is caused from food poisoning, rancid food, flu, bacteria, viruses, food allergies, traveling to foreign countries, and poor digestion. Lactase intolerance from milk products can also be a problem. Drugs can cause diarrhea; it's natures way of rejecting harmful substances from the body.

Chronic diarrhea can result from cancer, ulcerative colitis, or Crohn's disease. Giardia lamblia, a microscopic parasite, can cause severe diarrhea with fever, chills, muscle pain and intestinal bloating. It can also lead to chronic fatigue.

Giardia is the most common cause of water-borne infestation in America. Protozoa is a parasite, invisible to the eye. It causes frequent watery stools and forms a closed sac and it protects from hydrochloric acid. It creates a sodium and chloride loss.

Diarrhea is a form of constipation and is the way the body tries to regulate to a normal state. Diarrhea is the way the body has of eliminating toxins and cleaning the system.

NUTRITIONAL THERAPY

Stop eating and drink lots of liquids, especially herbal teas made from Red Raspberry, Ginger, Oak Bark, Gentian, Golden Seal or Slippery Elm Bark. These will soothe, heal and supply essential minerals. Carob powder drink will help stop diarrhea. Barley or rice water, or blackberry juice will soothe and stop diarrhea. Liquid chlorophyll drink, carrot juice, and plain yogurt will also heal. Acidophilus will help supply the natural bacteria.

An electrolyte formula drink will prevent mineral loss. Chopped apple and cinnamon with the fiber and pectin create a carminative effect upon the loose bowels and tighten up the muscles. Bananas absorb unhealthy bacteria, restores bowel balance, help correct irregularity, and are rich in potassium.

Herbs to help in diarrhea and dysentery are: Alfalfa supplies minerals, Burdock cleans the blood, Echinacea blood cleanser, Ginger settles stomach, Golden Seal eliminates toxins, Myrrh good for chronic diarrhea, antiseptic, Passion Flower relaxes nerves, Pau D'Arco cleans liver and blood, Psyllium cleans colon, Red Raspberry soothes and supplies minerals, Slippery Elm soothes, supplies protein, and White Oak Bark, an astringent which stops diarrhea.

HERBAL FORMULAS

Blood Cleansers—Colon Cleansers—(Parasite and worm formulas)—

VITAMINS, MINERALS AND SUPPLEMENTS

Vitamin A heals mucous membranes. B-complex vitamins help prevent digestive disorders. Potassium is essential and is lost in diarrhea. Calcium, magnesium and sodium also need to be replaced.

Chlorophyll will help eliminate diarrhea. Essential fatty acids, in flaxseed oil and salmon oil, are needed. Acidophilus is essential for supplying natural bacteria and strengthens and firms up looseness so diarrhea subsides.

DIVERTICULITIS

SYMPTOMS

Cramping—Tenderness on Left Side—Fever—Constipation alternate with Diarrhea—Nausea—Vomiting—Abdominal Swelling—Cramps—Pain—Hemorrhaging—Rectal Bleeding—

CAUSES

This is a common disease in the United States. It is estimated that half of Americans over age sixty have diverticulitis. It can go undetected for years until severe symptoms appear. Small pouches along the border of the colon are formed and can increase in considerable size. These are called diverticula. These pockets become filled with toxic feces which cause irritation and infections. This is caused by poor bowel function and auto-intoxication.

Constipation and straining from hard stools causes the pockets to develop. It can be serious and turn into cancer. Stress is another cause. The colon tightens up under emotional stress. Poor eating habits are an important factor especially a low fiber diet.

This disease causes malnourishment and other diseases throughout the body. It causes improper secretion of saliva in the mouth and prevents proper digestion and enzyme process.

Cataracts are formed, hearing is impaired because of starvation of nutrition and oxygen to the organs is lessened.

Toxic substances are absorbed into the bloodstream and cause many diseases such as liver damage, hardening of the arteries and strokes.

NUTRITIONAL THERAPY

A high fiber diet using whole grains, fruits and vegetables will provide natural bulk to clean the colon. Demulcent herbs are very beneficial to speed the healing along with lower bowel cleansing. Enemas, using slippery elm will sooth and speed the healing. Garlic enemas will help infections. In 1916, Dr. John Harvey Kellogg, M.D., author of *Colon Hygiene*, described diverticulitis as a newly-developed disease. It became limited to whole grains being replaced with white flour products, and increased meat eating, along with ingesting white sugar products.

Herbs that help in diverticulitis are: Aloe Vera healing, colon cleanser, Burdock, blood cleanser, Cascara Sagrada chronic constipation, Echinacea cleans blood, Ginger prevents cramping, and cleans, Golden Seal excellent to heal and clean colon, Kelp cleans and supplies minerals, Passion Flower relaxing, Pau d'Arco cleans blood, Psyllium cleans colon, Slippery Elm nourishing, White Oak Bark heals.

HERBAL FORMULAS

Blood Cleansers—Colon Cleansers—Digestive System — Immune Builders — Infection Fighters—Urinary System—

VITAMINS, MINERALS AND SUPPLEMENTS

Vitamin A is healing and B-complex is needed for a healthy digestive tract. Vitamin C with bioflavonoids heals and prevents infections. Vitamin E heals. Calcium and magnesium help in healing the colon. Minerals are necessary for healing and protecting the lining of the colon.

Acidophilus is a natural antibiotic and helps in assimilation of nutrients. Chlorophyll and blue-green algae will heal and provide essential nutrients.

Flaxseed oil and salmon oil are essential for a healthy immune system.

EAR PROBLEMS ————

SYMPTOMS

Sudden Hearing Loss—Itching—Pain—Insects—Objects in ear, (children put small objects in the ears)—Bleeding—Discharge from Ear—Infected Earlobe—Earaches—Babies Pull at ears—Restless—Irritable—Poor Equilibrium—

CAUSES

Earache (Otitis Media) is a common childhood infection. The child's eustachian tube is shorter than an adults and is more susceptible to ear infections. Dairy products increase ear infections causing mucus to collect in the ear canal inviting viruses and bacteria. Colds, childhood diseases, allergies, respiratory infections, and certain foods can irritate the sensitive mucous membranes and cause swollen tissues, which prevent proper drainage and cause collection of toxic material which invites bacteria. Excessive sweets and starches can cause a lower resistance of the nasal membrane and aggravates ear conditions.

One cause of ear infections is feeding babies cereal too early. Cereals will not assimilate until babies develop teeth for proper chewing. Saliva from chewing produces the enzyme for digesting cereals. This causes irritation to the mucous membranes.

Swimmer's ears is caused when water remains in the canal too long and macerates the skin causing bacteria or fungi to increase the risk of infections. A ruptured eardrum is serious. Put nothing in the ears until the eardrum is healed. Fomentation on the outside of the ear is healing. Avoid putting cotton swabs, bobby pins or any object in the ears. A severe ear infection, or a blow to the ear can cause eardrum rupture. If an infection is present, it causes intense pain as pus builds up in the ear. When the ear starts oozing pus, the eardrum has burst.

NUTRITIONAL THERAPY

Avoid cigarette smoke, for it can irritate the ear drums. Antibiotics create Candida, which produces toxic material and spreads to other parts of the body through the bloodstream. Keep the feet warm. Heat applied to the feet will draw blood from the head and improve circulation. Avoid sugar, dairy products, meat, and heavy meals until nature can take its course and heal the infection. Herbal teas such as peppermint, and herbal tinctures will help the body heal itself.

Herbs to help nourish the ears are: Bee Pollen strengthen the body, Blue Vervain antispasmodic, relaxes nerves, Burdock cleans blood, Cascara Sagrada, for constipation, Echinacea, an antibiotic, Ginger settles stomach, Golden Seal heals infections, Lobelia loosens mucous, Passion Flower relaxing, Pau d'Arco cleans blood, Red Raspberry helps in nausea, fevers, Slippery Elm is healing and nourishing.

HERBAL FORMULAS

Blood Cleansers—Colon Cleansers—Colds, Flu, Fever and Allergy—Digestive System—Infection Fighters—Nervous System and Brain—

VITAMINS, MINERALS AND SUPPLEMENTS

Vitamins A, and C with bioflavonoids will heal the mucous membranes. Vitamin C heals infections and catarrhal conditions that can settle in the ears. High levels of vitamin C with bioflavonoids prevents bacteria from invading the nose, throat and ears. Iron formulas containing yellow dock will build and clean the blood. Vitamin E will strengthen the immune system. Minerals are important for healing, especially selenium and zinc. Calcium and magnesium will relax the nerves. Potassium will protect the stomach while the body is eliminating toxins.

Acidophilus will heal and prevent candida. Chlorophyll and blue-green algae will heal and help in assimilation of all nutrients. Flaxseed oil and salmon oil will protect the immune system.

EPILEPSY _____

SYMPTOMS

Loss of Consciousness—Abnormal Motor Activity—Sensory Disturbances—Nervous System Disruptions — Involuntary Twitching—Sudden Onset and Short Duration—

CAUSES

Injury to the head, neck or spinal cord can cause epilepsy. Abnormal brain-wave patterns result in seizures which can range from mild twitching to violent convulsions that can cause unconsciousness. Brain injury before or during birth, high fevers during early childhood and infectious diseases can also cause epilepsy.

An incompetent ileocecal valve was seen by Dr. W. Curtis Brigham, D.O., Chief of Staff and Colon Specialist of the Monte-Sano Hospital as a possible cause. He found that many cases of epilepsy were caused by incompetency of the ileocecal valve. This causes powerful toxins to enter the blood stream and effect the delicate nervous system and the brain. (Rhodifer Leo M., LLB, Ph.D., *Epilepsy-The Strangest of Diseases*). Dr. Brigham did surgery and released adhesions and repaired the ileocecal valve and cleared up as many as fifty percent of his epilepsy cases.

Dr. Henry Lindlahr, M.D. a natural health doctor, made the following statement, "When the drainage system of the nose and the nasopharyngeal cavities has been completely destroyed, the impurities must either travel upward into the brain or downward into the glandular structures of the neck, thence into the bronchi and the tissues of the lungs." "If the trend be upward, to the brain, the patient grows nervous and irritable or becomes dull and apathetic. In many instances the morbid matter affects certain centers in the brain and causes nervous conditions such as hysteria, St. Vitus' dance, epilepsy, etc."

NUTRITIONAL THERAPY

Colon cleansing would be beneficial, making sure the ileocecal valve is working properly. When the colon is congested, the part of the colon called the cecum can press against the ileocecal valve and cause highly toxic poisons to enter the blood stream and cause numerous problems. A Naturopathic Doctor can help determine if this is the case.

A rotation diet is beneficial to determine if seizures are related to food. Chemicals and inhalants can also cause reactions. Stress management is important. Nutrition can help nourish and strengthen the nerves and brain. Food high in B complex vitamins such as brown rice, millet, oats, buckwheat, quinoa, and amaranth are high in fiber and nutrients. Fresh fruit and vegetable juices will supply vitamins and minerals to nourish the brain.

Avoid white sugar and white flour products, they destroy calcium and other minerals that help prevent brain problems. White flour contains chlorine, which can produce a toxin called alloxan.

Municipal drinking water contains chlorine.

Aloe Vera, helps to dissolve adhesions. Bee Pollen builds stamina. Black Walnut eliminates worms and parasites. Burdock cleans the blood. Cayenne is a great stimulant to provide nutrients to the brain. Echinacea cleans the blood. Ginseng builds immune response. Gotu Kola is food for the brain. Horsetail assists in calcium absorption. Ho-Shou-Wu improves resistance to disease. Kelp supplies essential minerals. Licorice feeds the adrenals glands for energy. Lobelia is a great relaxer and cleanser. Pau D'Arco cleans the blood and liver. Psyllium cleans the colon.

HERBAL FORMULAS

Blood Cleansers—Colon Cleansers—Digestive System—Glandular System—Immune Builder—Nervous System and Brain—Structural System—Urinary—

VITAMINS, MINERALS AND SUPPLEMENTS

Antioxidants vitamins A, C, E and minerals selenium and zinc increase circulation and supply oxygen and nutrients to the brain. Phenobarbital can cause deficiencies of folic acid, vitamins B12, B6, K and D. B complex vitamins are necessary for nerve and brain health and prevent toxins from accumulating.

Calcium and magnesium are essential for nerve health. A deficiency of manganese is seen in epileptic patients. Selenium and vitamin E were found beneficial in preventing seizures in rats.

Acidophilus detoxifies toxic substances and helps in digestion. Chlorophyll and blue-green algae supplies essential nutrients and oxygen to the brain. CoQ10 and germanium are needed for supplying oxygen and nutrients to the brain and building the immune system. Lecithin repairs brain and nerve damage. Flaxseed oil and salmon oil improve nerve and brain disorders.

EMOTIONAL FATIGUE SYNDROME

SYMPTOMS

Anxiety—Depression—Mental and Physical Fatigue—Fear and Panic Attacks—Constant Stress and Tension—Body and Muscle Aches and Pains—Digestive Problems—Loss of Interest—No Zest for Life—Cannot Cope With Everyday Problems—Loss of Confidence and Self Esteem—Sensitive to Criticism—Fear of Failure —Guilt—Hopeless Feelings—Loss of Sex Drive—Mood Swings—Muscle Spasms— Negative Attitude—Sensitive to Noise— Worry—(constant, about everything)—

CAUSES

People react in various ways when under emotional stress. Some people are very sensitive and take things and situations personally. They feel things deeply and when the immune system and nervous system become depleted, it is more than the body can cope with. When the nervous system is depleted, it affects their emotional stability. The main causes are constipation, autointoxication and nutritional deficiencies. When the liver is congested, the excess hormones (estrogen) can accumulate and enter the bloodstream and deplete the nervous system.

Drugs—Change in Life Style—Illness— Negative Thoughts — Frustration — Loneliness—Unresolved emotions—can all contribute to Emotional Fatigue—

NUTRITIONAL THERAPY

The nervous system and the immune system need to be strengthened. We do not have direct control over the autonomic nervous system. Exercise and relaxation therapy can help the autonomic nerves, and help deal with the stresses of life. Drugs prescribed for the stresses of life only cover up the problems and cause further damage to the nerves.

Positive thinking can be learned and is needed in emotional fatigue. Diet is important. High fiber foods, fruits, vegetables, juices, sprouts, grains, nuts, seeds, beans and supplements will all help build up the nerves and strengthen the immune system.

Herbs to help in fatigue are: Alfalfa, Bee Pollen, Horsetail, Kelp and Red Raspberry, which are nourishing to the blood and build immune response. Black Walnut, Burdock, Echinacea, Golden Seal, Pau d'Arco and Suma clean and heal the body. Hawthorn Berries, Lady's Slipper, Lobelia, Passion Flower, Valerian build and strengthen the nervous system.

HERBAL FORMULAS

Blood Cleansers—Colon Cleansers—Digestive System—Energy and Stamina—Glandular System—Nervous System and Brain—

VITAMINS, MINERALS AND SUPPLEMENTS

Vitamins A, D and a lack of C with bioflavonoids help prevent malnutrition. B complex vitamins, is associated with depression and nervous disorders. Vitamin E protects against free radical damage.

Calcium and magnesium nourish and protect the nerves. Phosphorus is needed for strong bones and is involved with transmission of nerve impulses and in healthy nerves. Potassium works with phosphorus in carrying oxygen to the brain and is essential for transmission of nerve impulses and contraction of muscles. Sodium works with potassium to maintain proper electrolyte balance. Sodium is also necessary for the production of hydrochloric acid in the stomach. Iron works with protein and copper for formation of hemoglobin. Manganese helps the nerve impulses between the brain, nerves and the muscles. Selenium and zinc

are natural antioxidants to help protect against radiation and disease. Chromium is a trace mineral important to help regulate blood sugar and sugar cravings.

Acidophilus increases the body's ability to absorb essential nutrients and provides friendly bacteria to prevent diseases. Blue-green algae helps to boost immunity by helping with interferon production. CoQ10 helps improve energy by improving heart function. Germanium provides oxygen to the cells and stimulates the immune defense to protect against toxins. Lecithin help protect the nerves from damage. Flaxseed oil and salmon oil are essential fatty acids which are necessary for every function of the body. They build immunity and protect against germs and viruses.

ENDOMETRIOSIS —————

SYMPTOMS

Abdominal Pain—Back Pain—Bleeding Between Periods—Cysts—Heavy Menstrual Periods—Infertility—Menstrual Cramps— (extremely Painful)—Painful Intercourse— Pelvic Pain—Constipation and Bladder Problems may exist—30% of women with Endometriosis have no symptoms.

CAUSES

Endometriosis develops when the cells in the lining of the uterus, called endometrium, accumulate outside and back up into the fallopian tubes and into the pelvic cavity. This can also occur in the ovaries, ligaments of the uterus, cervix, appendix, bowel and bladder. These can also invade the lungs or armpits.

The damage is done when the blood from the endometrial implants remain in the pelvis where it causes inflammation, cyst, scar tissue and other damage to the tissues and organs around the area.

An imbalance in the uterus could be caused by mucus forming food, hormones and antibiotics in meat and dairy products. A diet high in sugar and white flour products contributes to endometriosis. The colon and liver need to be kept clean and healthy. The liver becomes overloaded because the bowels are backed up and toxins enter the blood stream. Areas that are sensitive are where estrogen is present in the uterus, breasts, vagina and other related parts. When the immune system is depleted, it will invite imbalances in the body, usually in the weakest areas.

NUTRITIONAL THERAPY

Eliminate foods containing hormones and antibiotics such as dairy products, beef, chicken and introduce high fiber foods such as brown rice, buckwheat, millet, whole oats and rye. Whole grains are high in fiber, B complex vitamins, and vitamin E. They are rich in calcium and magnesium which help in muscle and nervous tension. Calcium helps reduce muscle cramps. Potassium helps eliminate excess water from the body. Whole grains contain protein for building healthy cells. Fiber in whole grains helps eliminate toxins and prevents constipation.

Beans, peas and lentils help in healing and nourishing the body. Yellow corn meal is excellent for the colon. Fruit, vegetables, and their juices, are healing. Green drinks will purify and nourish the blood.

Herbs that help in endometriosis are: Bee Pollen which is nourishing, Black Cohosh to balance hormones, Burdock a blood cleanser, Cayenne stops bleeding, Dong Quai builds blood and balances hormones, Echinacea eliminates infections, and build blood, Golden Seal heals, Gotu Kola, Ho-Shou-Wu, Ginkgo and Suma (will build the body for healing), Kelp, Red Raspberry and Slippery Elm provides nourishment, and Pau d'Arco protects the liver.

HERBAL FORMULAS

Blood Cleansers—Digestive System— Glandular System—Immune Builders— Infection Fighters—Urinary System—Female Formulas—

VITAMINS, MINERALS AND SUPPLEMENTS

Vitamins, minerals and supplements are important in helping the body heal itself. They help in balancing hormones, reduce bleeding and pain. They help in the prevention as well as in healing endometriosis.

Vitamin A, is necessary for healthy red blood cells, and to protect the immune system. The B-complex vitamins help eliminate bad estrogen from the liver, protect the nerves and brain, relieve fatigue, water retention and cramps. Vitamin C with bioflavonoids helps reduce bleeding by strengthening the capillaries. Vitamin C helps in iron absorption. It is also healing and helps in cramping. Vitamin E helps in regulating hormone balance and relieving breast tenderness.

Calcium and magnesium help relax nerves and eliminate pain. These also help with insomnia and muscle cramps. Potassium helps reduce cramps and water retention. Iron is essential to prevent anemia. Anemia is common in women during menstrual periods and causes fatigue and irritability.

Chlorophyll and blue-green algae will nourish and build the blood and provide nutrients essential for a healthy immune system. Acidophilus is considered nature's antibiotic and increases the body's ability to absorb nutrients. CoQ10 and germanium increase the body's ability to provide oxygen and nutrients to the cells. Lecithin helps protect and build the nerves. Flaxseed oil and salmon oil help regulate fertility, inflammation and immunity.

ENVIRONMENTAL POISONING

SYMPTOMS

Behavior Changes — Fatigue — Glandular Disturbances—Changes in Metabolism—Low Immune Function—(which can lead to all kinds of diseases)—It may take years for symptoms to manifest—Bone—Blood—Brain Cancers—

CAUSES

Toxins are in the air, water and food. They're filled with bacteria, viruses, fungi, dust, harmful chemicals, and protein in food that has not been properly digested. These foreign bodies have different ways of attacking the body and eluding the immune system. A healthy immune system with the help of the brain decides what would be harmful. It either neutralizes or destroys the foreign bodies. Herbicides and pesticide residue are everywhere. The air is full of cadmium and lead fallout. We are bombarded by electromagnetic radiation which has been linked to leukemia. More children than ever are contracting leukemia. Air pollution can cause asthma, chronic bronchitis, coughing, emphysema and chest pain. Polluted air can cause burning eyes and irritation of other mucous membranes. Respiratory cancer is significantly higher in high air pollution areas. The leading cause of air pollutants are: lead, ozone, carbon monoxide, nitrogen oxides, sulfur oxides, and fine particulates (PM 10).

Carbon Monoxide binds with hemoglobin in the blood stream and decreases the ability of the blood to transport oxygen and causes dizziness, headaches and slow reflexes. Long exposure could cause heart disease. Ozone can cause permanent lung scarring and decreased pulmonary function. It can cause eye irritation, wheezing and burning in the nose. Lead is toxic and can affect blood forming tissues, the reproductive and nervous systems and the kidneys. It can cause learning problems in children and nervous system disorders.

NUTRITIONAL THERAPY

Providing natural food in the diet will protect and prevent absorption of radiation, and environmental toxins in combination with vitamins, minerals and supplements. Short fasts, two to three days at a time, using fresh vegetable and fruit juices, herbal teas and distilled water are recommended. Water fasts are not recommended because they can drive toxins further in the body. Blood cleansers are beneficial.

Whole grains, beans, peas, nuts, seeds, sprouts, fresh fruit and vegetables will provide fiber (eliminate toxins), and nutrients. Eliminate white sugar and white flour products which counteract nutrients. Add grain and vegetable stews, bean and vegetable soups which are rich in fiber, minerals and vitamins.

Sea herbs such as Dulse and Kelp protect and eliminate toxins. Miso soup aids digestion and provides B-complex vitamins. Olive oil and lemon juice for salads are beneficial.

Single herbs to help protect against environmental toxins are: Alfalfa, Bee Pollen, Kelp, and Slippery Elm to provide nutrients. Aloe Vera, Black Walnut, Burdock, and Golden Seal, to clean and eliminate toxins from the blood. Gotu Kola is food for the brain. Hawthorn Berries protect the heart. Lobelia, Passion Flower, Lady's Slipper and Valerian protect and nourish the nervous system. Milk Thistle protects the liver from damage. Ginseng, Ginkgo and Suma protect and strengthen the body's defense system.

HERBAL FORMULAS

Blood Cleansers—Circulatory System—Colon Cleansers—Energy and Stamina—Immune Builders—Structural System—Nervous System and Brain—Structural System— Female or Male Formulas—

VITAMINS, MINERALS AND SUPPLEMENTS

Vitamin A and beta carotene protect against air pollution which irritates the eyes and lungs and all mucous membranes. They provide nutrients to the thymus gland to produce more T cells which fight toxins. A, D and B complex vitamins help eliminate strontium 90 from the bones and body. B-complex vitamins protect the nervous system and brain. The B vitamins also help the body produce antibodies for the immune system. Extensive animal studies have shown that the B complex vitamins protect against radiation and other pollutants. Vitamin C with bioflavonoids helps protect against radiation, air pollution and toxins in the food and water. Vitamin E is an antioxidant which protects the blood from toxin accumulation. It protects against X-rays and air pollution. It also helps in the assimilation of minerals.

Mineral supplements are important to protect the body against accumulation of environmental toxins. Calcium and magnesium protect the bones from lead, strontium 90, cadmium, lead, aluminum and mercury. Potassium protects the kidneys, reproductive organs and the muscles. Iron protects the red blood cells from accumulating pollutants. It protects the body from stress. Selenium is an antioxidant which protects the organs from free radical damage. It protects against cancer and the accumulation of lead, mercury, cigarette smoke and other heavy metals. Zinc is important to protect against heavy metal accumulation and to protect the immune system.

Acidophilus protects against bacteria and fungus and also detoxifies toxic substances and eliminates them. It helps produce some B-complex vitamins.

Cholorphyll and blue-green algae have been found to decrease radiation poisoning. Chlorophyll is similar in structure to blood and will enrich and nourish it.

Lecithin is an important nutrient in eliminating poisons from the body. It also repairs and protects the myelin sheath's that protect nerve fiber from damage due to toxic chemicals and heavy metals.

CoQ10 and germanium work as adaptogens, which stimulate the immune defenses to protect against toxins.

Salmon oil and flaxseed oil are essential fatty acids which are important for maintaining and regulating a healthy immune function.

Indoles, found in ordinary vegetables such as broccoli, cabbage, kale and brussels sprouts, belong to a group called the cruciferous family. They can clean and protect cells and internal organs. They protect against cancer and accumulation of toxins in the body.

EPSTEIN-BARR VIRUS

SYMPTOMS

Fatigue—Exhaustion—Recurrent Upper-Respiratory Tract Infections—Sore Throat—Swollen Lymph Nodes—Memory Loss—Achy Joints and Muscles—Low-Grade Fevers—Headaches — Night Sweats — Poor Concentration—Irritability—Deep Depression—

CAUSES

Chronic Fatigue Syndrome is another name for Epstein—Barr virus. It is a common virus and usually remains dormant in most people, unless the immune system is weak. This is considered an auto-immune disease. The virus also causes infectious mononucleosis, the "kissing disease" that often strikes young people. EBV is chronic and lingers for months and maybe years before a person realizes what it is. Mononucleosis strikes all at once, hits hard and may last two to four weeks or longer if the diet isn't corrected. EBV is invited when other diseases are present such as AIDS, cancer, arthritis, lupus, leukemia and Multiple Sclerosis.

NUTRITIONAL THERAPY

Recovering from EBS takes time, patience, rest and a nutritional program. A detoxification program to clean and support the blood, liver, colon, lymphatics and the nervous system is essential. Foods to support these systems are brown rice, whole grains, such as buckwheat, millet, whole oats, rye, and yellow corn meal, fruit and vegetables, sprouts, seeds, nut milks and vegetable juices. Cleansing the body with fasting and drinking lemon water, chlorophyll, vegetable broths and juices will help heal and strengthen the body.

Most people with EBV also have candida. A diet eliminating sugar, alcohol, mushrooms and all fungi, molds and yeast in any form, fermented foods such as sauerkraut, soy sauce, all dry roasted nuts, potato chips, soda pop, bacon, salt pork, pork, lunch meats and cheese of all kinds is recommended.

Single herbs that help in Epstein-Barr Virus are: Echinacea, clean the glands, Garlic, antibiotic, Golden Seal, clean and heal, Pau D'Arco, Red Clover blood cleansers, Saffron helps in aches and pains, Burdock, Scullcap, Horsetail, Lobelia and Yellow Dock also help.

HERBAL FORMULAS

Blood Cleansers—Colon Cleanser—Digestive System—Energy and Stamina—Glandular System—Nervous System and Brain—Urinary System—

VITAMINS, MINERALS AND SUPPLEMENTS

Vitamin A and beta-carotene build the immune system and stimulate interferon production. B-complex vitamins prevent fatigue and improve stamina and mental alertness. Vitamin C and bioflavonoids protect against germs and viruses and heal. It also supports adrenal function. Vitamin E protects the cells from damage.

Acidophilus improves digestion, heals candida and improves B vitamin production. Chlorophyll and blue-green algae help the body produce interferon for healing and restoring health.

CoQ10 and Germanium protect against germs and viruses. Lecithin helps dissolve plaque in the arteries and protects the nerves.

Flaxseed oil and salmon oil help the body make hormone-like compounds that control organs of the body.

EYE PROBLEMS

SYMPTOMS

Blood Spots—Blurred Vision—Bulging—Dark Circles—Double Vision—Dryness—Lumps on Eyelids—Itching—Yellow in Whites of Eyes—Pain—Redness—Twitching—Watering—

CAUSES

Eye problems can be caused by allergies, air pollution, tobacco smoke, household cleansers, and sprays. They can all cause dry, itchy, burning and bloodshot eyes.

Eye problems are usually an indication of problems in other areas of the body. In Chinese medicine, the liver is related to the eyes. When the liver degenerates the eyes will deteriorate. The spleen is also related to the eyes. Anger and hate will injure the liver. Emotions have a profound effect on the liver.

There are prescription drugs that can cause degeneration of the eyes and cause cataracts and glaucoma. Drugs that can increase intraocular pressure, like glaucoma, are: Cortisone like drugs, Epinephrine, Isosorbide Dinitrate, Phenylephrine, Tolazoline and Tricyclic antidepressants.

Macular Degeneration is the leading cause of severe visual loss in the United States and Europe. It usually hits persons aged 55 or older. It is associated with hardening of the arteries and hypertension. The cause is lack of blood, nutrients and oxygen to the eyes. The small blood vessels become constricted and hardened. Free radical damage is the main cause due to a high meat and fat diet. The liver and gall bladder cannot eliminate the excess oils and toxins because of constipation and autointoxication.

NUTRITIONAL THERAPY

Dealing with the health of the liver and gallbladder and using a good colon cleanse is essential. A change of diet is necessary. Eliminate margarine and vegetable shortenings. Use natural oils such as olive oil, safflower, and sunflower, etc.

Eliminate all fried foods, especially deep fried; they are usually rancid and can cause free radical damage.

Carrot, celery, parsley and endive juice will supply nutrients to the eyes. Juice fasting can help speed up the elimination of cholesterol along with colon cleansing.

Bilberry helps in cataracts, diabetic-induced glaucoma and myopia. It helps in arterial, venous and capillary problems. It strengthened capillaries and stimulates peripheral circulation.

Eyebright, Golden Seal, and Red Raspberry clean and nourish the eyes. Dandelion helps the liver to detoxify and Kelp supplies essential minerals.

HERBAL FORMULAS

Blood Cleansers—Circulatory System—Colon Cleansers—Digestive System—Immune Builders—Nervous System and Brain—

VITAMINS, MINERALS AND SUPPLEMENTS

Antioxidants will help eliminate free radical damage. They are vitamins A, E, C and minerals selenium and zinc. All vitamins are essential. B-complex helps eliminate toxins and builds up the nerves.

All minerals are necessary for circulatory health. Zinc is needed. The eyes along with the brain, require more nutrition and oxygen than any other single part of the body. Poor nutrition clogs up tiny arteries, veins and capillaries that support the visual system. The gradual clogging of the veins in the eyes, which have been traced to bad nutrition, can lead to eventual blindness.

Blue-green algae and chlorophyll will supply nutrients and clean the veins. Flaxseed oil and salmon oil help to keep the veins clean and prevent blood clotting. Germanium and CoQ10 will provide oxygen to the capillaries.

FATIGUE

SYMPTOMS

Anger—Frustration—Unable to Cope with Normal Situations—Loss of Sexual Desire—Lack of Energy—Tired after Sleeping all night—Negative Thoughts—

CAUSES

Common causes of fatigue are anemia, allergies, autointoxication, candida, Epstein-Barr virus, (and other auto-immune diseases), hypoglycemia, hypothyroidism, toxic metal poisoning, nutritional deficiencies and stress. Lack of exercise or lack of rest can also cause fatigue.

Stress can develop into serious health problems if it is not controlled. Colitis, high blood pressure, heart palpations, headaches, stiff neck and shoulders, and ulcers can all be problems.

NUTRITIONAL THERAPY

Learning to relax is necessary. Exercise will help the body relax. Chiropractic adjustments and massage therapy will help the muscles to relax. A nutritional diet will help relieve stress. B-complex vitamins, calcium, magnesium and nervine herbs have the ability to strengthen the nerves. Brown rice and millet are very nourishing. Millet is rich in calcium and magnesium, and is easily digested.

Carrot, celery, and parsley juice will help heal the nerves. Lots of steamed and fresh vegetables are rich in minerals.

Ginseng, Ginkgo, Gotu Kola and Suma are herbs that help the body cope with stress. They are called adaptogens, which nourish the brain and nerves and help the body adapt to stress.

HERBAL FORMULAS

Blood Cleansers—Colon Cleansers—Digestive—Energy and Stamina—Immune Builders—Nervous System—

VITAMINS, MINERALS AND SUPPLEMENTS

Vitamins A, D, C and E will strengthen the nerves and the immune system. B-complex vitamins are essential for strong nerves and proper digestion.

Calcium and magnesium are needed to maintain healthy nerves. Potassium is necessary for the circulatory system and protects the heart. Selenium and zinc will protect the body from stress. All minerals are needed for strong and healthy nerves.

Acidophilus is very helpful for digestion and the production of some of the B-vitamins. It protects the body from candida and other infections. Chlorophyll is rich in minerals and vitamins and helps to protect and nourish the blood. Blue-green algae is healing and nourishing and is needed when under stress. Essential fatty acids such as flaxseed oil and salmon oil help the body adjust to stress. Lecithin is needed to protect the nerves from damage. Germanium andCoQ10 are helpful in oxygenating the blood.

FEMALE STRESS SYNDROME

SYMPTOMS

Allergies—Amenorrhea (loss of menstruation)—Anorexia — Anxiety Neurosis — Bulimia — Depressive Psychosis—Frigidity—Infertility—Menopausal Melancholia — Postpartum Depression—Premenstrual Tension—

CAUSES

Female Stress Syndrome is very common, because women are more sensitive and emotional than men. Women have the unique honor of bearing and caring for children. They are unique because of their sensitivity. It is important for them to feel loved and wanted.

The stress of raising and caring for a family makes them more sensitive. Stress can effect them inwardly and cause many symptoms. Lack of nutrients and autointoxication makes it more difficult for women to cope and adjust to every day stress. They need more nutrients when pregnant, nursing and caring for a family. For example, they need more iron foods because of their menstrual cycle. They also need other nutrients to cope with the daily problems of consistently being with children.

NUTRITIONAL THERAPY

A nutritional diet to support the needs of a women's stressful life is important. Fresh juices made with carrots, celery, parsley and ginger are rich in calcium, vitamin, potassium, sodium, and iron. Whole grains will strengthen the nerves and body. Brown rice, buckwheat, millet, whole oats will supply protein, B-complex vitamins, and minerals. Thermos cooking will help maintain the enzymes for proper digestion. Fresh fruit, and fresh and steamed vegetables are high in minerals important for all body functions and buildup the body.

Gotu Kola, Ginkgo, Suma will strengthen and protect the body from stress. Hops, Scullcap, Chamomile, Lady's Slipper, Lobelia, Passion Flower and Valerian will protect and rebuild the nerves.

HERBAL FORMULAS

Blood Cleansers—Colon Cleansers—Energy and Stamina—Immune Builders—Nervous System—

VITAMINS, MINERALS AND SUPPLEMENTS

Antioxidants, Vitamins A, C, E, and minerals selenium and zinc, will protect the body from stress and free radical damage. Zinc nourishes the thymus gland, and it is destroyed under stress. When the body is under stress, it is more susceptibly to illness. B-complex vitamins are needed when under stress. They will strengthen the nerves and help in digestion and assimilation.

Calcium, magnesium and potassium are needed for nervous disorders. Iron is essential, and a deficiency can cause fatigue. All minerals work together to balance body functions and prevent depression and stress.

Blue-green algae and chlorophyll will clean the blood and provide vitamin K for rich blood. They also supply vitamins and minerals which fortify the body. Flaxseed oil and salmon oil are important to protect the nervous and immune systems. Dry skin and hair are indications of fatty acid deficiencies. Lecithin is an essential brain and nerve food. Germanium and CoQ10 are also beneficial.

FIBROCYSTIC DISEASE —

SYMPTOMS

Lumps In Breast—Soreness—Tenderness—Common in Women ages from 30 to 50 years of age. They could become chronic if diet change isn't adopted. It is common for women to feel lumps in the breast around their menstrual period.

CAUSES

Caffeine, theophylline and theobromine found in coffee, tea, cola drinks and chocolate have been linked with fibrocystic breast disease. Excess estrogen has a disturbing effect on cysts of the breast. It is also linked with cancer. Meat, chicken, and dairy products contain estrogen as well as antibiotics and can add more bad estrogen.

An excess of bad estrogen seems to be related to the formation of breast cysts. They rarely appear after menopause, when estrogen levels are less.

Constipation and autointoxication are the main causes of fibrocystic disease. The liver is supposed to filter the toxins and bad estrogen, but when it is congested from constipation, these are circulated in the blood stream and is attracted to the hormone part of the body, which consists of the breast and uterus.

NUTRITIONAL THERAPY

A change of diet has helped women who are prone to fibrocystic disease. Eliminating salt, sugar, caffeine products, sugar, meat and dairy products that contains hormones is recommended.

Eat more grains, such as buckwheat, millet, whole oats, brown rice and more fruit, vegetables, herbs, vitamins, minerals and supplements that strengthen the body.

Red clover will clean the blood, Dong Quai will help regulate hormone levels. Pau d' Arco will clean the blood and liver. Red Raspberry is rich in iron and calcium. Golden Seal will clean the digestive tract and heal any infections.

HERBAL FORMULAS

Blood Cleansers—Colon and Liver Cleansers—Digestive System—Immune—Nervous System—Structural System—Female Formulas—

VITAMINS, MINERALS AND SUPPLEMENTS

Vitamins A and C with bioflavonoids will build the immune system. Vitamin E is effective in preventing and treating cysts. Vitamin E is an antioxidant and helps prevent fat oxidation and the formation of free radicals. B-complex vitamins with extra B6 are effective to strengthen the body and eliminative excess estrogen from the liver.

Mineral supplement are necessary for vitamins and nutrients to help balance body chemistry. Iodine and iron are necessary to destroy toxins. Calcium and magnesium are calming and essential for strong bones and help protect against cancer.

Blue-green algae and chlorophyll help clean the liver and prevent formation of cysts. These nutrients will build the blood and clean the colon. Acidophilus will help digest nutrients and prevent yeast infections common in women. Germanium and CoQ10 provide oxygen to the cells and prevent free radical damage. Lecithin helps the body utilize oils and is essential for brain and nerve health. Salmon oil and flaxseed oil are necessary fats to prevent breast cancer.

FIBROSITIS
(CHRONIC MUSCLE PAIN SYNDROME)

SYMPTOMS

Anxiety—Chronic Muscle Aches and Pain—Depression—Fatigue (with no apparent reason)—Joint Swelling—Irritable Bowels—Lack of a Well-Being Feeling—Migraine Headaches—Sleep Disturbances—Stiffness—Tension—Poor Stress Tolerance—TMJ Syndrome—

CAUSES

Fibrositis is a syndrome and mimics other diseases. Stress is the main cause of fibrositis. It has been mistaken for arthritis, rheumatism or Epstein-Barr Syndrome. Emotions and frame of mind have a profound effect on physical health. The muscles and joints tighten up when under stress. Women seem to be more susceptible. This condition has been around many years and has been called by different names. Some of these include muscular rheumatism, fibromyositis, and tension myalgia. With fibrositis, shallow sleep is common and results in muscle spasms and pain in various parts of the body called tender body spots.

NUTRITIONAL THERAPY

A well balanced diet is essential. It should consist of fresh fruit, vegetables, grains such as millet, buckwheat, brown rice, whole oats, wheat, rye (strengthens muscles), beans, and herbs that relax and nourish the nerves.

Rest and relaxation are important. Learning to maintain emotional calmness, loosen up muscles, feel peace of mind, and relaxing from hard work, worry, and intense concentration is vital.

Learn about this disorder and what can be done to cope with this problem. Muscle relaxation in the form of exercise, stretching and massage therapy will help relax muscle pain and stiffness.

Avoid caffeine, found in coffee, tea, cola drinks, and in medications such as pain relievers. It can cause stress, insomnia, restlessness, and irritability. Caffeine and chocolate seem to have a very stressful effect on the mind and body.

Herbs that are beneficial are: Alfalfa, Comfrey, Dandelion, Kelp, Horsetail, and relaxing herbs such as Hops, Passion Flower, Scullcap, White Willow Bark, and Valerian.

HERBAL FORMULAS

Blood Cleansers—Colon Cleanser—Energy and Stamina—General Cleanser—Immune Builders—Nervous System and Brain—Structural System—

VITAMINS, MINERALS AND SUPPLEMENTS

The B-complex vitamins are very important. They strengthen the nervous system and help the liver eliminate the bad estrogen that most women have. Vitamin C with bioflavonoids will strengthen the connective tissues bones, muscles, tendons and cartilage.

The antioxidants, vitamins A, D and E, will protect the immune system. Deficiency in vitamin D can cause muscular weakness.

The antioxidant minerals selenium and zinc protect and heal the muscles. They also protect and build the immune system. Calcium and magnesium are essential for strong bones and muscles. They build and nourish the nervous system. Silicon is necessary for strong bones, tendons, cartilage and blood vessels. All minerals work together for healthy muscles.

Chlorophyll is healing and helps in absorption of essential nutrients. It purifies and heals blood vessel diseases. Blue-green algae is rich in vitamins, minerals and amino acids necessary for healthy bones and muscles. Lecithin improves nervous disorders. Flaxseed oils and salmon oil are involved in healing and repairing of tissues. They are especially effective for inflammatory muscles.

FOOD POISONING

SYMPTOMS

Vomiting—Pain—Cramping—Weakness—Diarrhea Dizziness—Symptoms usually come on quickly, between one and four hours after eating the contaminated substance. The symptoms of salmonella poisoning, pain, vomiting and diarrhea, can take several days to appear.

CAUSES

Salmonellosis is the most common form of food poisoning and has increased since the feeding of antibiotics to food animals to speed their growth. This promotes the development of antibiotic-resistant bacteria from the strains present in the intestinal tracts of all animals. It is also caused by the mechanical methods of evisceration, especially of poultry.

Giardiasis (a pathogen called giardia) is increasing. It is found in drinking water, and is found in surface drinking water, in lakes, reservoirs and mountain streams. It is not destroyed by water treatments including chlorination.

Trichinella is found in pork. Clostridium botulinum is found in improperly canned foods or in food left out overnight, Clostridium perfringens, is called "cafeteria germ," and grows rapidly in large portions of food or in meat or poultry dishes allowed to cool slowly. Staphylococcus is carried on human skin and easily transmitted.

Molds found on food can produce toxins and poisons. Moldy foods such as sliced lunch meat, grains, nuts, dried legumes, dairy products, bacon and soft vegetables should be destroyed. Potato sprouts should never be eaten, they have concentrated solanine, which can cause hallucinations even after recovery from food poisoning.

NUTRITIONAL THERAPY

Avoid contaminated food. Properly prepare meats, and cook them above 165 degrees Fahrenheit. Let frozen meats thaw in the refrigerator. Stuff chicken and turkey just before cooking. Never leave potato salad out of the refrigerator too long.

Acidophilus and yogurt increases the beneficial bacteria in the intestinal tract and produce B vitamins to protect against food poisoning. They destroy bad bacteria.

Golden Seal will also prevent food poisoning. Many people who travel to Mexico, take a capsule or two before eating. Ginger tea, ginger ale, or colas can reduce nausea and prevent dehydration. The body needs to eliminate the poisons without using nausea and diarrhea drugs. Herbs will help nature eliminate the poisons.

HERBAL FORMULAS

Blood Cleansers—(after symptoms subside)— Number 7 under Digestive System is a liquid drink that will supply essential electrolytes, also Ginger Formulas—Digestive Enzymes help to prevent food poisoning. They are decreased as we age.

VITAMINS, MINERALS AND SUPPLEMENTS

Vitamin A protects the immune system. The stronger a person's immune system, the less likely there will be severe reactions. The B-complex vitamins protect against bacteria growth. Vitamin C with bioflavonoids protects against bacteria invasion. All vitamins protect the immune system.

A mineral supplement will protect the immune system.

Acidophilus is beneficial to use as a preventive, especially when you are eating out. Yogurt is also beneficial. Chlorophyll and blue-green algae help the body produce natural interferon to fight poisons.

FRACTURES

SYMPTOMS

Deformity—Discoloration—Loss of Limb Function—Numbness—Pain—Pallor—Pulse Loss—Paralysis—Swelling—Tenderness— Tingling—

CAUSES

Accidents are the most common cause of broken bones. There could also be a weakening condition such as bone tumors, osteoporosis, and metabolic disease. With these types of weak bones, it doesn't take much to break a bone. A slight fall, a slip of the foot or a knock against an object will result in a fracture.

Weak bones could also be caused by a lack of nutrients, or the inability to assimilate minerals essential for healthy bone. Dr. Kervran, a European scientist, found that fractures or broken bones do not knit well when there are high amounts of calcium and little or no silica. They knit poor to fair however, when there are good amounts of both calcium and silica present, and the bones knit extremely well when there is an abundance of silica present with little calcium.

NUTRITIONAL THERAPY

Contact a doctor for proper healing of bones to prevent deformity. Calcium and minerals are found abundantly in natural foods such as green leafy vegetables, carrot juice, broccoli, almonds, millet, and herbs. White sugar products eliminate minerals from the body. White flour products contains chlorine which is harmful to the bones. Cola drinks, caffeine, chocolate, and alcohol will leach out calcium from the bones.

Exercise is essential to strengthen the bones. The bones are capable of supporting heavy loads and are a storehouse of calcium and other essential minerals. The red blood cells are found in the bone marrow. The bones protect the delicate body parts and create the joints that allows us to move about freely.

The herbs to help in strengthening the bone are: Comfrey, Horsetail, White Oak Bark, Kelp, and Alfalfa.

HERBAL FORMULAS

Blood Cleansers—Digestive System—Nervous System—(helps ease pain)—Structural System—

VITAMINS, MINERALS AND SUPPLEMENTS

Vitamins A and D will help the healing. The B-complex vitamins help make red blood cells. They help in the nervous system. Vitamin C with bioflavonoids helps the body handle physical and mental stress. Vitamin E is beneficial for its ability to protect vitamins A and C from oxidation and it increases their potency.

Calcium and magnesium are needed for the healing of bones, but silicon is the key to speed healing and increase bone mass. Selenium and zinc speed healing of bones and wounds. All minerals are essential for healthy bones. Liquid minerals will speed assimilation and healing.

Acidophilus helps the body absorb minerals. Liquid chlorophyll and blue-green algae increase healing.

Flaxseed oil and salmon oil help in the repair and healing process. Lecithin helps fight and prevent infections.

GALLBLADDER DISEASE

SYMPTOMS

Fever—Nausea—Pain—Vomiting—Symptoms appear suddenly after ingesting foods that irritate the gallbladder such as fried foods.

CAUSES

The cause of gallstones is cholesterol, toxic bile, or calcium and other minerals that have collected and hardened. Gallstones and gallbladder problems can be serious. Gallstones can move out and lodge in a channel called the cystic duct and cause inflammation. Gallstones are caused by poor diet and overeating.

The western diet is a major cause of gallbladder problems. Lack of fiber and too much fat (fried food) and too little organic minerals all contribute.

NUTRITIONAL THERAPY

Eliminate fried food, rancid oils, and eat small amounts of food at one meal. A high fiber diet is beneficial to eliminate excess toxins and oils from the liver and colon. Fruits, vegetables, grains, beans, sprouts and herbs will strengthen the body and prevent accumulation of heavy metals, inorganic minerals and toxins. Excess amounts of alcohol, meat, white sugar and white flour products increase the risk of gallbladder problems.

Olive oil in lemon or lime juice helps dissolve hard bile. The malic acid in fresh apple juice helps dissolve gallstones.

Herbs that help in gallbladder problems are: Aloe Vera, Burdock, Cascara Sagrada, Psyllium, Saffron and Slippery Elm.

GALL BLADDER CLEANSE

First day - No food to be taken
8:00 am 1 glass (8 oz) fresh apple juice
Then 2 glasses (16 oz) fresh apple juice at
    10:00 am, 12:00 am, 2:00 pm, 4:00 pm,
    6:00 pm.
Second Day - Same as first - at bedtime take 4 oz of olive oil in 1 8 oz glass of warm pure water with 1 juiced lemon or warm apple juice. Retire. It should start to work in the early morning. This helps to dissolve the stangnant bile and liquifies through the malic acid of the apple juice. The oil moves the residue.

HERBAL FORMULAS

Blood Cleansers—Circulatory System—Colon Cleansers—Digestive System—General Cleanser — Nervous System — Glandular System—(these are essential if the gallbladder has been removed)—

VITAMINS, MINERALS AND SUPPLEMENTS

The absorption of fat-soluble vitamins A, D, E, and K are reduced when inadequate bile production or gallbladder malfunction is present. Supplements are very essential in these conditions. B-complex vitamins will help improve digestion and gallbladder function. Vitamin C with bioflavonoids will help convert cholesterol into bile acids and prevent formation of gallstones.

Minerals work with vitamins. Magnesium stimulates liver production, sulphur aids the liver in bile secretion, and zinc aids digestion, and helps the acid-alkaline balance.

Chlorophyll and blue-green algae help nourish the spleen and liver to prevent accumulation of hard bile. Lecithin emulsifies fat and is important for the maintenance of soluble bile to prevent gallstones.

GOUT

SYMPTOMS

Lumps and Pain around the Joints— Especially around the big toe or other toes— Pain and lumps in the ear lobes could indicate gout—It can also appear on the hand, heel or any joint—Inflammation—Swelling—And Extreme Pain caused by buildup of needle-like uric-acid crystals.

CAUSES

Heredity may play a part. This is not surprising because we inherit weaknesses as well as strong points. How our ancestors have eaten in the past determines our strengths and weaknesses.

Too much uric acid in the blood and tissues causes gout. It crystallizes in the joints and creates swelling and pain from the abrasive action of the needle-like uric acid crystals. Gout has been associated with beer and wine drinking and a high meat diet. A by-product of meat is uric acid. Diets rich in fat and sugar also contribute to gout.

Gout is a type of arthritis and is seen primarily in adult men over the age of 30.

NUTRITIONAL THERAPY

A change of diet is necessary to eliminate and prevent the accumulation of uric acid in the blood. Distilled water will help eliminate toxins. A diet high in vegetables; fresh and steamed are rich in easily assimilated minerals. Millet is high in calcium and magnesium and is easily digested. Brown rice, buckwheat, whole oats, and wheat are high in fiber to eliminate toxins. Sour cherries consumed every day for several weeks are beneficial in lowering uric acid and preventing gout attacks. Carrot, celery and parsley juice is very beneficial. Liquids will help eliminate toxins.

Burdock is an herb that will clean and prevent deposits from accumulating in the joints and other parts of the body. Dandelion cleans the liver to filter uric acid. Devil's Claw cleans vascular walls and eliminates toxins from the blood. Kelp, Red Clover and Yucca are beneficial in eliminating uric acid and other toxins.

HERBAL FORMULAS

Blood Cleansers—Circulatory System—Colon Cleansers—Digestive System—General Cleanser—Structural System—

VITAMINS, MINERALS AND SUPPLEMENTS

The antioxidants vitamins A, D, C, E and minerals selenium and zinc, increase immune response. Vitamin C with bioflavonoids in 1,000 milligrams every hour at the onset of an attack and gradually lowering dosages to 1,000 a day will help eliminate uric acid. B-complex vitamins will help the liver convert uric acid into harmless compounds and also help relax the nerves. Vitamin E helps prevent uric acid accumulation.

Calcium and magnesium help in relaxing the body. Healing takes place when the body is relaxed. Potassium is the healing mineral and aids in waste elimination. All minerals are necessary in healing. Zinc is healing and protects the immune system. Silicon is essential for calcium absorption.

Chlorophyll and blue-green algae are beneficial for cleansing and healing the joints. Lecithin protects the nerves and helps eliminate toxins from the body. Acidophilus help vitamin and mineral absorption and increases the protective bacteria in the colon. CoQ10 and germanium help in pain and provide oxygen to the cells. Flaxseed oil and salmon oil are helpful in inflammation, and the repair process of the joints. They also helps in digestion.

GUILLAIN-BARRE' SYNDROME

SYMPTOMS

Neurological Weakness in Face—Arms—Legs—Muscle Weakness can Progress to Motor Paralysis—Respiratory Failure—It causes severe Anxiety—Fear— and Panic in the progressive phase. Because of slow convalescence and the possibility of permanent neurologic damage, depression occurs.

CAUSES

Guillain-Barre' syndrome affects the myelin sheath (protects the nerves) of the neuron, which leads to muscle loss and can lead to paralysis. Swine flu vaccine authorized by Gerald Ford, and introduced as a nation wide vaccination program in 1976-1977 was a disaster and caused Guillain-Barre' syndrome in some people. Other factors could be surgery, rabies, viral infection, Hodgkin's and lupus erythematosus.

NUTRITIONAL THERAPY

Daniel was told by his physicians that he had a severe case of Guillain-Barre' syndrome and was in critical condition. His recovery period would be 1 to 2 years with expected permanent muscle and nerve damage. He refused cortisone shots and decided to go the natural route. He went on herbal nervine formulas, B-complex vitamins, with extra pantothenic acid, licorice root, liquid chlorophyll, blue vervain extract, alfalfa, calcium herbal formula, multi-vitamin and mineral formulas, extra chelated minerals, and vitamin C with bioflavonoids. He also took green drinks, sprouts and herbal potassium formula. Within thirty days, he was back to work and has had no problems since. That has been about ten years ago.

A natural diet is very beneficial using fresh and steamed vegetables. Sprouted seeds, nuts, grains, thermos cooking of grains to retain enzymes, vitamins, minerals, fresh vegetable salads, millet which is rich in calcium and magnesium are excellent. Brown rice, whole oats, wheat, buckwheat, barley and rye, which are high in fiber, and nutrients to nourish the body will aid in the healing process.

Blue vervain is a natural tranquilizer, Chamomile contains tryptophan with sedative properties, Burdock and Echinacea clean the blood, and Ginkgo and Suma stimulates, brain function.

HERBAL FORMULAS

Blood Cleansers — Colon Cleansers — Digestion — Energy and Stamina —Immune Builders—Nervine and Brain—Structural System—

VITAMINS, MINERALS AND SUPPLEMENTS

Vitamins A, D, C, and E will strengthen the immune system and protect against nerve and free-radical damage. The B-complex vitamins are important for nerve repair with extra B5, pantothenic acid and B12.

A multi-mineral supplement for nerve repair with extra calcium and magnesium will help. An herbal calcium formula with horsetail and oatstraw will help speed nerve damage. Selenium and zinc will speed healing.

Acidophilus will protect against toxins and help in assimilation of essential vitamins and minerals. Blue-green algae and chlorophyll will speed healing and cleaning of the nerves and muscles. Germanium and CoQ10 will help in the healing of nerves and protect the circulatory system. Lecithin is vital for repair of nerve damage.

HAIR PROBLEMS

SYMPTOMS

Brittle, Dry Hair—Dandruff—Hair Loss— Loss of Lustre—Receding Hair Line—Split Ends—

CAUSES

Some of the causes for hair loss are hormonal imbalance, vitamin and mineral deficiency, the lack of assimilation of nutrients, stress, disease, X-ray therapy, anesthesia, medications, drastic reducing diets, pesticide poisoning, obesity, diabetes or other diseases.

Hair loss for men can be hereditary, (our ancestors lacked nutrients and passed them to their children), stress, protein deficiency and letting hair become too dry.

Hair loss for women can be due to a temporary drop in estrogen levels which occurs after giving birth and can cause traumatic hair loss. Hair loss usually starts 2-3 months after delivery and may continue for several months. It usually grows back.

During menopause, hormonal changes can cause scalp and hair problems including hair loss. Birth control pills can alter normal hair growth. They rob the body of vitamin A, folic acid, magnesium and zinc.

NUTRITIONAL THERAPY

The hair needs to be kept clean. Toxins are eliminated through the scalp. Dr. Henry Lindlahr, in his book, *Philosophy of Natural Therapeutics*, on page 70, said "Dandruff and falling hair are caused by the elimination of systemic poisons through the scalp. The thing to do is not to suppress this elimination and thereby cause accumulation of poisons in the brain, but to stop the manufacture of poison in the body and to promote its removal through the natural channels." One method he used was fresh, cold water and the comb.

A clean internal body is essential to prevent poisons accumulating in the head area. A natural food diet, fresh fruit and vegetables, whole grains, sprouts, vegetable juices, green drinks, seeds, nuts and eliminating sugar, white flour products and caffeine drinks is recommended.

Jojoba promotes hair growth and helps remove accumulated cholesterol from the scalp so that the new hair follicles can emerge unimpeded. Kelp is rich in minerals and works with vitamin E for assimilation. It also prevents dry, brittle, fading and falling hair.

Oatstraw and horsetail are rich in silicon and trace minerals for healthy hair. Rosemary helps prevent premature baldness and stimulates circulation in the head area. Sage is an astringent and acts as a scalp tonic and helps stimulate growth. Yarrow stimulates, cleanses and tightens pores in the head to prevent hair loss. It also helps in regulating liver function and healthy liver function is necessary for healthy hair.

HERBAL FORMULAS

Blood Cleansers—Colon Cleansers—Digestive System — Glandular System — Nervous System—Structural System—

VITAMINS, MINERALS AND SUPPLEMENTS

Vitamin A protects against a dry scalp, which can cause hair loss. Lack of B-complex vitamins can cause gray, dull, dry hair.

B6 and B12 are anti-stress nutrients, and prevent dry, dull, lifeless hair. A lack of folic acid can cause hair, eyebrow and eyelashes to fall out. It can help prevent gray hair. PAPA, biotin, folic acid and pantothenic acid assist gray to regain its normal color. Vitamin C with bioflavonoids protects vitamin A which is essential for healthy hair. Vitamin E improves circulation and protects essential fatty acids from free-radical damage.

Copper works with iron and zinc to help the hair retain its natural color. Magnesium and calcium help prevent hair from falling out and split ends. Manganese works with other minerals for vibrant, and healthy hair. Phosphorus stimulates growth of hair. If silicon and sulphur are lacking in the blood, the hair cannot be nourished properly and will fall out. Zinc is essential to help prevent baldness.

Flaxseed oil and salmon oil are essential fatty acids that help keep the hair lustrous without conditioners and oils. They are lacking in our diet which is obvious with all the hair preparations on the market today. Lecithin contains choline inositol which is vital to healthy growth. It creates thick and shiny hair.

HALITOSIS

(Bad Breath)

SYMPTOMS

Usually an unsuspected odor that other people notice. Your best friend may tell you. You can't taste it or smell it yourself.

CAUSES

One cause is fermenting plaque. Gum disease can also cause bad breath. Chronic sinus infection, indigestion, and lung problems can cause halitosis. Autointoxication can cause chronic halitosis. It is created from undigested food fermenting in the intestines and slowly eliminating gases.

NUTRITIONAL THERAPY

Strive for proper digestion. Avoid stress and learn to relax especially while eating. A raw food diet using mostly vegetable juices and fresh fruit will help balance the acid and alkaline content of the body. A cleansing diet with colon cleanse will help rid the body of toxins. Green drinks using parsley and wheat grass juice will clean the blood. Chewing on cloves will help with bad breath. A healthy diet, eliminating meat and using grains, beans, sprouts, salads, steamed vegetables and fruit will help with the problem. Eliminating white sugar products which can ferment in the intestines causing gas and bad breath is recommended. White flour products can also ferment and cause glue-like material to cling in the intestines.

Gentian and Golden Seal will clean and heal the digestive tract. Aloe Vera cleans the digestive tract. Peppermint sweetens the breath while speeding digestion. Fresh lemon juice in warm water first thing in the morning will help cleanse the liver. Tea Tree Oil used on tooth paste will help destroy germs.

HERBAL FORMULAS

Blood Cleansers—Colon Cleansers— Digestive—General Cleanser—Immune—

VITAMINS, MINERALS AND SUPPLEMENTS

The antioxidants, vitamins A, E, C, and minerals selenium and zinc will help protect the body from free-radical damage. The B-complex vitamins help prevent accumulation of toxins in the body. Minerals are essential for every function of the body along with vitamins. A multi-mineral supplement will prevent a lack of essential nutrients that can cause accumulation of toxins.

Liquid chlorophyll and blue-green algae will help purify and clean toxins that cause bad breath. Chlorophyll converts carbon dioxide to oxygen in the body and helps lubricate the digestive tract (i.e. esophageal, pyloric and ileocecal valves). These valves prevent gases and toxins from "backing up" through the digestive tract which can cause bad breath, sour stomach, heartburn, burping and body odors. Acidophilus will help in digestion and prevent bad bacteria from causing odors. Essential fatty acids found in flaxseed oil and salmon oil will help restore balance to the body and protect against the accumulation of toxins.

HAYFEVER

SYMPTOMS

Blurred Vision—Headaches—Itching Nose, Throat, and Eyes—Pain in Head and Sinuses—Runny or Stuffy Nose—Watery Eyes—Post Nasal Drip—

CAUSES

A weakened immune system can cause hay fever. When the sinuses are healthy, they are protected with moist mucous membranes similar to the skin inside the mouth. Healthy membranes are able to wash the pollen and other irritants out of the sinuses and down the throat and into the digestive tract where they are neutralized and eliminated from the body without doing harm.

Hayfever and all other allergic reactions are acute catarrhal symptoms trying to clean and purify the body of toxins. This is an elimination of toxins by way of the mucous membranes. Catarrh of the stomach is the first symptom, due to an abuse or overloading the stomach with wrong combining and overeating. Usually milk, ice cream sugar, white flour products as well too much meat should be eliminated.

Anger, hate, resentment or negative thoughts can increase symptoms. Protein and starch acids, which are created from the over-consumption of fried and rancid oils, cause irritation and inflammation of the stomach lining which leads to fermentation. The gas from the fermentation is passed directly by way of the stomach and colon and is also accumulated in the lungs. This gas elimination is irritating to the mucous membranes and is one cause of hay fever.

NUTRITIONAL THERAPY

A change of diet is necessary to change the health of the mucous membranes. Drink lots of pure water to help clean the toxins. An imbalance of nutrients can cause irritations to the mucous membranes. Constant eating or drinking of unnatural food will cause irritations to accumulate and weaken the inner organs of the body. Evaluate what you are eating and drinking every day and try to eliminate culprit foods for a variety of healthy foods.

Build up the immune system and clean the blood and colon.

Hydrochloric acid can help prevent irritating toxins from invading the mucous membranes. Healthy stomach acid prevents foreign invaders to accumulate. A vegetarian diet will help balance body chemistry and change the chemical reactions in the body.

Fenugreek will help eliminate hard mucus from the body. Garlic and onions work as an antihistamine. Golden Seal will help heal and clean toxins from the digestive tract. Ephedra will dilate the veins and prevent congestion. Scullcap has anti-inflammatory action.

HERBAL FORMULAS

Blood Cleansers—Colds, Flu, Fever and Allergies—Colon Cleansers—Digestive System — General Cleanser — Immune Builders—Nervous System and Brain—

VITAMINS, MINERALS AND SUPPLEMENTS

Vitamin A or beta carotene help heal and prevent infections and are essential for healthy mucous membranes. B-complex vitamins with extra B6 and B12 help the body eliminate toxins through the liver and prevent hay fever reactions. Vitamin C with bioflavonoids helps the body produce interferon to protect the body against allergens. Vitamin E prevents the formation of irritating substances and prevents free-radical damage to the cells.

Calcium and magnesium have an anti-hayfever effect and can help repair damage done to cell membranes. Potassium protects the cells from leaking and causing the reactions typical of hay fever. Selenium and zinc are healing to the mucous

membranes. All minerals are essential for healthy mucous membranes.

Chlorophyll and blue-green algae help to digest and eliminate toxins from the body. They will purify the blood and supply essential nutrients for the immune response to allergies. Acidophilus aids in digestion. It reduces the toxic wastes in the large intestine to prevent hayfever.

HEADACHES

SYMPTOMS

Back of Neck Pain—Frontal Head Pain—Sinus Headaches—Migraine—Tight, sore feeling in Scalp—

TENSION- *Headaches occur when muscle contracts and they are believed to be emotional or psychological in origin. They are usually felt on both sides of the head as well as at the back and come with aching and severe discomfort. Anxiety, depression and muscle spasms can trigger this kind of headache.*

VASCULAR-*This is a throbbing headache which hits the front and sides of the head. It is called a classic migraine. This can cause altered vision, light-headedness, confusion, nausea, and vomiting.*

CLUSTER-*This is called migrainous cranialneuralgia. It causes a stabbing or burning pain, which concentrates on the eye area, with pain traveling to the face or temples.*

Watch for various types of headaches, which may be serious such as headaches in children that recur, daily headaches, one following a blow to the head, one associated with fever, a sudden headache and one associated with convulsions. Also watch for a headache that would cause one to faint or lose consciousness, one that is associated with pain in the eye, ear, nose, or in other parts of the body. The work place may be causing headaches, if you work under fluorescent light or sit at a computer all day.

CAUSES

The main causes of headaches are constipation and impure blood which create irritation to the nerve centers causing intense pain. The pain is caused by the dilation or expansion of the cranial arteries putting pressure on the nerves and pain receptor sites in the head area. This can be caused by tension, allergies, or a weak nervous system.

Samuel Thomsen, an herbalist in the 1800's said that headaches proceed from the stomach, the bile loses its powers, the food clogs, by not being digested and the effect is felt in the head. He said that sometimes there is sickness in the stomach; when this happens, it is called sick headache and vomiting follows and the headache is relieved. He suggested the composition powder formula using Bayberry, Ginger, Cayenne, Cloves, and Lobelia.

Headaches from emotional causes are real and need to be addressed. Inner emotions and feeling need to be dealt with. If the reason is tension or stress from work, or an unhappy relationship, the inability to resolve upsets could manifest itself as a headache. It could be feelings that are uncontrollable, anxiety and fear, or the inability to face an issue or other unresolved problems.

NUTRITIONAL THERAPY

Changing the diet is important, using more natural food.

Cooking grains or rice in a thermos overnight retains the nutrients such as B-vitamins, and enzymes necessary for proper digestion and assimilation. The B-vitamins protect the nervous system.

Eating fresh or lightly steamed vegetables is important. At least 6 to 8 vegetables a day, two fruits, one starch and one protein will help achieve a balanced diet.

Chiropractic treatments have helped many people. Bone and nerve supply could be a problem and adjustment by a chiropractor can very beneficial. This is especially beneficial for preventing disease.

Formulas with Black Cohosh or Blue Vervain are natural tranquilizers. Hops contain tonic and nervine properties. Passion Flower, Scullcap, and St. Johns Wort act as gentle tranquilizers, and are useful in cases of depression. White Willow Bark is a safe, natural source of aspirin-like constituents without the side effects. Wood Betony is considered one of the best herbs for headaches and nervous tension. Dong Quai helps prevent spasms and excessive contractions and has been used successfully for headaches for both men and women. Feverfew is an herb found useful for alleviating migraine headaches and pain.

HERBAL FORMULAS

Allergy—(under colds and flu)—Blood Cleansers—Colon Cleansers—Digestive System—Energy and Stamina—Immune Builders—Nervous System—

VITAMINS, MINERALS AND SUPPLEMENTS

Vitamin A protects the immune system. B-complex vitamins with extra B12, B15 and pangamic acid will relax the muscles. A deficiency of vitamin B5 or pantothenic acid results in headaches and depression. Vitamin C with bioflavonoids help constrict and clean the veins. Vitamin E supplies oxygen to the brain.

Potassium and sodium balance are important to prevent water retention which could put pressure on the brain. Calcium and magnesium are important for the nerves. Selenium and zinc protect the immune system. All minerals work together for better health.

Lecithin is important for the brain and nerves. Liquid chlorophyll and blue-green algae provide minerals and vitamins to help the veins constrict.

Essential fatty acids are vital; deficiencies are related to immune system disorders and mental illness. Flaxseed oil and salmon oil help supply EFA. Germanium and CoQ10 are beneficial to dilate and feed the veins.

HEARING PROBLEMS ——

SYMPTOMS

Hearing loss may be a problem when: Complaints That You're Not Listening— Speaking Too Loudly—Confuse Words You Hear—Ask People To Repeat—Understand Men's voices better than Women's—Difficult to hear a ticking watch, crickets or running water—

CAUSES

The ears are organs which gradually change and degenerate, therefore it is not readily noticed when hearing loss occurs. It may take 20 years to develop and be obvious. When the ear drums become hardened, this usually accompanies hardening of the arteries. Poor ear circulation is one problem.

Catarrhal deafness develops over a period of years. It starts when acute diseases such as cold and flu are suppressed and are not allowed to run their natural cleansing course.

Gradual deafness develops when acute diseases are treated with aspirin, quinine (which was widely used in the past), barbiturates, aureomycin, streptomycin, cocaine, opium and their derivatives. These push the toxins further in the body and create chronic disease.

Diets heavy in table salt (sodium chloride) contribute to ear problems. This causes an imbalance in minerals. Smoking and caffeine drinks cause spasms and narrowing of the blood vessels. Mineral imbalance is caused by poor nutrition and toxic substance such as lead, mercury, cadmium,

etc. They accumulate over a period of years and if the diet is poor, they stay in the tissues.

Excessive noise puts a stress on the ear drums and has a destructive effect to hearing. It causes constriction of the blood vessels which increases blood pressure, faster heart beat, tension in the muscles, and increased adrenal gland activity, action of the kidneys and liver, increased breathing rate, and dilation of the pupils of the eyes. Noise along with poor nutrition and the suppression of acute diseases can speed up hearing loss.

NUTRITIONAL THERAPY

A colon and liver cleanse and a change of diet will to help clean the arteries. This will help dissolve catarrh and eliminate toxins so the body can absorb nutrients to feed and nourish the head area.

A high fiber diet using whole grains, beans, fresh salads, steamed vegetables, sprouts, fresh fruit and vegetable juices will help.

Fresh juice with carrot, celery, parsley, and fresh garlic will help eliminate cholesterol. Exercise will speed up the circulatory cleanse.

Eliminate sugar products they leach out the important B-complex vitamins, calcium and other minerals. Eliminate white flour products, for they are void of nutrients and contain the bleach, chlorine which is detrimental to the organs of the body.

Ginkgo increases circulation in the head area and supplies nutrients, improves memory and mental alertness. It helps to reduce anxiety, tension and vertigo. Gout Kola is a brain food. It helps balance the right and left sides of the brain and increases stamina. Ginseng and Suma increase circulation and lower cholesterol. They are nourishing for the entire body.

HERBAL FORMULAS

Blood Cleansers—Circulatory System—Colon Cleansers—General Cleanser—Immune Builders—Nervous System—Urinary System—

VITAMINS, MINERALS AND SUPPLEMENTS

The antioxidants will help feed and provide essential nutrients to the ears. Vitamins A, D, E, C, and the minerals selenium and zinc are beneficial. The B-complex vitamins are associated with hearing problems. They fight stress and strengthen the nerves. Extra pantothenic acid prevents over-stimulation of the adrenal glands.

Niacin is a vasodilator and drives blood to the head area. Vitamin E provides oxygen to the tiny ear arteries. Vitamin C with bioflavonoids strengthens the capillaries and cleans toxins. It also acts as an antihistamine and natural diuretic.

Minerals are lacking in the head area because of circulatory problems. A multi-mineral supplement will help increase the absorption of nutrients and eliminate heavy metals from the system. Liquid chlorophyll and blue-green algae will help in absorption of nutrients, as well as help clean the arteries. Lecithin, along with germanium and CoQ10 will dissolve fatty deposits on the blood vessel walls. Choline found in lecithin is a principal component of the ears' nerve fiber and is essential for the transmission of nerve impulses.

HEMORRHOIDS

SYMPTOMS

Bleeding with Bowel Movements—Burning and Itching in Rectum—External and Internal Swelling and Protruding Veins in the Rectum and Anus—

CAUSES

Internal hemorrhoids can be present for some time before they are discovered. Bleeding may be the first sign of internal hemorrhoids. Continual bleeding for too long can cause anemia.

The main cause is constipation and straining during a bowel movement. Circulatory weakness of the veins is the cause of hemorrhoids, along with constipation. Liver congestion can be a contributing factor. Hemorrhoids are common in pregnancy, in junk food diets and low fiber diets, lack of exercise, sitting while working, heavy lifting and obesity.

NUTRITIONAL THERAPY

A high fiber diet will help heal and prevent hemorrhoids. Drink a lot of liquids using pure water. Vegetable juices will provide enzymes and minerals for healing. Carrot, celery, parsley with a clove of garlic will help heal. Apples, pomegranates, grapes, oranges, carrots, cabbage, salads using green leafy lettuce and endive are beneficial. Endive will help in the digestion of food.

Whole grains will provide bulk and prevent constipation. Use millet, buckwheat, brown rice, rye, barley, wheat, yellow corn (good for constipation), and whole oats. These can be cooked in a thermos for better assimilation and nutrient content.

Herbs that help for hemorrhoids are: Butchers Broom, Capsicum, Cascara Sagrada, Golden Seal, Horsetail, Kelp, Oatstraw, Pau D'Arco, and White Oak Bark.

HERBAL FORMULAS

Blood Cleansers—Circulatory System—Colon Cleansers—Digestive System—Immune Builders—

VITAMINS, MINERALS AND SUPPLEMENTS

Vitamin A will promote healing. B-complex vitamins help in digestion and strengthen the nerves. Vitamin C with bioflavonoids strengthens and heals the capillaries. Vitamin E is healing for hemorrhoids. Vitamin E can be used externally for healing.

Minerals are essential for healing. Calcium and magnesium are healing as well as zinc.

Chlorophyll contains vitamin K and iron to

prevent anemia and excessive bleeding. Blue-green algae is healing and nourishing to strengthen the veins. Germanium and CoQ10 speed healing and provide oxygen to the veins. Lecithin rebuilds nerve fiber. Flaxseed oil helps soften stools and rebuilds damaged capillaries.

HEPATITIS _____

(Liver Problems, Jaundice)

SYMPTOMS

HEPATITIS—Fever—Flu-Like Symptoms—Loss of Appetite—Nausea—Muscle Aches—Weakness—Vomiting—Abdominal Discomfort—Drowsiness—LIVER CONGESTION—Digestive Disturbances—Headaches—Insomnia—Sluggish Feeling when Waking—Yellowed Skin—Emotional symptoms of Liver Stagnation is Anger—Arrogance—Aggression—Frustration—Hate—Impatience—Violence—

CAUSES

Toxic overload is the main cause of liver problems. Constipation prevents the liver from eliminating toxins. When the liver is congested, the toxins circulate in the bloodstream and can enter the brain, nervous system or other organs and cause numerous symptoms. When the liver tries to expel the poisons forced on it, it burdens the kidneys and causes further congestion.

Liver congestion is also caused by blood stagnation, caused by excessive amounts of fat, sugar (converts to fat in the liver), alcohol, white flour products and chemicals found in water, food and air.

The liver overload also affects the eyes and the heart. Cataracts, night blindness, near or far-sightedness, glaucoma, and other eye problems are caused by the liver. Liver congestion causes circulatory problems.

Goiter is a sign of liver congestion. Growths such as cancer or tumors are caused by liver and colon congestion, lack of fiber and eating rich, junk food.

NUTRITIONAL THERAPY

The liver is vital to overall health. Most diseases are caused by colon and liver congestion. It pays to take care of the liver. A fasting diet using juices will help cleanse the liver. Raw food will speed the healing of the liver. Carrots, celery, parsley and apple juice is rich in vitamin A and healing for the liver. Green leafy vegetables and sprouts are healing.

A half lemon or lime juice in warm water first thing in the morning will clean and heal the liver. Vegetables and fruits such as artichokes, broccoli, parsley, leaf lettuce, cauliflower, collards, endives, green pepper, pomegranate, raspberries, strawberries, tangerines, apples, cherries, cranberries, and plums should be eaten.

Olive oil in lemon juice helps dissolve hard bile. Short juice fasts helps restore liver function. Eating the last meal of the day around 2 or 3 will help the liver restore and rest for faster healing. Squash of all kinds are rich in vitamin A and very healing.

Miso, pickles, and endive lettuce will help in digestion and assimilation and lift the load off the liver. Sour cherries and sour apples will also help in liver function.

Eliminate meat, excessive fat, refined foods, white sugar and flour products, and alcohol from the diet. Give the liver a chance to restore itself.

Burdock restores function to the liver and cleans blood. Milk Thistle helps repair the liver. Dandelion and Cascara Sagrada clear obstructions from the liver. Gentian is a bitter herb and helps in digestion and liver function. Pau D'Arco protects the liver from damage.

HERBAL FORMULAS

Blood Cleaners—Circulatory System—Colon Cleansers and Liver—Digestive System—General Cleanser—Immune Builders—Nervous System and Brain—Urinary System—

VITAMINS, MINERALS AND SUPPLEMENTS

Vitamin A is healing. B-complex vitamins help the liver eliminate toxins. A deficiency in vitamin C causes liver problems. Vitamin E speeds healing and prevents scarring.

A multi-mineral supplement will help the liver to detoxify. Zinc is healing. Deficiencies in chromium, manganese, magnesium, potassium, and selenium are seen in liver disorders.

Flaxseed oil and salmon oil heal the liver and eliminate cholesterol. Chlorophyll and blue-green algae help heal and clean the liver.

HERPES
(Simplex and Genital Herpes)

SYMPTOMS

Fever—Aches—Pain—Inflammation on Skin—Symptoms disappear but the Virus does not die.

CAUSES

Three Common Viruses of the Herpes Family: Herpes Simplex 1 (affects the mouth and causes "Fever Blisters" and "Cold Sores")— Herpes Simplex 2 (causes Genital Herpes)— Herpes Zoster (well known to cause Chicken pox, and, as a secondary infection, Shingles).

Herpes is a virus; a parasite that enters the body through the skin and resides deep inside the body in the nerve group at the base of the spine and doesn't go away. Herpes can lay dormant and then recur when the immune system is lowered by stress, diet, autointoxication, illness, overexposure to sunlight, some foods and drugs. The initial infection can go away but not the virus.

Recurrence of genital herpes is caused by sexual intercourse from irritation caused to the skin. The sores may appear on the cervix, anus, buttocks, thighs, or the vaginal walls in women and on the penis, scrotum, perineum, buttocks, thighs, anus, and the urethra in men.

The secondary infection of herpes zoster is not called "chicken pox," but is known as "shingles."

NUTRITIONAL THERAPY

A diet including grains, beans, fresh vegetables, fruit, some fish and poultry excluding sugar, chocolate, nuts (contain the amino acid arginine), white flour, caffeine products, cigarettes, alcohol and drugs is recommended.

Eliminate red meat and animal fat, because the virus lives in these foods. When an outbreak occurs, a short cleansing diet would help speed the healing. Carrot, celery, parsley will provide vitamin A and zinc.

Exercise will build resistance to the disease. Exercise in fresh air if possible.

Foods high in the amino acid lysine should be eaten for short periods. They control the herpes virus. Eat fish, chicken, beans, cabbage, alfalfa, sprouts, papaya, apples, apricots, pears, grapes, avocados, bananas, cantaloupe, grapefruit, and oranges to help with herpes.

Echinacea, Golden Seal and Burdock are antiseptic and blood cleansing. Kelp seems to help in herpes. Iodine content helps kill the virus. Myrrh is also an antiseptic and is healing. Aloe Vera is healing to put on sores.

HERBAL FORMULAS

Blood Cleansers—Colon Cleansers—Digestive System—Immune Builders—Infection Fighting—Nervous System—

VITAMINS, MINERALS AND SUPPLEMENTS

Beta carotene is healing, and 25,000 i.u. twice a day for two weeks is recommended. B-complex vitamins are essential for the nerves. Extra B12 helps in pain. Vitamin C with bioflavonoids, taken in 1,000 mg. increments throughout the day helps heal and increase immune response. Vitamin E is healing internally and externally, and will prevent scarring.

Calcium and magnesium taken throughout the day will heal and build up the nerves. The amino acid, L-lysine inhibits viral function if taken when symptoms appear. Bee pollen is high in amino acids and cuts the craving for sugar and raises the blood-sugar levels.

Chlorophyll and blue-green algae will clean and purify the blood. They will help heal and eliminate the symptoms.

HIATAL HERNIA

SYMPTOMS

Acid in Throat—Belching—Bloating— Diarrhea—Discomfort in Chest Area— Constipation—Heart Burn—Intestinal Gas— Nausea—Vomiting—It can even Mimic a Heart Attack—

CAUSES

A small portion of the stomach slips through an opening (hiatus) in the diaphragm forcing the stomach to push into the chest. This is a common cause of discomfort in the elderly.

Leakage of acid in the lower esophagus is the reason for the discomfort and burning feeling. This can be caused from a low fiber diet, constipation (straining when eliminating), lack of exercise (lack of muscle tone in the stomach), eating wrong combinations of food which causes fermentation, and gas that protrudes the stomach upwards. Anger, hate and negative feelings effect the stomach.

NUTRITIONAL THERAPY

A calm atmosphere when eating will help prevent hiatal hernia and lessen its symptoms. Eating small meals and chewing well will prevent swallowing air which causes heartburn. Avoid drinking liquids with meals, because it dilutes the enzymes and hydrochloric acid and prevents proper digestion.

Foods high in fiber such as whole grains, beans, seeds, sprouts, vegetables and fruit will help keep the colon clean. Fiber will help prevent constipation and straining when eliminating which will aggravate a hiatal hernia. A high fat diet slows digestion and causes irritation to a hiatal hernia.

A chiropractor can manipulate the hiatal hernia back where it belongs. Drinking two 8 ounce glasses of water and bouncing on the heels 12 times may help jar it into place.

Loose weight if that is a problem. Avoid tight clothes. Eliminate alcohol, cola and drinks that contain carbonation. Eat small meals and wait at least three hours before lying down. Avoid coffee and chocolate because they weaken the esophagus. Avoid drugs; they only aggravate heartburn.

Hiatal hernia is linked with clogging of the arteries. It can also cause damage to the esophagus. The juices from the acidic stomach wash back into the esophagus causing inflammation and irritation. If this continues, it can cause ulceration, scarring, and even blockage of the esophagus requiring surgery. Aspirin can be very harmful and injure the esophagus.

Aloe Vera is healing and prevents scarring. Gentian, Ginger and Golden Seal are healing for the digestive tract. Slippery Elm is nourishing and healing.

HERBAL FORMULAS

Blood Cleansers—Colon Cleansers—Digestive System — Immune Builders — Nervous System — Structural System — Urinary System—

VITAMINS, MINERALS AND SUPPLEMENTS

Antioxidants will strengthen the immune system as well as heal the mucous membranes of the digestive tract. These include vitamins A, D, C, E, and minerals selenium and zinc. B-complex vitamins are essential for stomach and nerve health.

A multi-mineral is needed for stomach health with extra calcium, magnesium, potassium, sodium and silicon.

Aloe vera juice and chlorophyll will heal the esophagus and stomach. Chlorophyll helps the body produce interferon to fight infections.

Germanium and CoQ10 are healing to the circulatory system and provide oxygen to the cells. Lecithin is healing to the nerves.

HIGH BLOOD PRESSURE

(Hypertension)

SYMPTOMS

No Symptoms at the Beginning—As the Disease Progresses it can cause Dizziness—Energy Loss — Fatigue — Headaches — Insomnia—Irritability—Nervousness—Blood Pressure Reading should be taken frequently to determine how The Blood Pressure is—

CAUSES

High blood pressure is a chronic degenerative disease caused by incorrect living habits, eating and attitude towards life. It is the most common cardiovascular disease in the United States. It can lead to stroke, heart attack, kidney damage, pancreatic damage, and eye diseases.

Hypertension occurs when cholesterol, plaque and toxins deposit in the walls of the arteries. They harden and constrict the blood vessels compressing the blood into a smaller volume thereby raising blood pressure.

The major cause is toxic blood and colon. High meat and fat diet, with little fiber collects on the colon wall and creates autointoxication in the blood. Excess salt can cause water retention and put extra pressure on the veins. Being overweight and a lack of exercise can contribute to its symptoms. Stress is also a factor in high blood pressure. Heavy metals in the blood can also increase blood pressure.

NUTRITIONAL THERAPY

Diet changes can be a positive factor in lowering blood pressure. Eliminate table salt (sodium chloride) and add more potassium foods such as potatoes, avocados, lima beans, white and pinto beans, dried peas, dried apricots, almonds, parsley, yams, bananas, carrots, celery and green leafy vegetables. Eat less meat and fat, adding more grains, vegetables, fruit and natural food. Herbs have helped with blood pressure with their high content of minerals. Carrot, celery, parsley and garlic will benefit the blood.

An exercise plan, along with stress reduction will help in lowering blood pressure. Sugar can cause retention of salt in the body and increase blood pressure. Coffee, tea, chocolate and many soft drinks contribute to high blood pressure.

Garlic and Onions have lipid lowering and blood pressure lowering activity. Hawthorn Berries are beneficial for dilating and strengthening the blood vessels. It nourishes the heart. Mistletoe lowers blood pressure (used in formulas). Parsley is a natural diuretic.

HERBAL FORMULAS

Blood Cleansers—Circulatory System—Colon Cleansers—Digestive System—General Cleansers—Immune System—Nervous System and Brain—Structural System—(calcium formulas)—Urinary System—

VITAMINS, MINERALS AND SUPPLEMENTS

B-complex vitamins help the liver detoxify and prevent fatty deposits in the arteries. Vitamin C and bioflavonoids nourish the veins and improve arterial function. Vitamin E supplies oxygen in the blood to improve heart function.

Calcium and magnesium are beneficial, and are often lacking in those with HBP. Potassium protects the heart and blood vessels, and an herbal potassium formula is beneficial. Silicon, found in herbal calcium formulas helps improve circulatory problems. Zinc along with all minerals improves circulatory diseases.

Flaxseed oil and salmon oil improve arterial function. These are lacking in the typical American diet. Chlorophyll and blue-green algae clean and build the blood and veins. Germanium and CoQ10 are nutrients that provide oxygen to the vessels and reduce high blood pressure.

HODGKIN'S DISEASE ____

SYMPTOMS

Painless Enlargement of Lymph Nodes and Spleen—Fatigue—Fever—General Unwell Feeling—Night Sweats—Weight Loss— Weakness—Itching can be an early symptom—

CAUSES

This is also called Hodgkin's lymphoma, a form of cancer that affect the lymph glands. It is most common in young adults. It is a malignant disorder found in the lymph nodes and spleen. The spleen is part of the immune system and when it becomes congested, it throws toxins back into the lymph system and the blood. The spleen is sometimes removed and causes more problems of congestion.

If the tonsils and appendix are removed, this also causes problems with the immune system.

These are organs that help the body remove toxins and protect against bacteria and germs.

NUTRITIONAL THERAPY

A vegetable juice fast for 2 to 3 days to start is recommended. Then every few days as the body gains strength use periodic fasts. Changes need to be made in the diet in order to clean the blood. Eliminate sugar, refined oils, margarine, caffeine, milk and all dairy products, meat, peanut butter, alcohol, fried and smoked foods. A little fish is acceptable.

Drink wheat grass juice, chlorophyll, and juices using carrots, celery, parsley and garlic and potassium broth soup. Simmer potatoes, carrots, celery, parsley, onions and garlic and drink the juice.

The cells contain the food we are used to eating in the past and cravings for those kinds of foods are very common. It may take a lot of cleansing before the desire for these foods are gone.

Burdock cleans the blood, Echinacea is beneficial for cleaning the lymphatics and Red Clover formulas will neutralize the poisons in the blood. Pau D'Arco tea protects the liver and cleans the blood. The colon needs to be kept clean so the toxins are eliminated when the blood is cleaned.

HERBAL FORMULAS

Blood Cleansers—Colon Cleansers—Digestive System — Glandular System — Immune Builders—Nervous System and Brain—

VITAMINS, MINERALS AND SUPPLEMENTS

The antioxidants, A, C, E, selenium and zinc help inhibit cancer growth. Vitamin C with bioflavonoids detoxifies cancer causing compounds.

Every cell contains potassium. Kelp, alfalfa and parsley contain potassium. These are necessary in releasing energy from carbohydrates, fats and proteins and for the formation of glycogen. Calcium and chromium are seen as deficiencies in cancer. All minerals are essential for improving blood and eliminating toxins.

Germanium boosts interferon production in the body. CoQ10 is a powerful antioxidant. Chlorophyll stimulates interferon and detoxifies toxins from the blood. Acidophilus provides friendly bacteria while the body is cleansing. Flaxseed oil and salmon oil are potent in increasing the production of antibodies which destroy cancer cells.

HIVES

SYMPTOMS

Skin Develops Red, Itchy Bumps—They sometimes have a white center and join together in large irregular patches. Hives are a very common disorder. They are harmless but irritating—Allergic reactions can occur within 30 minutes to foods such as shellfish, strawberries, monosodium glutamate—

CAUSES

Allergies are the most common cause of hives. Drugs such as penicillin, aspirin, codeine, and many others can cause a hive reaction. Stress can make hives worse. Bug bites or stings are one cause. Food additives, strawberries, shellfish or preservative that are added to food can all cause hives.

Hives can be caused by serious diseases such as lupus erythematosus, hepatitis, infectious mono-nucleosis or upper respiratory diseases.

If hives cause breathing difficulties, swelling or cover the entire body, with a rapid pulse, shock may occur and medical attention is required.

Echinacea, Burdock, and Red Clover are beneficial for hives. They clean the blood to help eliminate the hives. When the skin breaks out, the inside mucous membranes can also be affected.

NUTRITIONAL THERAPY

An elimination diet would determine if food is causing the hives. Fresh vegetable juices would speed the healing. Fasting, using pure water, chlorophyll and juices would help clean the blood.

Eliminate cured meats, alcohol, cheese, chocolate, shellfish, citrus fruits, milk, eggs, sugar and white flour products.

A lack of hydrochloric acid may prevent the allergens from being destroyed. Sun bathing for short periods will speed the healing. Black Walnut and Aloe Vera externally are healing.

Millet is easy to digest, and is rich in calcium, magnesium, silicon and other minerals. Brown rice will supply B-complex vitamins, which are necessary for strong nerves and helping the liver to eliminate toxins.

HERBAL FORMULAS

Blood Cleansers—Colon Cleansers—Colds, Flu and Allergies—Digestion—Immune System Builders—

VITAMINS, MINERALS AND SUPPLEMENTS

Vitamin A is healing for the mucous membranes and is necessary for healthy skin. Vitamin C with bioflavonoids and vitamin A together help to decrease the symptoms of skin eruptions. B-complex helps in detoxifying the cause of hives. The need for these important vitamins is increased when hives occur.

Minerals help in preventing and healing, especially selenium and zinc. Calcium and magnesium help in the absorption of B12 and improve nerve function.

Acidophilus helps in digestion and in the prevention of allergies. Blue-green algae and chlorophyll help clear the blood of allergens.

HYPERACTIVITY
(Attention Deficit Disorder)

SYMPTOMS

Hyperactivity is now termed "Attention Deficit Disorder." Some symptoms are: cannot sit Still—Short Attention Span—Runs rather than Walks—Impulsive—Acts before Thinks—Forgets Easily—Moody—Irritated and Indifferent when Disciplined—Temper Tantrums—Determined to get their Way— These symptoms are not limited to children— Many adults have these symptoms.

Mental hyperactivity is common in our computer age. Our brains receive excess material because of the easy access, through computers, television,and videos.

CAUSES

Hyperactivity is diet related especially with the wide use of sugar. Sugar is abundant in our food and is addictive and has a profound effect on the mind, body and emotions. Children can react very quickly to sugar and food additives. Allergies to milk, wheat, chocolate, oranges, yeast, food additives and antibiotics are common.

Wheat causes reactions because it becomes rancid very fast. Oranges, are not picked ripe, and this can cause allergies. Lead poisoning has been linked with hyperactivity. Lead attacks the brain and nervous system. Lead is inhaled in the lungs, and is assimilated into the blood faster than when we ingest it in food.

NUTRITIONAL THERAPY

Find the cause, whether it is allergies, sugar, or toxic metals. Diet change can only improve the brain and nervous system.

A lazy colon can also be a problem. The brain is sensitive to toxins and if the colon is sluggish, it can affect the brain and nerves. Sugar depletes nutrients from the body especially B-vitamins and calcium which are critical to mental and emotional health.

Grains and vegetable soups are excellent, because they are rich in minerals vital for eliminating heavy metals from the body. Brown rice, millet, and whole oats are excellent for the nerves and brain. Millet is rich in calcium and magnesium. Rice is rich in B-complex vitamins. Thermos cooking will retain all the B-vitamins and minerals in the grains. Raw vegetables and salads are excellent. Fruit is cleansing and provides energy when children are taken off sugar.

The combination of Gotu Kola, Bee Pollen, and an herbal formula containing: Siberian Ginseng, Gotu Kola, Bee Pollen and Capsicum is beneficial. Another formula containing: Valerian Root, Scullcap, Hops, Thiamine, Riboflavin, Nicotinamide, Calcium, Pyridoxine HCL, Ascorbic Acid, Choline, Inositol, Schizandra, Folic Acid, and other ingredients is also good.

Single herbs to help are Black Walnut, which kills parasites, Burdock, to clean the blood, Gotu Kola for brain food, Hops to relax, and Scullcap to build nerves.

HERBAL FORMULAS

Allergies—(under colds, Flu, Fevers)—Blood Cleansers—(Eliminates sugar from the body)—Colon Cleansers—Energy and Stamina—Nervous System and Brain—

VITAMINS, MINERALS AND SUPPLEMENTS

Vitamins A, D, and C, will help prevent lead absorption and build the immune system. Vitamin E, flaxseed oil, and salmon oil are beneficial in hyperactivity in adults and children. They produce prostaglandins for positive immune response.

Calcium and magnesium eliminate lead and are essential for nerves and brain, and protect against anxiety. Multi-mineral contain selenium and zinc and help strengthen the body and eliminate toxins.

Chlorophyll and blue-green algae are nourishing and build the blood. They clean toxins from the blood. Lecithin protects the nerve sheath and neutralizes toxins.

HYPERTHYROID AND HYPOTHYROID

SYMPTOMS

Some symptoms of hyperthyroidism are Fatigue—Insomnia—Intolerance—Rapid Heartbeat—Sweating— Weakness—Some symptoms of hypothyroidism are—Anemia— Bruising (easy)—Cold Feeling—Depression— Fatigue—Hair Loss—Low Back Pain—Muscle Cramps—Muscle Weakness—Recurrent Infections—

CAUSES

Hyperthyroidism occurs when too much thyroxine is produced by the thyroid gland causing an overactive metabolism.

Hypothyroidism occur when the thyroid gland produces too little hormone. An overactive thyroid gland can result in Graves's disease.

Kelp has been found to slow an overactive thyroid. Symptoms of Graves's disease are rapid and irregular heartbeat, increased appetite but steady weight loss, anxiety, insomnia, and frequent bowel movement. As it gets worse, there is muscle weakness and a general wasting. Supplements are essential to build and strengthen the glands.

The thyroid is a small, butterfly-shaped gland located in the neck and weighs less than an ounce. The thyroid gland is very important and controls metabolism, which is the process by which food is transformed into energy and many vital chemical changes take place. Every organ, tissue and cell is affected by the hormone secretions of the thyroid.

A lack of iodine can cause hypothyroidism and the gland may become as large as a tennis ball. Myxedema, a disease of the immune system, is another cause. The body's own immune system slowly destroys the thyroid. Other causes are diseases of the pituitary gland and hypothalamus which normally produce substances called thyroid stimulating hormone, and thyrotropin releasing hormone which stimulate the thyroid gland for sufficient thyroid hormone production.

NUTRITIONAL THERAPY

Natural iodine is essential and is found in Kelp. The soil in the United States is low in iodine. A diet high in fiber is important. A diet using a variety of foods such as grains, fruit, vegetables, sprouts, seeds and nuts is good. Brown rice and miso soup once a week are beneficial. Don't overeat. Obesity can occur with hypothyroidism. Watch weight gain and exercise at least three times a week.

Eliminate meat except fish for a while. A low fat diet helps to regulate metabolism.

Kelp and Alfalfa help to regulate the thyroid gland.

HERBAL FORMULAS

Blood Cleansers—Colon Cleansers—Digestive System—Glandular—Immune Builders— Nervous System—Male and Female—

VITAMINS, MINERALS AND SUPPLEMENTS

Vitamin A is necessary for iodine to be properly absorbed. B-vitamins work together to nourish the thyroid. B2 is necessary for ovaries and testes to secrete their hormones. If there is a lack of vitamin B6, the thyroid cannot use it's iodine effectively in hormone production.

B12 helps the thyroid gland work properly. Deficiencies of vitamin C and E can cause overproduction of the thyroid hormone. They help to regulate hormone function.

Minerals are necessary in proper glandular function. All minerals work together for glandular

329

function.

Liquid chlorophyll works with Kelp and Alfalfa for proper assimilation. Blue-green algae feeds and cleans the glands. Essential fatty acids help in glandular metabolism and are found in flaxseed oil and salmon oil. Germanium and CoQ10 provide oxygen to the cells.

HYPOGLYCEMIA _____

SYMPTOMS

Some common symptoms are: Anxiety—Antisocial Behavior — Confusion — Depression — Emotional Instability — Exhaustion—Headaches—Impatience—Inability to Cope—Intense Hunger—Nervousness—Phobias—Irritability—Sugar Craving—Faintness—Dizziness—Mental Confusion—

CAUSES

The adrenals become exhausted from stress, worry, and the toxic accumulation of undigested starches, sugars, proteins and dairy products. This depletes the cortin hormone and the ability to digest properly.

Dietary choices are the main cause of hypoglycemia. A diet high in refined food and excessive sugar intake exhausts the adrenals. Glandular dysfunction and mineral deficiencies are other causes. Heavy metal poisoning can produce hypoglycemia. Addictions are linked to hypoglycemia.

White sugar is not a food; it is a chemical which wears out the glandular system. The adrenals and pancreas are over-stressed when refined starches, sugars, and a high meat diet are eaten. Sugar is an addictive substance, and the low blood sugar state, which you get from eating it makes the cravings more intense. The food industry has discovered that increasing the sugar content in products increases the amount a person will eat, which will increase sales.

NUTRITIONAL THERAPY

The following should be eliminated from the diet: nicotine, caffeine, theobromine, theophylline, and purines found in animal products, coffee, meat, and tea. Chocolate contains toxic alkaloids, that damage the pancreas. They interfere with glandular function and create addictions.

Carbonated drinks interfere with digestion. Stomach problems are common with hypoglycemia. Avoid heavy fat diets and fried foods. They cause a lowering of blood sugar and a reduction of sugar in the urine. Avoid an excess of dairy products; they are constipating and are high in lactose (mild sugar).

Read labels when purchasing food. The following are forms of sugars: Dextrose, dextrin, maltose, lactose, sucrose, fructose, modified food starch, cornstarch, corn syrup, corn sweetener, natural sweetener, honey (use in small amounts), and molasses (use in small amounts). The following are forms of alcoho and react in the body as with refined carbohydrates: sorbitol, mannitol, hexitol and glycol. Also avoid too much table salt. It creates adrenal exhaustion and causes a loss of potassium which leads to a drop in blood sugar.

Eat natural foods and eliminate the ones that caused the problems in the first place. White flour and white sugar products, refined and processed foods, fast foods cooked in rancid oils, heavy meat diets, ice cream, pastries, cookies, candy, processed cereals, soft drinks, and caffeine products should be eliminated.

Eat small meals through out the day. Learn stress reduction. Increase the intake of whole grains, (millet, buckwheat, rye, wheat, barley, amaranth and quinoa). Use raw seeds, nuts, beans, vegetables and fruit. Sprouts are rich in nutrients. Grains digest slowly and release sugar into the blood stream gradually for as long as 6 to 8 hours after the meal. Grains help to keep blood sugar level constant for a long period of time.

Licorice root acts in the body like the cortin

hormone and protects the gland by helping to cope with stress. It allows the blood sugar level to remain normal and provides a feeling of well-being. Alfalfa provides vegetable protein which is essential for the glands. Cedar berries heal and nourish the pancreas. Golden Seal helps to regulate blood sugar levels.

HERBAL FORMULAS

Blood Cleansers—Circulatory System—Colon Cleansers—Digestive System—Glandular System — Immune Builders — Nervous System—

VITAMINS, MINERALS AND SUPPLEMENTS

Vitamin A assists in maintaining normal glandular function. B-complex vitamins are necessary to control the highs and lows in hypoglycemia. They build the adrenals and calm the nerves. Vitamin C with bioflavonoids helps to prevent low blood sugar attacks. It plays an important role in sugar metabolism. Vitamin E protects the B vitamins from rapid oxidation and reduces cholesterol. It is necessary for rebuilding the adrenal and pituitary glands.

Minerals are vital to rebuild the adrenals. Calcium and magnesium help prevent adrenal instability. They work with A, C and E, zinc and inositol for proper absorption. Chromium is essential for correct sugar metabolism. Iodine regulates hormones to control metabolism. Manganese assists in pancreatic development and in maintenance of healthy nerves.

Acidophilus is beneficial for improving digestion. Blue-green algae and chlorophyll are cleansing and healing. Germanium and CoQ10 help in providing oxygen to the veins and cells. Essential fatty acids found in flaxseed oil and salmon oil are necessary because the body cannot make them. They serve as precursors to hormone-like substances that help regulate every body function.

IMMUNE SYSTEM DISORDERS

SYMPTOMS

Some common symptoms are: Colds (frequent)—Flu—(catch every virus)—Mental Depression—Susceptible to many Auto-Immune Diseases such as—AIDS—Bacteremia—Cancer—Candida Albicans—Chylamydial Diseases—Legionnaires' Disease—Leprosy—Lupus Erythematosus—Reye's Syndrome—Many others.

CAUSES

Autoimmune diseases have increased since drugs and vaccinations were introduced. Aspirin is linked to Reyes' syndrome, asthma, low birth weight and birth defects. If over-the-counter drugs can cause such serious conditions, what are the stronger drugs doing to the immune system?

The typical American diet, lack of proper rest, inherited weakness and stress all contribute to a weakened immune system. Drinking alcohol, smoking, drugs and eating a high sugar diet weaken the immune system. Air pollution contains toxins that weaken the lungs. The air is thick with lead, cadmium, and other toxins. The lungs absorb toxins much faster than ingesting them.

Meat contains antibiotics, hormones, and microbes which cause diseases. Heavy meat eating weakens the immune system. It overstimulates the nerves, endocrine system and overloads the liver and kidneys. Meat is lacking in fiber and minerals.

Viruses and germs enter the body of healthy individuals and remain dormant and harmless unless the immune system is weakened.

NUTRITIONAL THERAPY

Eat a lot of fresh fruit and vegetables; six vegetables a day, two to three fruits, one protein, and one starch. The fruits and vegetables help neutralize toxins and move them from the body. Meat causes fermentation in the intestines and produces indole, skatole and other gases. These toxins dissolve in the water and enter the bloodstream through the intestinal wall.

The body needs amino acids (made from protein), and they can be easily obtained from a combination of plant foods. Grains, beans, vegetables, fruit, seeds, nuts, sea vegetables, and sprouts are high in essential nutrients including protein.

Fish, beans, and grains contain argentine, an amino acid which stimulates immune response. The T-cells of a healthy immune system will destroy cancer cells, bacteria, germs and viruses.

Organic foods are recommended if you can get them. If not, supplements are a must. Broccoli, cauliflower, brussels sprouts, cabbage, onions, garlic, leeks, and chives will enhance the immune system.

Herbs that help build up the immune system are: Burdock, Dandelion, Echinacea, Golden Seal, Horsetail, Kelp, Pau D'Arco, Red Clover, Ginkgo, Suma, and Bee Pollen.

HERBAL FORMULAS

Blood Cleansers—Circulatory System—Colon Cleansers—Digestive System—Energy and Stamina—Immune Builders—

VITAMINS, MINERALS AND SUPPLEMENTS

Antioxidants protect the immune system; vitamin A, D, C, E selenium and zinc. The B-complex vitamins enhance immunity and help the liver to detoxify the toxins.

Calcium and magnesium regulate lymphocyte function. Manganese, magnesium, copper, calcium, selenium and zinc increase immune response. A multi-mineral is necessary for assimilation of vitamins.

Acidophilus will improve digestion and colon health. It helps in the assimilation of all nutrients. Blue-green algae and chlorophyll help in eliminating toxins and nourishing the blood.

Germanium and CoQ10 help in providing oxygen to the blood and improving immunity. Salmon oil and flaxseed oil are essential for protecting the immune system.

IMPOTENCE AND INFERTILITY

SYMPTOMS

Impotence is the lack of power or virility in the Male—Becoming very common—Infertility is the inability of couples to conceive a child, when they are doing everything possible—Also becoming very common.

CAUSES

Impotence can be a physical or emotional problem, It could be caused by fatigue or stress. Depression, stress and fatigue cause hormonal changes to take place. There are medications that can cause this problem. Antidepressants, tranquilizers, anti-hypertensive drugs and anti-ulcer drugs are some drugs that can cause impotence.

The following ailments can cause impotence: arteriosclerosis, hypertension, diabetes, cancer, and brain and spinal cord injuries.

The cause of infertility in males could be low sperm count, prostate infections, loss of interest in life (dietary problems), and job dissatisfaction. Caffeine consumption can lower fertility.

NUTRITIONAL THERAPY

Diet changes in both the male and female have helped many people conceive and bear children. Eliminating a high meat diet, which contains artificial hormone supplements, will help balance hormones. Decreasing or eliminating eggs, chicken, and dairy products which also contain antibiotics and hormones will help clean and rebuild the glandular system. Adding grains, rice and beans will supply amino acids. Fresh fruit and vegetables will supply vitamins and minerals to build up the hormone levels in the body.

Herbs contain mini nutrients and constituents that stimulate body functions. Siberian Ginseng, increases male function. Sarsaparilla is considered a male tonic. Saw Palmetto stimulates glandular function. Pumpkin seeds are rich in zinc. Bee Pollen is a complete food.

HERBAL FORMULAS

Blood Cleansers—Circulatory System—Colon Cleansers—Digestive System—Energy and Stamina—Glandular System—Immune Builders—Nervous System—

VITAMINS, MINERALS AND SUPPLEMENTS

Vitamin E is considered the fertility vitamin and a lack of it can cause premature births. Vitamin A and C are antioxidants to protect the cells against damage and increase immune function. B-complex vitamins are important to provide energy and prevent depression. They are utilized as coenzymes in almost all parts of the body.

Pantothenic Acid, a B vitamin is important. A deficiency in male animals has caused sterility and in females miscarriages or deformities. Folic acid deficiencies may cause hemorrhaging, miscarriage, premature birth, and infant death. Both men and women need this nutrient.

Minerals are very important in the male glandular system. A lack of zinc can cause a low sperm count and prostate problems. A lack of iodine can cause retardation in the growing fetus.

Essential fatty acids, found in flaxseed oil and salmon oil are missing from the diets of most people. It has increased conception in some people. Acidophilus will help in assimilating vital nutrients for strengthening the glandular system. Chlorophyll and blue-green algae help to build the blood, nourish the stomach, and provide vitamin K and other essential nutrients for a healthy glandular system. Germanium and CoQ10 provide oxygen to increase nutrients absorption and strengthen the immune system.

INDIGESTION
(Dyspepsia)

SYMPTOMS

Most common symptoms are Belching—Full Uncomfortable Feeling after Eating—Gas—Heartburn—Pain in Stomach—Regurgitation—

CAUSES

The main causes of indigestion are dietary habits and stress. Eating when under stress upsets the stomach. The stomach is the seat of emotional problems and is seen as the beginning of chronic disease. Eating under stress upsets the stomach and may cause indigestion.

Lack of hydrochloric acid and enzymes are a major cause of indigestion. Lack of enzymes prevents hormones, vitamins and minerals from doing their job. Not enough live food and too much cooked food puts a stress on the liver, gallbladder, pancreas and other organs and causes them to overwork. Lack of fiber causes constipation and autointoxication and results in toxins entering the blood stream and can lead to all kinds of disease. It pays to take care of the stomach.

NUTRITIONAL THERAPY

Fresh and raw foods are rich in enzymes that help digest and assimilate the nutrients. Enzymes are destroyed when heated to temperatures over 120 degrees F (49° C), and during food processing.

Kouchadoff, a Russian scientist, experimented with cooked food and found when eaten, white blood cells increase in the intestines. The white blood cells are part of the immune system and protect us. They increase in number when there is a need to eliminate hostile invaders. Their extra concentration indicates the start of an inflammation or disease. Cooked food is seen as a hostile invader and puts a strain on the immune system. This is one reason we have so many auto-immune diseases.

Eating raw foods protects the immune system and does not cause an increase in white blood cells. Dr. Bircher-Benner, a Swiss nutritionist, found that eating raw vegetables before cooked food prevents the formation of white cells in the intestines. He adopted the eating of fresh raw salads first before eating cooked food in his sanatorium.

Eat a lot of raw vegetables before meals. Thermos cooking for rice and grains such as wheat, buckwheat, rye, millet, and others helps retain their enzymes and protects the stomach from digestive problems.

To heal the stomach, chew food slowly, and create a positive attitude. Eat one food at a time. Fiber is important for the entire digestive tract and not just the colon.

Coffee can cause indigestion. Pineapples contain a protein-digesting enzyme called bromelain. A half fresh lemon or lime juiced in a glass of water before meals will help in digestion.

Carrot juice, celery and cabbage with ginger are healing for the stomach. Ginger is a natural carminative and will protect the stomach from damage.

Papaya, Fennel, Fenugreek, Catnip and Peppermint are helpful in digestion. Gentian and Golden Seal are healing to the entire digestive tract. Aloe Vera juice is healing and nourishing.

HERBAL FORMULAS

Blood Cleansers—Circulatory System—Colon Cleansers—Digestive System—Immune Builders—Nervous System—

VITAMINS, MINERALS AND SUPPLEMENTS

Vitamins and minerals are depleted quickly when under stress and when the wrong diet is eaten. They are important for proper digestion.

Vitamins A and E are healing for the mucous membranes of the stomach and prevent free-radical damage. B-complex vitamins help in the digestion of food. A supplement would help, because they are destroyed in cooking. Vitamin C with bioflavonoids helps in the assimilation of nutrients, especially calcium. It also protects the immune system.

Calcium and magnesium aid in digestion and help relax the stomach for better absorption. Iron and zinc are healing for digestive problems. A multi-mineral supplement will help provide proper digestion.

Acidophilus helps in the digestion of food to prevent stomach upsets. It also protects against bad bacteria in the colon. Blue-green algae and chlorophyll are healing and nourishing to the stomach. Flaxseed oil and salmon oil are essential for digesting and assimilating nutrients. Germanium and CoQ10 help in oxygenating the cells.

INFERTILITY AND FRIGIDITY
(Women)

SYMPTOMS

Infertility is very common and is the inability of women to conceive when not using prevention and trying for at least a year without success—Frigidity is when women lack sexual desire.

CAUSES

Some of the causes of infertility are infections, venereal disease, inherited disorders, mishandled abortions, bacterial organisms, endometriosis, drugs, plugged fallopian tubes or nutritional deficiencies. Emotional trauma can also be a cause.

NUTRITIONAL THERAPY

Nutrition plays a vital role in the ability to conceive and in the health of the baby. Kidney problems can cause reproductive imbalances. Cleaning the kidneys would be beneficial. Ginger, fennel and fenugreek are good for the kidneys.

Adopting a natural health diet eliminating sugar, meat, white flour products, caffeine drinks, fried foods and any unnatural food will strengthen the female glandular system. Grains, rice, beans, sprouts, vegetables, fruit, seeds, nuts and sea vegetables will build up the female glands.

Herbs that help infertility and build up the sex glands are: Black Cohosh, Blessed Thistle, Burdock, Cramp Bark, Dong Quai, False Unicorn, Feverfew, Horsetail, Red Clover, Red Raspberry, Sarsaparilla, Wild Yam, and Yellow dock. Nervine herbs are also important: Chamomile, Hops, Passion Flower, Scullcap, St. John's Wort and Valerian are recommended.

Black Cohosh balances hormones. Red Raspberry is rich in iron and calcium. Kelp is rich in minerals. Dong Quai contain vitamin E for fertility. False Unicorn helps in conceiving. Wild Yam is useful for infertility.

HERBAL FORMULAS

Blood Cleansers—Circulatory System—Colon Cleansers—Digestive System—Energy and Stamina—Glandular System—Immune Builders — Nervous System — Urinary System—

VITAMINS, MINERALS AND SUPPLEMENTS

Vitamin A will protect the lining of the reproductive organs. Vitamin C and bioflavonoids are needed every day to protect the immune function and help regulate menstrual flow. Vitamin E is important for production of the sex glands. B-complex vitamins are important for regulating the bad estrogen in the liver. This estrogen can cause all kinds of female problems.

Calcium is important along with magnesium. Calcium levels in the blood drop ten days before menstruation. This is one reason for cramps, and calcium can help prevent the pain. Phosphorus helps prevent emotional problems and depression. Magnesium is important and helps increase B-complex absorption and aids in the elimination of bad estrogen from the liver. Iron is important for women because of their monthly periods. Anemia can result along with fatigue, weakness and depression. Iodine prevents water retention and helps regulate estrogen levels.

Silicon is very important for strong bones and nerves. Manganese and silicon help prevent osteoporosis. Potassium helps regulate water in the body. Selenium and zinc are healing and improve immune function.

Chlorophyll and blue-green algae clean the blood and nourish at the same time. This will help prevent toxemia. Flaxseed oil and salmon oil along with vitamin E increase chances for conceiving and nourish the female glandular system. Acidophilus helps in the assimilation of nutrients and protects the female organs. Germanium and CoQ10 increase immune function and the chances for conceiving.

INSOMNIA

SYMPTOMS

Unable to Falling Asleep—Wakeful Periods—Waking up in the Middle of the Night and Unable to go Back to Sleep—When it goes on for weeks at a time, it could be serious—

CAUSES

Some causes of insomnia are anxiety, stress, lack of nutrients, worry, hypoglycemia, nervous tension, physical aches and pains, and eating heavy meals late at night. Stimulants will cause the brain to be active and unable to relax. Caffeine found in coffee, tea, chocolate or cola and some soft drinks are all stimulants. Sugar is a stimulant and can increase anxiety.

One main cause is autointoxication. Chronic constipation can effect the nervous system and the brain. Nutritional deficiency is a major cause.

Avoid drugs to induce sleep. They can cause you to wake up feeling dull and are addictive.

NUTRITIONAL THERAPY

Research has shown that people with chronic insomnia are lacking in key nutrients such as B-complex vitamins, Vitamin C, and the minerals calcium, magnesium, manganese, potassium and zinc.

A diet change using food rich in B-complex vitamins such as brown rice, almonds, green leafy vegetables, millet, beans, sunflower seeds, alfalfa, kelp, parsley, avocado, bee pollen, potatoes, asparagus, broccoli, and carrots is encouraged.

Chamomile tea before going to bed is calming and relaxing. Nervine herbs an hour before going to bed are also calming. Hops, Lady's Slipper, Lobelia, Passion Flower, Scullcap, Valerian Root, St. John's Wort and Wood Betony are all beneficial for the nervous system.

HERBAL FORMULAS

Blood Cleansers—Circulatory System—Colon Cleansers—Digestive System—Immune Builders—Nervous System—

VITAMINS, MINERALS AND SUPPLEMENTS

B-complex vitamins are important for the nervous system. Studies have shown that niacin, B3, helps reduce tension, fatigue, depression and insomnia. B5, pantothenic acid reduces anxiety and induces sleep. B6 relieves tension and calms the nerves. B12 helps to prevent depression. Vitamin C in large doses of 1-2 grams daily relieves tension and insomnia.

Calcium has a sedative effect on the nervous system. Magnesium works along with calcium. Silicon helps calcium remain in solution to prevent building up in the joints. A multi-mineral supplement is beneficial for balancing the brain and nervous system and in preventing break down in that system.

Acidophilus is necessary in our day and age with all the chemicals, antibiotics, and hormones in our food. It protects against many ailments such as candida.

Chlorophyll and blue-green algae serve as protections for the nervous system helping to eliminate toxins or heavy metals that can accumulate and destroy the myelin sheath around the nerves. Salmon oil and flaxseed oil eliminate cholesterol from the circulatory system. Germanium and CoQ10 build the immune system.

IRRITABLE BOWEL SYNDROME

SYMPTOMS

Abdominal Pain—Alternating Constipation and Diarrhea—Anorexia—Bloating—Gas— Nausea—Fatigue (from diarrhea and loss of vital minerals—Depression—

CAUSES

The main cause of irritable bowel syndrome is a low fiber diet causing excess mucus and toxins to remain in the bowels too long. Excess fat consumption causes the liver to produce more bile salts in trying to break down the fat in the intestines. The acids from the excess fat increase toxicity and can even cause cancer. Fat also causes secretions of excess estrogen which is known to cause tumors. Toxins are also absorbed into the bloodstream and cause other problems. Food allergies can be another problem.

Stress and emotional upsets can cause irritable bowel syndrome.

NUTRITIONAL THERAPY

A diet high in fiber prevents these problems. Whole grains, especially millet and buckwheat, are easy to digest yet high in fiber and nutrients to heal the colon. Vegetable and fruit juices will help heal the colon.

An electrolyte drink will help prevent an imbalance in minerals. Brown rice and barley drink will help ease diarrhea. A low fat diet will help heal the colon. Carrot, celery, and parsley juice will provide minerals especially calcium and vitamin A.

Aloe Vera, Alfalfa, Dandelion, Garlic, Hops, Kelp, Marshmallow, Myrrh, Cascara Sagrada, Psyllium, and Slippery Elm are herbs which can help heal and strengthen the intestinal tract.

HERBAL FORMULAS

Blood Cleansers—Colon Cleansers—Digestive System—Drinks—Under Energy and Stamina— Immune System — Nervous System—Urinary System—

VITAMINS, MINERALS AND SUPPLEMENTS

Vitamin A is necessary for healing and tissue repair. B-complex vitamins are necessary for proper digestion and for preventing the formation of excess estrogen. The mucous membranes will heal faster with Vitamin C and bioflavonoids and will help prevent infection. Vitamin E is healing for the mucous membranes.

A deficiency of Vitamin K is often seen in this disorder. It is found in chlorophyll and blue-green algae, which are very healing. Calcium and magnesium promote relaxation. A multi-mineral supplement is essential for colon health. Selenium and zinc help to promote healing.

Germanium and CoQ10 help promote a healthy colon. Flaxseed oil and salmon oil help in supplying oxygen to the cells in the colon.

LEGIONNAIRES' DISEASE

SYMPTOMS

Aches in joints and muscles—Appetite Loss—Confusion—Cough—first dry and later watery—High Fever—Chills—Nausea—Sore Throat—Vomiting—

CAUSES

This disease is caused from a bacteria called Legionella Pneumophila. The original Legionnaires' disease was found in the air conditioning in the building where a meeting was held in Philadelphia during the summer of 1976. It is considered a disease of a weakened immune system.

NUTRITIONAL THERAPY

The immune system needs to be strengthened. A natural diet, eliminating sugar, salt, white flour products, meat, fried food, (they create free-radicals and suppress the immune system), and any processed food is recommended. Flour products can be rancid and cause damage to the immune system.

A high fiber diet, stressing grains, beans, sprouts, fruit and vegetables is beneficial for strengthening the immune system. Supplements are essential to augment health building nutrients.

Vegetable juices help to build the immune system. Carrot, celery, apple and parsley contain vitamins A, C, calcium and potassium in quantities to nourish and build the body.

Thermos cooking using rice and grains will help in the assimilation of nutrients. Green salads provide fiber and are rich in minerals and vitamins.

Herbs to build the immune system are: Burdock, Echinacea, Golden Seal, Hops, Red Clover, Ginkgo, Suma and Bee Pollen.

HERBAL FORMULAS

Blood Cleansers—Colon Cleansers—Digestive System Builders—Nervous System—Urinary System—

VITAMINS, MINERALS AND SUPPLEMENTS

The antioxidants are important to build the immune system. Vitamins A, D, C, E, and the minerals selenium and zinc are beneficial. They can be taken individually along with a multi-vitamin.

A multi-mineral supplement will help in the digestion and assimilation of nutrients and food.

Germanium and CoQ10 help strengthen the circulatory system and build immunity. Flaxseed oil and salmon oil will build immunity.

LEPROSY

(Hansen's Disease)

SYMPTOMS

Leprosy is an insidious disease, similar to AIDS, as it develops slowly and without warning. It is a slow growing disease with an incubation period from two up to ten years. It progresses slowly. The body appears to decay in the typical leprosy called lepromatous. Another form is called tuberculoid leprosy, which mainly attacks the nervous system. Patches of discolored skin appear first and than sensation to physical stimuli is lost.

CAUSES

Leprosy is caused by a very unusual, slow growing bacteria. There are billions of bacteria in each cell, yet the leprosy patient feels well. With leprosy, the nerves are deadened in the extremities and rats have been known to bite off toes in victims living in poverty conditions while they sleep. Affected areas are easily infected and victims don't realize it because of the lack of sensation.

Leprosy is making a comeback, and there are an estimated ten million cases around the world. It is found in Europe, South America and in the United States and is increasing. The drug Thalidomide is also back and is being used on Leprosy and T. B. patients. It is manufactured and used in Brazil for leprosy. It is an extremely dangerous drug because of its effects on unborn children. There are deformed babies and children aged 3 to 13 in Brazil and Europe. Women during pregnancy are contracting leprosy and taking the drug. The babies whose mothers took Thalidomide often have body deformities. One doctor said that there are other drugs to use, but it is cheap and easy to distribute.

NUTRITIONAL THERAPY

When leprosy is treated with drugs, it kills the bacteria, and they come back when the drug is stopped. It is felt that the bacteria may change into a viral form and hide in the cells where the antibiotics are ineffective.

Researchers in Hawaii have discovered that Vitamin C prevents the leprosy bacillus from utilizing one of the nutrients needed for its growth. Additional tests need to be conducted before it is proven. It seems logical however that nutrients may be of more use than drugs.

The wrong diet and congestion of the colon and liver can be one cause. A cleansing diet, using fresh vegetable juices, herbal teas, blood cleansers, and urinary cleansers can be beneficial. The skin becomes congested when the colon and urinary tract are not eliminating toxins.

Nervine herbs are beneficial to relax the body and speed the healing process. Hops, Chamomile, Scullcap, Valerian Root, Passion Flower, Wood Betony, and St. John's Wort are herbs that can help.

HERBAL FORMULAS

Blood Cleansers—Circulatory System—Colon Cleansers—Digestive System—Glandular System—Immune System—Nervous System— Structural System—Urinary System—

VITAMINS, MINERALS AND SUPPLEMENTS

The antioxidants, vitamins, A, D, C, and E, and minerals selenium and zinc will help clean and purify the cells. The B-complex vitamins are essential for healthy nerves, skin, hair, eyes, liver and mouth and for the entire digestive system.

A multi-mineral supplement is important for maintaining health of the entire body. Iron, iodine, potassium and zinc are healing and necessary to protect the skin and mucous membranes.

Essential fatty acids play an important role in healing the skin, mucous membranes and nervous system. Lecithin will help repair the nerves. Chlorophyll and blue-green algae will clean the cells and nourish the blood. Germanium and CoQ10 help in the healing process by supplying oxygen to the cells. Bee pollen is rich in nutrients to build the immune system especially the amino acids and B-complex vitamins.

LOU GEHRIG'S DISEASE

(Amyotrophic Lateral Sclerosis)

SYMPTOMS

This is the most common motor neuron disease of muscular atrophy. Motor weakness is progressive—Atrophy of the muscles—Weakened respiratory muscles predispose to pneumonia—Difficulty chewing and swallowing—Cramping—Stiffness—Involuntary quivering of small muscles—

CAUSES

ALS is seen as an inherited disease, an autosomal dominant trait, in about 10% of the cases. In noninherited ALS, it hits persons whose occupations require strenuous physical labor. This can result for various reasons such as nutritional deficiency of motor neurons related to a disturbance in enzyme metabolism.

A deficiency of vitamin E and F can cause damage to the cell membranes and a metabolic interference in nucleic acid production by the nerve fibers and autoimmune disorders.

Factors that can precipitate it include trauma, viral infections and physical exhaustion. (*Professional Guide To Diseases*, P. 634-36).

Diseases that hit the nervous system could be caused by heavy metals, or some kind of toxic poison, (the air is filled with toxins). The lungs are sensitive and absorb toxins quicker than when they are digested. Lack of nutrients that protect the nerves could be another cause.

NUTRITIONAL THERAPY

A diet high in freshly ground grains cooked in a thermos will protect the enzymes and B-vitamins from destruction. Rancid whole grains can add to the destruction of the cells.

Vegetable juices will provide nutrients to the cells in large amounts. Juices made from carrots, celery, and parsley are rich in calcium, vitamin A and other essential minerals. Bee pollen will help nourish the nerves.

Soups made with grains, rice, and vegetables are rich in minerals to build up the immune system. Fresh vegetables and fruit provide nutrients. Eliminating dairy products, meat, sugar and white flour products will speed the healing.

Herbs can strengthen the muscles such as Alfalfa, Black Cohosh, Blue Vervain, Boneset, Buchu, Burdock, Comfrey, Devil's Claw, Cornsilk, Echinacea, Ginkgo, Gotu Kola, Horsetail, Kelp, Saffron and Suma.

HERBAL FORMULAS

Blood Cleansers—Circulatory System—Colon Cleansers—Digestive System—Immune Builders — Nervous System — Urinary System—

VITAMINS, MINERALS AND SUPPLEMENTS

Vitamins A, C, D, E and the minerals selenium and zinc can protect the cells and prevent damage. A deficiency of vitamin E is seen in Lou Gehrig's disease. Vitamin C with bioflavonoids will help build up the nerves.

Calcium and magnesium will support the nerves. Potassium will strengthen the muscles. Silicon is needed for the nerves and muscles.

Flaxseed oil and salmon oil are essential for the healing and repairing process. It is needed for the digestive, and immune system. Bee pollen, germanium and CoQ10 are nourishing.

LUPUS

SYMPTOMS

Some symptoms are: Fever—Malaise—Joint Pains—Joint Swelling—Tenderness in the Joints—Allergic-Like Skin Eruptions— "Butterfly" rash on Face—Hair Loss— Spontaneous Bruising—Fatigue—Depression—

CAUSES

Lupus is an inflammatory disease of the connective tissues. It is an autoimmune disease; an abnormal reaction of the body to its own tissues. A weakened immune system is one cause. "Physical or mental stress, viral infections, immunizations and pregnancy may all affect the development of Lupus." (*Professional Guide to Diseases*, pp 561-2).

Parasites are involved with Lupus. The droppings they excrete in the body are poisonous and prevent healing until they are eliminated. The blood carries these toxins along with ones we breathe, eat and drink. Until the bloodstream is cleaned and parasites removed, healing cannot take place.

In *Guess What Came To Dinner* by Ann Louise Gittleman, she explains the damage parasites create—

1. They produce toxic substances that are harmful to the body. In cases of chronic infection, the body's immune response can be pushed into overdrive, producing elevated levels of eosinophils. Eosinophils are specialized white cells that normally combat any microscopic pathogen, but when their level is elevated, they themselves can cause tissue damage that results in pain and inflammation.

2. The presence of parasites irritates the tissues of the body, inducing an inflammatory reaction on the part of the host.

3. The presence of parasites depresses immune system functioning while activating the immune response. This can eventually lead to immune system exhaustion.

Lupus victims have a high level of antibodies which turn on their bodies and attack the nerves, tissue and internal organs. The kidneys are often affected, the adrenals are weakened and a minor heart attack is possible with systemic lupus erythematous.

Allergies can be involved with Lupus. The immune system is so weak, the mucous membranes cannot tolerate all they come in contact with. The most common cause of allergies from food seem to be beef, cow's milk, corn and wheat. Wheat becomes rancid very quickly unless it is ground at once or refrigeratored.

There can also be sensitivity to ammonia, formaldehyde, hair spray, ethanol, perfume and pesticides. The symptoms of chemical sensitivity are chest pain, arthritic pain and severe headaches. Food additive testing found backache, headache, and painful myalgia. Toxins can build up when the immune system is weak and can take months to clear from the body.

Stress is often linked with Lupus. Stress weakens the adrenal glands producing a pseudo-hypoglycemic effect on the body.

NUTRITIONAL THERAPY

Eliminate fat from the diet especially fried foods. They become rancid very quickly and are harmful to the connective tissue. They will wear away the myelin sheath covering the nerves. Animal fat, especially beef and pork are harmful. Dairy products create excess mucus in the body where toxins and parasites feed and live.

A diet high in vegetables, fruit, grains, brown rice, sprouts, and green salads will strengthen the immune system and clean the blood.

Vegetable juice fasting using wheat grass juice and liquid chlorophyll will rest the immune system and clean the blood.

The colon needs to be cleaned, for that is where the toxins accumulate and are redistributed in the bloodstream causing many diseases. Parasite formulas will kill the parasites, and colon and blood cleansers will eliminate them.

Ginkgo, Suma, Cayenne, Ginseng, and Gotu Kola will boost immunity and allow the body to heal faster. Nervine herbs are essential along with the immune formulas. They are: Hops, Valerian, Wood Betony, Scullcap, Black Cohosh, Mistletoe, Lobelia, Capsicum and Lady's Slipper.

HERBAL FORMULAS

Blood Cleansers—Circulatory System—Colon Cleansers—(include parasite formulas)—Digestive System—Glandular System—Immune Builders—Nervous System—Structural System—Urinary System—

VITAMINS, MINERALS AND SUPPLEMENTS

Antioxidants are vital and include vitamins A, D, C, E, selenium and zinc. Free radical damage is involved with Lupus. The high intake of rancid oils can destroy connective tissue. Vitamin C with bioflavonoids are essential for connective tissue health.

B-complex vitamins strengthen the nerves and are essential for stress. Extra B12 and pantothenic acid are needed.

Calcium and magnesium are necessary for the health of the nerves and connective tissue. Herbal calcium formulas contain silicon which boost absorption into the areas they are needed. All minerals are essential to sustain a healthy body. They are needed for every function in the body.

Omega-3 fatty acids, found in flaxseed oil and salmon oil, produce significant drops in inflammation and blood cholesterol in Lupus. Acidophilus is nature's antibiotic and increases the body's ability to absorb essential nutrients. Chlorophyll and blue-green algae help in the absorption of nutrients and boost immunity. They also clean the blood of toxins. Lecithin is essential for repair of connective tissues, brain and nerves. Bee pollen boosts immunity and contains amino acids for tissue repair.

MALABSORPTION SYNDROME

SYMPTOMS

Anemia—Diarrhea—Dry Skin—Fatigue—Hair Loss—Muscle Weakness—Painful Abdominal Bloating—Weight Loss—

CAUSES

This syndrome can cause anemia and osteoporosis. Malabsorption syndrome can be caused by a lack of hydrochloric acid, enzymes, poor diet, deficiency in essential nutrients, and diseases of the pancreas, liver and bile ducts. Diarrhea and constipation can also disrupt the natural flora. Candida can contribute to this syndrome.

Improper digestion of food and malabsorption go together. This is the cause of many diseases. Incomplete digestion of proteins causes many problems in the body. Toxic materials are produced during the breakdown of protein by bacteria resulting in toxins multiplying in the bloodstream.

Tension can interfere with nutrient absorption. Digested food usually passes through the system with natural wavelike motion. With stress and tension, the foods can move too fast or too slow, and with uneven motion so the food is poorly digested and cannot be absorbed.

When emotional stress causes diarrhea, it creates a loss of vital minerals and causes nutritional problems.

NUTRITIONAL THERAPY

The small intestine is designed for correct absorption. All the food necessary for energy, for growth and the maintenance of all biochemical processes depend upon the small intestine.

Good nutrition will help improve proper absorption. The lining of the small intestine, vital for absorption, can degenerate when adequate nutrients are not present. The lack of vitamins and minerals can impair absorption.

One cause of premature aging is a decline in secretions of stomach acid and digestive enzymes. When poor absorption exists, it creates poor nutrition.

A positive attitude toward physical, mental, emotional and social outlook are important for proper digestion. Exercise provides oxygen to the cells which aids in digestion and assimilation.

A good diet is important. Millet, buckwheat, and brown rice should be on the top of the list. They are easy to digest and provide vitamins and minerals for absorption, especially if they are cooked in a wide mouthed thermos, which contains B vitamins and enzymes. Raw fruit and vegetable juice are live foods for assimilation. Fresh vegetables eaten at the beginning of a meal will help assure proper digestion. When cooked foods are eaten first, the white blood cells come to the stomach thinking they are toxins. Eat a lot of fresh and steamed vegetables which are rich in minerals essential for absorption.

Gentian, Golden Seal and Oregon Grape are healing and improve digestion. Chamomile is calming for a nervous stomach. For an acid stomach or heartburn, use Raspberry Tea, Slippery Elm or Ginger in warm water. Aloe Vera is healing for the digestive tract. Marshmallow reduces inflammation. Papaya, Peppermint and Parsley are healing. The nervine herbs help for a nervous stomach. They include: Hops, Passion Flower, Scullcap and Valerian.

Taking care of the colon will help protect the small intestine from absorbing toxins which can cause irritation to the lining of the digestive tract.

HERBAL FORMULAS

Blood Cleansers—Colon Cleansers—Digestive System—Immune Builders—Nervous system and Brain—

VITAMINS, MINERALS AND SUPPLEMENTS

Calcium and magnesium are important supplements. It is estimated that only about half the calcium we eat in food is absorbed. Iron, zinc and chromium are also absorbed in small amounts.

Vitamin C and calcium should be taken together for calcium absorption. Vitamin C is also important for iron absorption. Vitamins and minerals aid in the absorption of each other. Vitamins A and E are absorbed better when essential fatty acids are present as well as minerals.

B-complex vitamins are important for proper digestion. They are involved and utilized as coenzymes in almost all parts of the body. They promote energy and are necessary for the metabolism of carbohydrates, fats and proteins.

Acidophilus is important for proper digestion. It helps in keeping the bacteria in balance; preventing the bad bacteria from taking over. Chlorophyll is an aid in proper digestion, along with blue-green algae. Aloe vera is healing for the digestive tract and will help prevent scarring. Bee pollen helps in digestion, and provides nutrients essential for a healthy body.

MEINIERE'S SYNDROME

SYMPTOMS

Loss of Balance—Hearing Loss—Ringing in the Ears—Violent Dizziness—Nausea—(Could last from 10 minutes to 8 hours)—Reeling Sensation—Unsteadiness—Whirling Vertigo—

CAUSES

Meiniere's syndrome is seen as one of the most incapacitating disorders affecting man. Because of the unsteady feelings, it prevents activities necessary for everyday life.

Drugs may be responsible for contributions to the disease. Aspirin poisoning is one example. Other causes include: infections, thyroid disease, heavy metal poisoning, diabetes, hypoglycemia, injuries, noise exposure, nerve deterioration, and malnutrition. It can also be associated with cholesterol levels in the blood, which can decrease blood supply to the ear mechanisms. The nervous system could be defective. The vessels supplying blood to the inner ear go into spasms and cause vertigo and deafness.

NUTRITIONAL THERAPY

A change of eating habits needs to be considered. This has improved hearing levels in some people with reduction of ringing in ears and controlled dizziness. Carbohydrates should be limited to fruits, vegetables, seeds, nuts, sprouts and whole grains. Baked potatoes, millet and brown rice are excellent. They can even be eaten for breakfast. Almonds are great for snacks. Raw vegetables, a little fish and chicken will supply protein. Six small meals throughout the day are best.

Eliminate white flour products. They contain chlorine, which causes many problems. White sugar and all foods that contain sugar should be eliminated. Table salt (sodium chloride) can build up in the body. Smoking and drinking should be stopped, and limit fat intake.

Potassium foods such as almonds, dried apricots, avocados, and endive are beneficial. Nutrition may be essential to effectively control this disorder.

Herbs to help in increasing circulation are Cayenne, Ginger, Ginkgo, Gotu Kola, Suma, and Hawthorn Berries.

Exercise, massage therapy and warm, sauna baths will contribute to good vasomotor tone, which helps control attacks.

HERBAL FORMULAS

Blood Cleansers—Circulatory System—Colon Cleansers—Digestive System—Energy and Stamina—Immune Builders-Nervous System and Brain—Structural—Female and Male —

VITAMINS, MINERALS AND SUPPLEMENTS

Vitamins and minerals are important for supplying nutrients to the head area. A deficiency of vitamin A is seen in loss of hearing. B-complex vitamins help relieve spasms. Niacin opens blood vessels and increases circulation to the head area. A deficiency of B6 and pantothenic acid (B5) can cause dizziness and painful throbbing in the ears and Meniere's symptoms. The B vitamins build up the adrenal glands and help the blood develop its natural cortisone for stress.

A lack of vitamin C is seen in Meniere's syndrome. The tissues of the middle ear stores vitamin C. It heals damage done to the ear area and eliminates fatty deposits in the veins. It also prevents swelling and adhesions. Vitamin E can prevent calcification that causes build-up in the small capillaries of the head area.

Minerals are as important as vitamins. Calcium is necessary for bones, cartilage (inner ears) and hormone formation. A lack of manganese can cause deafness, dizziness and ear noises. A lack of magnesium can cause nerve twitching and sensitivity to noise.

Phosphorus builds new tissue and provides energy. A lack of potassium can cause nerve impulses and muscle contraction. An iodine deficiency can cause enlarged glands, headaches and can lead to dizziness, dull hearing and poor equilibrium. Zinc assists in the digestion of carbohydrates.

Germanium and CoQ10 can improve circulation to the head area. Acidophilus and chlorophyll will clean and nourish the veins. Bee pollen will build up the nerves and provide nutrients such as amino acids and B-complex vitamins.

MENINGITIS

SYMPTOMS

Sore Throat—Fever—Chills—Malaise— Headaches—Vomiting—Nausea—Delirium— When a child is listless a doctor should be consulted. Stiff Neck—Convulsions—A Child can hurt when picked up—

CAUSES

Meningitis is an inflammation of the membranes that cover the brain and spinal cord. It is a contagious disease and is an infection in the brain. Some causes could be a virus, such as the one which cause measles or poliomyelitis, a yeast infection, or bacteria.

A depleted immune system along with throat and nose infections can cause toxins which enter the blood stream and spread to the brain. The nervous system and brain are very sensitive to toxins.

The flu can develop into meningitis if treated improperly. When infections are neglected, such as ear, sinus or throat, they can develop into meningitis. Taking drugs and eating heavy meals when acute diseases are present can drive them deeper into the system and allow them to enter the brain and head area.

NUTRITIONAL THERAPY

If meningitis is suspected, medical treatment should be sought. It can be serious and cause permanent damage to the brain or death. Antibiotics have reduced the mortality rate. After antibiotic treatment, steps can be taken to clean the blood and build up the immune system.

When acute diseases attack the body, stop eating. The toxins are being squeezed from the tissues and are sent to the stomach to be eliminated. When we eat heavy food, it stops the elimination in order to digest the food. This suppresses the toxins and throws them further into the organs which may cause serious damage later.

Drink citrus juices, such as lemons, oranges, limes and grapefruit, diluted with pure water. Herbal teas will help eliminate the toxins. An herbal tea will help clean the bowels and kidneys eliminating toxins.

Herbal teas or extracts containing Garlic, Black Walnut, Mullein, Scullcap, Comfrey, Lobelia, White Oak Bark, and Marshmallow are beneficial.

Fenugreek will help eliminate even hard mucus. Golden Seal, Echinacea, and Burdock are healing and cleansing.

HERBAL FORMULAS

Blood Cleansers—Colds, Flu, Fevers and Allergies — Colon Cleansers — Immune Builders—Infection Fighting—Nervous System and Brain—

VITAMINS, MINERALS AND SUPPLEMENTS

Vitamins and minerals are very important in preventing disease. Children cannot eat enough to get the required vitamins and minerals. Vitamin C is needed every day. It helps the body produce its own interferon to fight infections. Vitamin A prevents infections of the mucous membranes and builds immunity. The B-complex vitamins are usually missing in the diet, and they protect the body. Folic acid, part of the B vitamins, helps the body produce white blood cells which fights germs. Vitamin E is an antioxidant that protects the cells from damage.

Calcium and magnesium will help protect the nerves. Potassium helps with nausea and vomiting. Deficiencies can cause listlessness, muscle weakness and heart failure. Selenium and zinc are healing. Iron will protect the blood and increase energy.

Acidophilus will help protect the body from bacteria and germs. It is nature's antibiotic. Chlorophyll cleans, heals and provides essential nutrients for protection. Essential fatty acids are necessary for immune function. They are usually missing from children's diets.

MENOPAUSE

SYMPTOMS

Hot Flashes—Night Sweats—Depression—Dizziness—Headaches—Heart Palpitations—Difficult Breathing—Fatigue—Nervousness—Vaginal Disorders — Chills — Emotional Instability is one of the most disturbing symptoms. It causes attacks of mild anxiety to severe bouts of "black" depression.

CAUSES

Menopause is the physical and emotional transition that marks the permanent cessation of menstruation. The symptoms are mainly caused by a poor diet and living habits. Women who have good health find the menopausal syndrome is nonexistent. They express joy, freedom and energy with a new life style before them.

The main cause of symptoms associated with menopause are constipation and liver congestion. The liver is the main cause of hormonal imbalances. It is supposed to eliminate blood levels of estradiol, which is the "unfavorable" type of estrogen. When estradiol enters the bloodstream, it can travel to the brain and other parts of the body and cause depression and bizarre mental manifestations. When the diet is correct and the liver is healthy, it is eliminated through the kidneys and colon.

Following menopause, a small amount of estrogen is produced by the ovaries. In a hysterectomy, when the ovaries are removed, the adrenals begin to form a type of female hormone which takes the place of estrogen. When one gland is unable to function properly, the other glands take over if they are given the proper nutrients. Many women have adrenal exhaustion and will have problems during menopause.

NUTRITIONAL THERAPY

This is one time in life when the body needs to be nourished properly. Less food is needed, because this is the time in life when the chance of weight gain is increased with the glandular changes taking place.

A low fat diet is stressed. Animal fat, rancid fats, and fried foods are discouraged. Sugar should be avoided, for it leaches calcium from the bones. What you eat is one of the most important decisions you can make. Meat, sugar, caffeine, white flour products, fried food, coffee, alcohol, salt, chocolate, and dairy products all leach out minerals from the body and cause bone loss. Dairy products and meat contain antibiotics and hormones which create an imbalance in estrogen levels. Phosphoric acid in soft drinks interferes with calcium absorption or increase its excretion.

Increase the intake of vegetables, fruit, grains, nuts, seeds, and sprouts. Millet is rich in calcium and magnesium. Almonds contain protein, calcium, and magnesium. Brown rice contains B vitamins. All grains help build health and aid the body in balancing nutrients.

Whole grains do not interfere with mineral absorption. Many dieticians and doctors have the mistaken belief that the phytic acid content in grains interferes with the metabolism of calcium in the body and often caution women not to eat too many grains.

In some USDA studies, volunteers eating whole wheat in normal amounts exhibited good mineral absorption. Dr. Eugene Morris said, "The whole wheat actually contributed to the body's absorption of minerals rather than subtracting from it".

Use whole grains such as millet, buckwheat, oats, wheat, yellow cornmeal, and rye. Beans, lentils, and brown rice are very nutritious. Pre-soaking and low-heating of grains have a beneficial effect on the body's utilization of all nutrients. Thermos cooking retains all the enzymes and nutrients. A high fiber diet is essential, as it will aid in the elimination of bad estrogens from the liver and through the colon.

The herbs beneficial for menopause are Dong Quai, Black Cohosh, Ginkgo, and Suma, (produces a safe estrogen production. It contains sitosterol, an ingredient that increases the natural estrogen and eliminating any excess). Wild Yam, False Unicorn, and Red Raspberry help the body produce natural estrogen and eliminate symptoms of menopause.

Exercise for 20 to 30 minutes a day either brisk walking, cycling, rowing machine, or rebounding on a mini trampoline will burn fat, strengthen bones, and relieve depression.

HERBAL FORMULAS

Blood Cleansers—Circulatory System—Colon Cleansers—Energy and Stamina—Glandular System—Immune Builders—Nervous System and Brain—Urinary System—Female Formulas—

VITAMINS, MINERALS AND SUPPLEMENTS

Antioxidants will help prevent cell damage which include vitamins A, D, C, E, and the minerals selenium and zinc. Vitamin A protects the mucous membranes of the uterus, vagina, ovaries, and breast. Vitamin E helps the body produce its own estrogen. Vitamin C is involved with bone metabolism and helps the body utilize iron. B-complex are very important during menopause. When the B vitamins are present in the liver, it can eliminate the bad estrogen, and without the B vitamins, the bad estrogen enters the bloodstream and causes problems.

Calcium and magnesium are important. Magnesium is necessary to help the body eliminate excess estrogen from the bloodstream. Calcium builds the nerves and strengthens the bones. Fats found in fried foods, fatty meats and hydrogenated oils interfere with magnesium absorption.

A multi-mineral supplement will help the body utilize all the nutrients in the diet. Acidophilus helps in the absorption of all nutrients. Chlorophyll protects and nourishes the body. It also helps in digestion. Blue-green algae is rich in nutrients. Germanium and CoQ10 help the body utilize oxygen and increase immune function. Flaxseed oil and salmon oil help the body produce natural hormones. An herbal bone formula, containing silicon will help the body use calcium.

MENTAL ILLNESS

(Manic-Depressive Disorder, Schizophrenia)

SYMPTOMS

Anxiety—Depression—Delusions— Nervousness—Panic Attacks—Loss of Interest in School or Work—Sleep Pattern Changes— Withdrawal from Society—Irritability— Sudden Rages—Lack of Enthusiasm—

CAUSES

Women are twice as likely to suffer from mental illness as men. Nutritional deficiencies have a strong effect on mental health. Autointoxication and constipation are contributing factors in mental illness.

At an annual meeting of the American Medical Association in 1917, a scientific report was shared stating that 517 cases of mental problems were relieved by eradicating intestinal toxemia. These symptoms ranged from mental sluggishness to hallucinations. (Sprince, H., "Biochemical aspects of indole metabolism in normal and schizophrenic subjects", *Annals New York Academy of Sciences.* Vol 96. 1962).

More recently, schizophrenia has been added to the list of mental disorders which improved when toxemia was eliminated. Nutrition plays an important part in preventing mental illness.

NUTRITIONAL THERAPY

A high carbohydrate diet stimulates the presence of L-tryptophan in the brain and creates a calm and peaceful feeling. Grains such as millet, buckwheat, corn. oats, quinoa, amaranth, wheat, and rye provide L-tryptophan. Short fasts, will help eliminate toxins from the blood. Eat in abundance foods such as fruit, vegetables, sprouts, seeds, chlorophyll rich foods, almonds, and fresh oils.

Eliminate or reduce dairy products, eggs, meat, sugar, peanuts, white flour and sugar products.

They cause a build-up of mucus, toxins and cause a glue like material in the colon.

Exercise and relaxation therapy are very beneficial for relieving mental illness. Cleaning the colon and liver, adding herbs, vitamins, minerals and supplements will strengthen the nervous system and allow the body to handle mental disturbances.

Chamomile tea is calming, and contains calcium. Hops, Scullcap, Passion Flower, Wood Betony, Valerian and Schizandra to help calm and nourish the brain.

HERBAL FORMULAS

Blood Cleansers—Circulatory System—Colon Cleansers—Digestive System—Energy and Stamina—Glandular System—Immune Builders—Nervous System and Brain— Urinary System—Male or Female formulas—

VITAMINS, MINERALS AND SUPPLEMENTS

All nutrients work together to create a balance in the brain and nervous system. Vitamin A protects against germs and viruses. Vitamin C deficiency can cause copper retention which accumulates in the brain and liver. Zinc and manganese flush out excess copper. Vitamin B-complex is important for eliminating excess estrogen from the liver and preventing it from causing mental problems, especially B3, B6, B12 and folic acid.

Manganese helps in the absorption of essential fatty acids. Calcium and magnesium protect the nerves from damage.

Chlorophyll helps the liver to detoxify and regenerate. Blue-green algae builds the immune system and eliminates toxins. Acidophilus helps in digestion of all nutrients. Bee pollen provides energy and nutrients. Germanium and CoQ10 provide oxygen to the cells and protect the circulatory system. Flaxseed oil and salmon oil are involved in every function of the body.

MONONUCLEOSIS

SYMPTOMS

It has been called the Kissing Disease and Glandular Fever. Extreme Fatigue— Headaches—Chills—Fever—Sore Throat— Swollen Glands—Weakness—

CAUSES

It effects the liver and spleen. The Epstein-Barr virus causes mononucleosis, which is a member of the herpes family. It is an acute infectious disease that spreads easily. Those with low immune system function suffering from improper nutrition and exhaustion are the most vulnerable. It can be transmitted by blood transfusions and has been reported after cardiac surgery. This is a disease where the virus lays dormant in the body until the immune system becomes weakened. This is another disease that could be the result of the mass inoculation that is highly advertised and pushed in our society.

One main cause is nervous and physical exhaustion due to lack of nutrition and excess stress.

NUTRITIONAL THERAPY

This is an acute disease that needs to be treated properly in order for the body to recover completely. Bed rest is recommended as long as the fever lasts which is from 1-2 weeks. It is found that those who return to their activities early usually get over their weakness and tired feelings much faster than those who curtail their activities.

The lymph nodes in the neck, armpits and groin become swollen and painful when the colloid gel accumulates with infection. It is important to keep the fluid in the lymph glands circulating in order to remove the toxins. This is why normal activities are important, especially walking, exercise on a mini trampoline and any mild exercise until strength is back. The lymphatic capillaries help remove the excess build-up of poisons from the body, and whenever the body accumulates more toxins than the lymphatics can process and eliminate, the nodes become enlarged and painful.

Eliminating heavy protein, dairy products, and sugar and white flour products will help speed healing. Using digestive enzymes such as hydrochloric acid and pancreatic enzymes will help the cleansing of the glands and give the digestive system a rest.

A simple diet or a juice fast will help clear out the lymph glands. Vegetables are important, both lightly steamed and fresh. They contain vital vitamins and minerals for building and healing.

Baked potatoes with the skin on, potassium broths, using potato peelings, celery, parsley, onions and cabbage makes an excellent healing broth. Brown rice and millet are easy to digest and are very healing.

Herbal combinations will help eliminate toxins, such as Red Clover blends. Garlic, Echinacea, Golden Seal, Burdock, and Myrrh act like antibiotics for natural healing. Pau D'Arco is cleansing and healing.

HERBAL FORMULAS

Blood Cleansers—Colds, Flu, Fevers and Allergies—Colon Cleansers—Digestive System— Glandular—Immune Builders—Infection Fighters—Nervous System and Brain—

VITAMINS, MINERALS AND SUPPLEMENTS

Vitamin A heals and protects against infections. Vitamin C kills bacteria and viruses. B-complex vitamins protect the nerves and brain, and improve digestion. Vitamin E protects vitamins A and C from oxidation and keeps them potent. It also increases the production of an enzyme called superoxide dismutase which protects our bodies from free radical damage.

Calcium is essential for aiding in the absorption of many nutrients, including vitamin B12. It is used with magnesium in regulating the contraction and relaxation of muscles. Phosphorus is important for its involvement in processes which store and produce energy. It makes the B vitamins effective. Zinc is important for healing and to prevent free radical damage. Iron deficiency can cause an increase susceptibility to infections and impaired antibody production. It can also contribute to high fat levels in the liver and blood.

Manganese is important for proper nerve function. It is essential for bone growth and has many functions in the body such as immune function. Selenium is an antioxidant protecting the immune system. It is involved in eye, hair and vascular health. Iodine is necessary to regulate hormone metabolism. These hormones influence the nervous system, circulatory function and the metabolism of nutrients.

Bee pollen helps speed healing and supplies amino acids and essential vitamins and minerals. Acidophilus protects against the bad bacteria, especially if antibiotics are used. Germanium and CoQ10 protect the immune system and supplies oxygen to the cells. Chlorophyll cleans the blood, improves digestion and supplies nutrients.

MORNING SICKNESS

SYMPTOMS

Nausea—Usually in the morning—It can also happen in the Evening or anytime—Or all the time—

CAUSES

Morning sickness could be a result of hormone imbalance or low blood sugar. One of the main causes is the body preparing for a clean environment for the baby and forcing the body to cleanse. This causes toxins to form in the blood stream and this results in nausea. Incomplete digestion can also cause nausea.

NUTRITIONAL THERAPY

Prevention is the best method. Cleanse the body before conception. Few women think of preparing for a baby before they get pregnant.

Keep the bowels clean. Eat a lot of raw fruits and vegetables, plain yogurt, whole grains, raw carrots, celery and an apple every day. Psyllium hulls and a lower bowel formula are useful for keeping the bowels moving. Constipation in the beginning of pregnancy is common because the same hormone that maintains your pregnancy also makes the intestines less active in order to increase absorption of nutrients for the growing baby.

Tips to help ease nausea: Lemon and warm water first thing in the morning to cleanse the stomach. Ginger tea made in a thermos and put by the bed to drink before arising will ease nausea. Freeze in an ice cube tray the following: 16 Tab. water, 8 Tab. fresh orange juice, 4 tea. lemon juice and 2 tea. honey. Suck on the cubes to ease nausea. Keep small snacks at the bedside, and chew slowly before getting out of bed. Nibble small amounts during the day, chewing thoroughly.

Red raspberry tea supplies calcium which relaxes the stomach. Chamomile tea is relaxing. Ice packs at the base of the neck and skull and one over the solar plexus (area of belly just below breast bone) can be helpful. Leave on for 20 minutes for severe nausea.

Liquid chlorophyll in water is cleansing and healing. It contains vitamin K, which is calming. Yogurt is good because it aids in digestion and helps prevent nausea.

Warm peppermint tea with a dash of nutmeg is also calming for nausea. Be sure and take in small sips to prevent vomiting. If vomiting does occur, peppermint tea will calm and ease spasms.

HERBAL FORMULAS

Blood Cleansers—Colon Cleansers—Digestive System—Immune Builders—Nervous System and Brain—Female Formulas—

VITAMINS, MINERALS AND SUPPLEMENTS

Vitamins C and K together can calm nausea within one hour. Vitamin K is found in chlorophyll. Low magnesium levels have been associated with nausea and vomiting.

B-complex vitamins help in digestion and calm nausea. Vitamin B6 is beneficial take 200 mg. for 7 days and 5 mg. a day until nausea is over. Digestive enzymes, papaya, and alfalfa tea are all helpful.

Minerals are very important, not only to help balance hormones, but are vital in preventing birth defects. A growing fetus needs minerals. Calcium, magnesium and potassium are calming for the nerves.

Vitamins A and E help to prevent nausea in pregnancy. Essential fatty acids found in flaxseed oil and salmon oil also help balance hormones.

Acidophilus helps in the digestion of food and helps prevent nausea. Liquid drinks containing electrolyte minerals can be beneficial.

MOTION SICKNESS

SYMPTOMS

Mild to severe could be Nausea—Cold Sweats—Excess Salivation—Vomiting—Sleepiness—Dizziness—Vertigo—Fainting in some cases—Symptoms occur when traveling in a car, bus, boat, plane or even the swaying in a swing or rocker. Queasy and uneasy feeling—Churning of the stomach—

CAUSES

Some people are sensitive to over stimulation of the labyrinthine receptors of the inner ear by motion. Predisposing factors include tension, fear, offensive odors, and sight, sound or feelings associated with a previous attack. The eyes and inner ears contribute to the sense of balance. An imbalance is created when these two systems send different messages to the brain. Nausea occurs when the brain cannot figure out what to tell the body to do.

Congestion and mucus in the stomach can cause nausea as well as autointoxication. There is weakness in the stomach when nausea is a problem.

NUTRITIONAL THERAPY

Ginger has been found to prevent motion sickness. It absorbs acids and prevents nausea. It should be taken at least one half hour before traveling. For severe nausea and vomiting, cola syrup can be used in an emergency. Learn to stare at stationary things when traveling.

Cleansing of the stomach will help prevent nausea. The stomach can become congested with mucus and toxins, and this can cause nausea. Lemon juice in water, lobelia, chlorophyll, red raspberry, and mint teas will all help cleanse the stomach.

The colon and the bloodstream will help eliminate nausea and stomach weakness. Eat more vegetables, fruit, grains, beans, sprouts, nuts, seeds, less white sugar and white flour products, meat and fried foods.

Pau D'Arco tea has a cleansing effect on the liver, blood and stomach. The stomach accumulates toxins that the cells eliminate, and if there is too much accumulation, the body reacts by stomach upset. Cleansing diets are important to rid the body of toxic wastes. See remedies under morning sickness.

A nervous stomach is another cause of motion sickness. The nervine herbs help to strengthen the nervous system. Hops, Passion Flower, Scullcap, Chamomile, Valerian Root, and Lady's Slipper are all beneficial.

HERBAL THERAPY

Blood Cleansers—Colon Cleansers—Digestive System — Glandular System — Immune Builders—Nervous System and Brain — Urinary System—(the kidneys need cleaned)—Female Formulas—

VITAMINS, MINERALS AND SUPPLEMENTS

Vitamin A is necessary for the health of the mucous membranes. The B-complex vitamins are vital for the health of the stomach, especially for digestion and eliminating toxins. Vitamin C is cleansing and protects against germs and viruses. Vitamin E is necessary for a healthy blood stream.

Minerals are necessary for proper digestion and elimination. Selenium and zinc protect against free radical damage. Calcium and magnesium protect the stomach and the nervous system. Potassium promotes healing and prevents germs from accumulating.

Acidophilus helps in the digestion of food. Chlorophyll and blue-green algae clean the blood and stomach. Germanium and CoQ10 help in many bodily functions.

MUSCLE AND JOINT INJURIES

SYMPTOMS

Sore—Swollen—Bruised ankles, wrists, finger, knees, back and hips.

CAUSES

A strain can happen when muscles are used too long and hard causing them to tighten. When ligaments are stretched beyond their capacity, they can tear and cause a sprain. Unexpected twisting, when playing sports such as basketball, where turns and twists are common can result in muscle injuries. A hard fall can cause breaks, sprains and stretched ligaments. They are very common in athletes.

A diet high in sugar weakens the bones and can cause unnecessary injuries.

NUTRITIONAL THERAPY

The diet should consist of whole grains such as whole wheat, whole oats, buckwheat, brown rice, millet, barley, and yellow corn meal. There are new grains such as amaranth, spelt, and quinoa which are very nutritious. Salads, using leafy green vegetables are rich in calcium and other minerals necessary for strong bones. Steamed vegetables, sea weed, sprouts, seed, nuts, and vegetables juices, using carrots, celery, parsley are rich in minerals.

Milk products are high in protein and are not good sources of calcium. They also contain antibiotics and hormones which weaken the immune system. Silicon is essential for strong bones. It is found in Oatstraw and Horsetail. Calcium with silicon produces strong bones.

HERBAL FORMULAS

Digestive System—Energy and Stamina—Immune Builders—Structural System—Female or male formulas—

VITAMINS, MINERALS AND SUPPLEMENTS

Vitamin A protects against antioxidant damage. It is also necessary for healing bones and cartilage. Vitamin D deficiency causes muscle weakness. Vitamin E protects against muscular disorders. Vitamin C aids in the assimilation of calcium. It is also healing for injuries.

Minerals speed healing of bones and muscles. Zinc speeds healing of bones. Manganese and silicon help in assimilation of calcium.

Acidophilus helps in mineral absorption. Chlorophyll is rich in minerals and speeds healing. Lecithin protects the nerves from damage. Germanium relieves pain in injuries. CoQ10 supplies oxygen to the cells and speeds healing.

MULTIPLE SCLEROSIS —

SYMPTOMS

Numbness in the tips of the fingers and limbs—Weakness in the limbs—Loss of bladder or bowel control—Slurring of speech—Tremors—Blurred or Double vision—Mood Swings—Irritability—Depression—The symptoms can be mild and can come and go.

CAUSES

This is considered an autoimmune disease; a break down of the immune system. The immune system considers the myelin sheath as foreign material and attacks it. Scar tissue is formed preventing nerve impulses from flowing along the nerve tissue. Some doctors believe this is caused from a virus attacking the myelin sheath protecting the nerves.

Another possible cause is metal poisoning such as lead and mercury. There is a high lead content in the air and mercury fillings are very common. Breathing toxins causes them to be absorbed much faster than ingesting them. Mercury vapor can leak out of fillings when chewing food and breathing it is a possibility. Both metals interfere with the nervous system. These metals collect easily when the diet is deficient in essential nutrients such as selenium, zinc, vitamin E, lecithin and essential fatty acids.

Emotional stress, overwork, fatigue, pregnancy and acute respiratory infections are known to precede the onset of multiple sclerosis. This could very well indicate a low immune system. A bad diet with lack of essential nutrients, along with the added burden of toxic metals, can deplete immune function. Vaccinations effect the nervous system and the myelin sheath around the nerves.

Diet seems to be the main cause of this disease. There is a strong evidence that a diet heavy in meat, sugar, refined grains and rancid oils may be the main cause of MS.

NUTRITIONAL THERAPY

Eliminating animal foods, such as meat, milk, eggs, and all dairy products may help. Sugar has a negative effect on the nerves. It leaches out essential minerals such as calcium. White flour products contains chlorine, which produce toxins in the colon and can be circulated in the bloodstream. Use only natural foods without pesticides if possible. Avoid rancid oils, especially fried foods. Flour products are often rancid which causes free radical damage. MS is linked to low levels of the antioxidants. Rancid oils, and grains can actually destroy cells.

A diet high in vegetable and fruit juices is beneficial. Raw and steamed vegetables supply minerals for a healthy immune system. Use millet, buckwheat, and brown rice. Use thermos cooking to supply enzymes along with B-complex vitamins to feed the nerves.

Aloe Vera can help dissolve fatty deposits on the nerves. It can also heal and dissolve scar tissue. Burdock and other blood cleansers will help prevent toxins from accumulating in the body. Ginkgo, Gotu Kola, Suma, and Kelp all help along with the nervine herbs. Hops, Scullcap, Chamomile, Passion Flower, Lady's Slipper, and Valerian will feed and nourish the nerves.

HERBAL FORMULAS

Blood Cleansers—Circulatory System—Colon Cleansers—Digestive System—Glandular System—Immune Builders—Nervous System and Brain—Structural System—Urinary System—

VITAMINS, MINERALS AND SUPPLEMENTS

The antioxidants are essential since studies show that they are lacking in MS patients. Vitamins A, C and E and the minerals selenium and zinc are important. A good chelating combination containing vitamins, minerals and herbs will help dissolve toxins from the circulatory system. B-complex vitamins nourish the myelin sheath that protects the nerves.

Calcium and magnesium along with a multi-mineral will help heal and nourish the nerves and prevent deterioration of the myelin sheath.

Lecithin helps repair and restore myelin sheath around the nerves. Flaxseed oil, and salmon oil, and essential fatty acids are seen lacking in MS. Candida is frequently seen in MS, and acidophilus will help restore the friendly bacteria. Chlorophyll and blue-green algae will help clean the blood and speed healing along with supplying nutrients to a depleted immune system. Germanium and CoQ10 will provide oxygen to the cells and speed healing.

MUSCULAR DYSTROPHY

SYMPTOMS

Muscle Weakness and Atrophy—All muscles eventually become involved and lead to terminal condition. The muscles gradually shrivel and weakens. The muscles contract gradually and causes severe pain and disability.

CAUSES

It strikes chiefly in young children and teenagers. It affects the muscles especially in the trunk of the body. Inactivity causes constipation which creates a build-up of toxins.

This disease is believed to be inherited. There is a weakening and wasting of muscle tissue which usually isn't noticed until there is substantial deterioration, as much as 50%. It isn't noticed because it is replaced by fat and hard fibrous scar tissue. Adelle Davis tells in her book, *Let's Have Healthy Children,* that every variety of animal given a vitamin E deficient diet develops muscular dystrophy. She also said that muscular dystrophy could be wiped out if vitamin E were given to all

expectant mothers and bottle fed babies. Mother's milk contains six times as much vitamin E as cow's milk and almost twice as much selenium. So nutrition could play a big role in muscular dystrophy prevention.

NUTRITIONAL THERAPY

A natural diet is vital; a weak body builds toxic waste and needs building foods. Fresh whole grains contain fiber and nutrients. Rye builds muscle and wheat contains vitamin E necessary for muscle development. Buckwheat and barley contain rutin for healthy capillaries. Millet is rich in calcium and magnesium. Brown rice is rich in B-complex vitamins for healthy muscles.

Raw and lightly steamed vegetables are rich in minerals and build the immune system. Carrot juice is high in vitamin A and calcium. Use asparagus, beets, cauliflower, cabbage, leafy green vegetable salads, artichokes, beans, broccoli, onions, leeks, and squash. Use all fruits and vegetables.

Alfalfa and Kelp are rich in minerals. Parsley is rich in copper and chlorophyll. Burdock cleans the blood and prevents toxins from accumulating. Lady's Slipper relaxes and helps relieve pain. Pau D'Arco will protect the liver and relieve pain.

HERBAL FORMULAS

Blood Cleansers—Circulatory System—Colon Cleansers—Digestive System—Glandular System—Immune Builders—Nervous System and Brain—Structural—Urinary System— Female and male formulas—

VITAMINS, MINERALS AND SUPPLEMENTS

The antioxidants are beneficial. A and C are natural antioxidants that block the oxidation of fats at the cellular level and limit their ability to form harmful peroxides. Muscular dystrophy began increasing at the same time vitamins in the diet were declining. Whole wheat flour was bleached and destroyed the main source of vitamin E. It is estimated that 96% of Americans are deficient in vitamin E.

Americans eat a lot of sodium chloride which causes a loss of potassium in the body. Potassium is essential for muscle contraction and nerve impulse transmissions.

Vitamins and minerals are essential. Because the typical diet, drugs, chlorinated water, and pesticides, vitamins and minerals are depleted from the body. It is usually the lack of nutrients that causes disease.

Lecithin is necessary for healthy muscles and nerves. Chlorophyll cleans and nourishes the blood. Essential fatty acids are lacking in the American diet. Flaxseed oil and salmon oil can help alleviate symptoms. Germanium and CoQ10 provide oxygen to the cells.

MYASTHENIA GRAVIS

SYMPTOMS

Fatigue—Muscle and Skeletal Weakness—May be severe enough to cause paralysis—Worse after Menses—Emotional Stress—Droopy Eyelids—Difficulty in Swallowing, speaking and breathing—When it involves the respiratory system it could be fatal.

CAUSES

Myasthenia gravis is considered to be an autoimmune disease that causes malfunctioning of the enzyme acetylcholine, which is responsible for inducing muscles to contract. It often attacks adolescents and young adults. It is more common in women than men. It is also seen in new born babies and adults over the age of 40 (with tumor of the thymus).

It is caused by a failure in transmission of nerve impulses at the neuromuscular junction. It occurs from an autoimmune response, ineffective acetylcholine release or inadequate muscle fiber response to acetylcholine.

Autointoxication could be one main cause. Toxins can accumulate in the blood and destroy the muscles and effect the skeletal system. It can be caused by the cecum (part of the colon), pressing against the ileocecal valve, and causing it to open and allow toxins to back up into the small intestine, which absorbs toxins faster then from the large intestine. Chronic constipation causes congestion of the cecum.

NUTRITIONAL THERAPY

Cleaning the colon will protect against autointoxication and allow nutrients to assimilate which will protect the muscles and nervous system. A diet eliminating the glue foods, such as white flour, white sugar, fried oils, animal fats, and dairy products, will help protect the body. Cheese and eggs are also considered glue foods. These foods lack fiber and cause congestion in the colon.

Buckwheat and millet are easy to digest and high in fiber. Vegetables are high in minerals and will help build muscles. Rye builds and nourishes the muscles. Potato broth is used to feed the muscles. Use red potatoes peelings, distilled water (two quarts), add 6 medium carrots, 10 stalks celery, and parsley. Simmer for about 15 to 20 minutes. Drink the broth throughout the day.

Solanine, found in the nightshade family, can interfere with the neurotransmitter acetylcholine. Some people have improved after eliminating tobacco, tomatoes, white potatoes, peppers and egg plants which all contain small amounts of solanine.

Relaxation is important in helping the assimilation of minerals and other nutrients to improve muscle health. Most people do not know how to relax. Many do not have good sleep habits.

Exercise is important. Start gradually walking in the fresh air, or jumping on a trampoline.

Herbs for building muscles are Comfrey, Oatstraw, Horsetail, and Slippery Elm. Nervine herbs will relax muscles for faster healing. Hops, Scullcap, Passion Flower, Chamomile, Lady's Slipper, Valerian, Wood Betony, Mistletoe, Dong

Quai and Lobelia all are relaxing.

HERBAL FORMULAS

Blood Cleansers—Circulatory System—Colon Cleansers—Digestive System—Energy and Stamina—Glandular System—Immune Builders—Nervous System and Brain—Structural System—Urinary—Female or Male Formulas—

VITAMINS, MINERALS AND SUPPLEMENTS

A deficiency in vitamin A can cause muscular and spinal cord degeneration and retarded growth and development particularly in the bones. The B-complex vitamins protect the muscles, nervous system, brain and the heart. They help the liver detoxify and clean. Vitamin C with bioflavonoids helps to maintain collagen, a protein necessary for formation of skin, ligament, muscles and bones. A deficiency of Vitamin E is seen in muscle weakness. It provides oxygen, thins the blood and allows normal heart function.

Minerals are necessary for healthy muscles, nerves and bones. Calcium and magnesium are directly responsible for activating normal muscle contraction. Potassium is necessary in muscle contraction. Relaxation speeds the assimilation of potassium. Silicon and manganese help in the assimilation of calcium. Manganese strengthens connective tissue and muscles. Zinc is healing and protects against muscle cramps.

Lecithin is essential for every cell in the body. It protects the arteries, so they can supply nutrients to the cells. Chlorophyll is important for the assimilation of nutrients. It contains sodium, magnesium and potassium which help tone and firm the muscles.

Germanium and CoQ10 provide oxygen for the cells. Germanium helps the body produce its own interferon to protect against germs and viruses.

OSTEOPOROSIS

SYMPTOMS

Stooping Shoulders—Loss of Height—Widow's Hump—Backache—Spontaneous Fractures in Hip—Bone loss in Jaws causing loose teeth—

CAUSES

Osteoporosis is a bone-thinning disease. It is a metabolic bone disorder which slows down the rate of bone formation and accelerates the rate of bone reabsorption, which causes loss of bone mass. This is prevalent in the jaws causing teeth to loosen. The bones affected by this disease lose essential calcium and phosphate salts and become porous like a honeycomb.

The main cause of osteoporosis is the intake of sugar, coffee, caffeine, high meat diet and cigarette smoking. The lack of minerals will cause bone loss.

Lack of hydrochloric acid prevents calcium and other minerals from absorbing properly. A high sugar diet causes calcium to excrete in the urine. Sugar robs calcium from the bones, muscles, arteries, veins, capillaries and tissues. Excess sodium causes the loss of large amounts of calcium in the urine. Chocolate contains oxalic acid and prevents the absorption of calcium.

Research shows that women with osteoporosis drink more coffee and soft drinks than women with normal bones. Loss of calcium is related to heavy use of coffee and drinks high in phosphorus.

Drugs, such as diuretics, inhibit calcium assimilation. Excess protein, meat, alcohol, and the solanum genus of vegetables such as tomatoes, potatoes, eggplant, bell peppers and tobacco contain the calcium inhibitor solanine.

NUTRITIONAL THERAPY

Sea vegetables are rich in calcium and essential minerals for assimilation. Kelp, dulse, blue-green algae, hijiki, and kombu, wheat grass juice and liquid chlorophyll are rich in minerals.

They also assist in the assimilation of nutrients. Millet is rich in calcium and magnesium. Almonds are high in calcium. The grains amaranth and quinoa are rich in minerals.

A diet rich in vegetables, raw and steamed, is beneficial. Pinto beans, salmon, brown rice, turnip greens, hazelnuts, kale, spirulina, collard greens and sesame seeds are foods high in calcium.

Suma and Dong Quai are effective in regulating hormonal imbalances. Suma contains sitosterol, an element which increases the natural estrogen production without stimulating an excess. Horsetail and Oatstraw are rich in silicon. When silicon is present, the bones assimilate calcium more effectively. Alfalfa, Comfrey and Slippery Elm are excellent for healthy bones.

HERBAL FORMULAS

Blood Cleansers—Circulatory System—Colon Cleansers—Digestive System—Glandular System—Immune Builders—Nervous System and Brain—Structural System—Urinary System—Female and Male Formulas—

VITAMINS, MINERALS AND SUPPLEMENTS

Vitamin A is necessary for proper digestion and assimilation of nutrients. Vitamin C and D help in the body's assimilation of calcium. Vitamin K, found in alfalfa and chlorophyll is necessary to synthesize osteocalcin, a unique protein matrix which attracts calcium to the bones. Deficiency is seen in those with osteoporosis.

B-complex vitamins help in bone mass formation. Folic acid helps prevent the formation of a toxic compound called homocysteine from the essential amino acid methionine, which may cause osteoporosis. Folic acid deficiency is seen in those who use oral contraceptives, alcohol and tobacco. B6 increases the strength of the connective tissues in the bones. All B vitamins help prevent the toxins from accumulating in the liver.

Minerals are essential for healthy bones. Boron is one trace mineral necessary for healthy bones.

Silicon, found in horsetail and oatstraw is necessary for calcium absorption.

Acidophilus produces enzymes for digestion of food. It also is involved with the production of vitamins B-6, B12, and folic acid which are important for bone mass growth. It feeds the colon and eliminates putrefying bacteria. It can also protect against viruses. Chlorophyll and blue-green algae are rich in minerals and vitamins for building strong bones. They eliminate toxins and nourish the blood.

Salmon oil and flaxseed oil are necessary for the production of hormones in the body. It assists in assimilation of nutrients and helps in the repair of tissues. Germanium and Co Q10 help the body utilize oxygen. They increase energy and improve circulation. It also protects the immune system.

PANCREATITIS

SYMPTOMS

Acute—produces a sudden attack of severe upper abdominal pain—Nausea—Vomiting—Pain may spread to the back and is made worse by moving—Chronic—Excessive gas—Fever—Muscle aches—There can be permanent damage to the pancreas because of constant inflammation which can cause fibrosis to the pancreas. It can also cause diabetes, digestive problems and cancer.

CAUSES

Acute pancreatitis is usually caused by gallstones, alcohol abuse, a viral infection or injury. It is an inflammation of the pancreas. It can cause hearing, kidney and respiratory failure. Chronic pancreatitis is usually caused by alcohol, drug abuse, or cancer. It is one of the leading cancers.

A diet rich in fats, sugar and meat contributes to pancreatitis.

NUTRITIONAL THERAPY

Whole grains and vegetables are vital for their ability to metabolize in the body slowly as energy is needed by the body. Chewing food thoroughly helps the saliva contribute to the digestion of grains.

Millet, yellow corn meal, buckwheat, barley, oats, and brown rice help build and nourish the pancreas and spleen. Vegetables that can help build the pancreas include: asparagus, squash of all kinds, broccoli, brussels sprouts, cabbage, cucumber, cauliflower, celery, green beans, and leafy green vegetables including endive. Sweet potatoes, chickpeas, and lentils are nourishing. Miso soup will help repair the pancreas and spleen. Carrot, celery, garlic and ginger juice is healing and building.

Eliminate sugar, fruit juice and dried fruit from the diet.

Golden Seal helps regulate blood sugar. Cedar Berries helps in the healing of the pancreas. Buchu, Mullein, Garlic, Dandelion, Marshmallow and Licorice are good for the pancreas. Burdock, Golden Seal, and Garlic will help heal inflammation. Saffron helps in the digestion of oils.

HERBAL FORMULAS

Blood Cleansers—Circulatory System—Colon Cleansers—Digestive System—Glandular System — Immune Builder — Infection Fighters—Urinary System—

VITAMINS, MINERALS AND SUPPLEMENTS

Vitamins A and C with bioflavonoids help in the healing of the pancreas. B-complex helps fight stress and aid in digestion. Vitamin E is an antioxidant and helps heal infections. Vitamin K, found in chlorophyll, is essential for healthy blood to kill infections.

Chromium is an essential component of the glucose tolerance factor. Copper is also vital. All minerals are needed for healing and nourishing the body. Selenium and zinc are healing. Calcium, magnesium and potassium will help glandular problems.

Digestive enzymes are important to take the load off the pancreas. Lecithin helps in the assimilation of fats. Chlorophyll and blue-green algae aid in digestion and help the body produce interferon. Germanium helps in the body's natural production of interferon. CoQ10 helps in supplying oxygen to the cells for healing.

PARKINSON'S DISEASE

SYMPTOMS

Slight tremor of one hand—Arm—Leg—Later causes stiffness—Weakness—Trembling of the muscles—Stiff shuffling—Trouble walking—Increased trembling of the hand shows more marked at rest—Depression—Permanent Rigid Stoop—Eating, washing and dressing all become difficult—

CAUSES

This disease causes a degeneration of/or damage to nerve cells within the basal ganglia in the brain. Nutritional deficiencies, (especially the lack of antioxidants) and autointoxication are thought to be the main causes. Heavy metal poisoning can also be a cause. Mercury accumulates in the body over the years in toxic amounts. It is stored in the brain and attacks the nervous system.

Some drugs can cause this disease by blocking dopamine and causing a form of secondary parkinsonism. They include: Droperidol, Chlorprothixene, Thiothixene and Lithium to name a few. Drugs destroy the nervous system and prevent the assimilation of essential nutrients for brain and nerve function.

Parkinson's is seen when there is an imbalance of two chemicals, dopamine and acetylcholine. Chemicals in the brain can be restored with proper nutrients if there is no permanent damage.

NUTRITIONAL THERAPY

A high fiber diet will help eliminate toxic, carcinogenic substances in the colon and prevent them from entering the blood stream and brain. Grains such as wheat, whole oats, yellow corn meal, millet, amaranth, quinoa, and brown rice are high in fiber. Cook them in a thermos to retain the enzymes. Vegetables are rich in minerals which are needed to protect against metal poisoning.

Eat raw foods, nuts, sprouts, and seeds in the diet to help repair the nerves and brain. Vegetable juices assimilate fast and are rich in vitamins and minerals. Carrot, celery, and parsley are very beneficial.

Herbs to help in brain function are Garlic, Ginkgo, Gotu Kola, Kelp, and Suma. Alfalfa, Burdock, Dandelion, Comfrey, Onions, Watercress, Horseradish, Kelp, Echinacea, and Parsley will help clean the blood. The nervine herbs will help repair the brain. They include: Hops, Scullcap, Ppassion Flower, Chamomile, Valerian and Lobelia.

HERBAL FORMULAS

Blood Cleansers—Circulatory System—Colon Cleansers—Digestive System—Energy and Stamina—Glandular System—Immune Builders—Nervous System and Brain—Urinary System—Female and Male Formulas—

VITAMINS, MINERALS AND SUPPLEMENTS

The antioxidants protect against free radical damage. They are Vitamins A, D, C, E, selenium and zinc. They are implicated in Parkinson's disease. Free radicals are caused by air pollution, tobacco smoke, some drugs, and a poor diet such as rancid oils found in fried foods and stale wheat products. B-complex vitamins help in digestion and help the liver to detoxify toxins.

Minerals are vital to protect the brain from damage. Deficiency is seen when the brain and nerves are damaged. Calcium and magnesium are necessary for nerve impulse transmission. Potassium helps prevent the accumulation of toxins in the arteries. Phosphorus builds the brain and nervous system. Sodium dissolves poisons in the body.

Lecithin increases acetylcholine production in the brain which conveys impulses from one nerve cell to another. Deficiencies are seen in Parkinson's disease. It is necessary to feed the nerves and and protect them from damage.

Chlorophyll and blue-green algae are high in calcium, magnesium and potassium to nourish the blood. It helps in the assimilation of nutrients. Germanium and CoQ10 helps in brain repair by supplying oxygen to the cells. It improves circulatory disorders.

PARASITES AND WORMS

SYMPTOMS

Constipation—Diarrhea—Gas and Bloating— Anemia—Allergies—Irritable Bowel Syndrome— Nervousness—Sleep Disturbances—Chronic Fatigue—Teeth Grinding—Possible Problems caused by Parasites and Worms: Arthritis— Back and Neck Pain—Bruxism (grinding of teeth)—Cancer—colitis—Fatigue—Diabetes— Headaches—Hypoglycemia—Indigestion— Lupus—Mineral Imbalance—Nausea—Sinus Troubles—Thyroid Imbalance—

CAUSES

A poor diet lacking in hydrochloric acid, which can destroy parasites and worms, is one problem. Ingestion of larvae or eggs from handling meat or eating partially cooked meat is a problem. Pork is often contaminated with parasites even when it is cooked. Walking barefoot on contaminated soil can pick up larva or eggs.

Giardia lamblia, a microscopic organism, is found in our drinking water. It is found in the streams and introduced to the water supplies by animals. Antibiotics and immune-suppressing drugs reduce the beneficial intestinal flora and provides an environment for parasites and worms.

NUTRITIONAL THERAPY

Parasites and worms feed off toxins and waste material in the body. If the body is clean, the scavengers have nothing to live on. The danger of having them in the body is that their waste is extremely poisonous and parasites produce toxic substances harmful to the host. Some worms rob the host of serious amounts of blood and large tapeworms deprive it of digested food.

The body can be cleansed from these scavengers. Colon cleansing is essential. A diet high in fiber helps eliminate parasites and worms. Pomegranate, figs and pumpkin seeds are beneficial. Garlic, onions, cabbage and carrots contain sulphur, which expels parasites and worms. Citrus seed extract inhibits some microbes and parasites such as amoebas, bacteria, viruses as well as candida.

Eliminate sugar, and junk food on which they live and grow. A change of diet is essential to protect the body from infestation.

Herbs to expel worms are Burdock, Cascara Sagrada, Black Walnut, Wormwood, and Echinacea kill parasites in the digestive tract. Garlic kills worms. Horsetail kills parasite and worm eggs. Golden Seal destroys parasites and worms.

HERBAL FORMULAS

Blood Cleansers—Colon Cleansers—(parasite and worm formulas)—Digestive System— Immune Builders—Urinary System—

VITAMINS, MINERALS AND SUPPLEMENTS

The antioxidants help protect the immune system. Vitamins A, D, C with bioflavonoids, E, and minerals selenium and zinc are recommended.

B-complex helps in digestion and detoxifies the liver.

Iodine, which is found in kelp, kills parasites and worms. Iron enriches the blood. Vitamin and mineral supplements will help protect and prevent parasites and worms from invading the body.

Acidophilus provides friendly bacteria which protect the body. Chlorophyll and blue-green algae help food to digest and are rich in calcium, magnesium and potassium.

PERIODONTAL DISEASE

SYMPTOMS

Bleeding Gums—Red Gums—Swollen Gums—Bad Breath—Pain—Abscesses—Inflamed gums is known as Gingivitis—

CAUSES

A lack of proper nutrients and nutrient absorption, poor oral hygiene and smoking contribute to the demise of teeth and to their underlying support structures. Lack of vitamin C can cause scurvy-like symptoms which includes bleeding gums.

Plaque, which is a film on the teeth where bacteria will flourish, can harden into a rock-like substance known as tartar. Tartar accumulates at the base of the tooth where the gum line meets if the plaque isn't brushed off daily. The tartar irritates the gums further and causes more bleeding. The bacteria loosen the teeth from the gums and migrate lower where they form pus pockets. This extremely dangerous condition is known as "pyorrhea."

Pus will discharge into the mouth itself and the teeth actually loosen from the sockets. The roots are destroyed, and so the teeth are extracted... hence, the need for dentures.

The main cause in tooth loss is not plaque and gingivitis, but osteoporosis of the jaw, which causes the teeth to loosen and the gums to recede.

NUTRITIONAL THERAPY

Good oral hygiene is necessary for healthy gums and teeth. Flossing daily and brushing from the base of the teeth (near the gums) toward the crown, can do much to clean away plaque.

The main key to good dental health is to build a dense bone mass in the dental structure. Even people who have dentures need a strong bone mass. A strong bone mass is possible no matter how old your are.

Eliminate smoking. It definitely contributes to periodontal disease. Periodontal disease is rarely seen in non-smokers. Smoking causes osteoporosis in women. Smoking hinders calcium and other vital mineral absorption.

Eliminate soft drinks, for they contain high amounts of phosphorus and contribute to an imbalance of calcium-phosphorus ratio.

Tea tree oil on toothpaste brushed onto the teeth will act as an antiseptic and germicide. A herbal bone formula containing horsetail, oatstraw, comfrey and pan pien lien can build bone mass. It is rich in silicon which is essential for the assimilation of calcium. It is the key to increasing bone mass and preventing periodontal disease.

A diet rich in whole grains, beans, sprouts, nuts, seeds, raw and lightly steamed vegetables will build strong bones. Fruit, and vegetable juices are rich in vitamins and minerals. Proper digestion is necessary and adding digestive enzymes and hydrochloric acid may be needed. Cooking in a thermos is a slow way of cooking grains to maintain the enzyme and vitamin B content for digestion.

White Oak Bark Powder is useful as an astringent for bleeding, spongy gums. Applied directly, it will help heal the gums and strengthen the teeth. Comfrey is high in calcium and is excellent for bone structure.

HERBAL FORMULAS

Blood Cleansers—Circulatory System—Colon Cleansers—Digestive System—Immune Builders—Infection Fighters—Nervous system and Brain—Structural—Female and Male Formulas—

VITAMINS, MINERALS AND SUPPLEMENTS

Vitamin A is necessary for healing infections. Vitamin C with bioflavonoids protects the gums and prevents infections. Vitamin D works with calcium for strong bones. Vitamin E provides oxygen to the cells to prevent free radical damage. The B-complex vitamins are necessary for energy and are vital for the metabolism of carbohydrates, fats, and proteins.

Minerals are vital to strong bone growth and mass. Silicon plays an important role in calcium metabolism, bone formation, normal growth and prevention of osteoporosis and jaw bone loss. Zinc and selenium are healing for infections. Calcium, magnesium, and manganese are necessary for healthy bones. Potassium prevents germs from accumulating.

CoQ10 has proven to be very effective in treating periodontal disease. It works through the immune system in re-energizing the gums and reversing periodontal disease. Germanium has the ability to stimulate interferon to protect against infections. Chlorophyll used internally and as a mouth wash will clean the blood and mouth to prevent gum disease. It is also useful after dental extraction to clean and protect against infections.

PNEUMONIA

SYMPTOMS

Fever—Chills—Fatigue—Sore Throat—Cough—Muscle Aches—Chest Pain—Breathing Difficulties—Walking pneumonia is slow and causes fatigue and general weakness—It is the fifth leading cause of death in the United States. It is serious for the elderly and is common in hospitals after surgery.

CAUSES

Pneumonia is an inflammation of the lungs including the bronchial tubes, bronchiolus, and alveoli. The infection is caused by bacteria, viruses and fungi. Weak kidneys and colon will cause toxins to eliminate from the lungs. The lungs are very sensitive to these irritants and are not supposed to eliminate them.

Air pollution is high in toxins that weaken the lungs. Breathing in toxins assimilates them faster into the bloodstream than ingesting them. Fine particulate matter (PM 10) can cause and worsen respiratory illnesses including asthma, bronchitis, and pneumonia. PM10 suppresses the body's immune system and may even cause cancer.

Lung scarring is caused by air pollutants and can lead to pneumonia and other diseases. The six leading air pollutants we breath are lead, ozone, carbon monoxide, nitrogen oxides, sulfur oxides and fine particulates.

Pneumonia is a serious acute disease and needs to be treated naturally. Other causes are aspiration under anesthesia and malnutrition. Allergies can weaken the lungs and cause pneumonia. Chemical irritations can eventually weaken the lungs. These pollutants stay in the lungs unless proper treatment is taken to protect them with supplements.

Lung problems are associated with hypoglycemia as well as food allergies. Sugar products and dairy products are very harmful on the lungs.

NUTRITIONAL THERAPY

The first step in healing is to stop eating. The body is trying to eliminate the toxins and pushes them from the cells and into the stomach to be eliminated through the colon. If you eat with any acute disease, the cleansing is stopped in order to digest the food. Drinking citrus juices, such as grapefruit, orange, lemon and limes will help nature heal. Using herbal teas and extracts will also help nature cleanse.

Lower bowel cleansing is essential to assure that the toxins are eliminated and not absorbed into the blood stream. The colon is the main cause of health problems.

In order to prevent pneumonia, eating foods to build the lungs are important. Fresh fruit and vegetables are rich in nutrients. Sprouts, whey, plain yogurt, seeds, nuts, onions and garlic are strengthening for the lungs. Brown rice and millet are strengthening.

Ginger, Licorice, Horseradish, Fenugreek, Comfrey, Lobelia, Slippery Elm, Alfalfa, and Aloe Vera are healing for the lungs.

HERBAL FORMULAS

Blood Cleansers—Circulatory System—Colds, Flu and Allergies—Digestive System—Energy Stamina—Immune Builders—Infection Fighters—Nervous System and Brain—Urinary System—Female and Male Formulas—

VITAMINS, MINERALS AND SUPPLEMENTS

Vitamin A is essential for healthy lungs. It is usually lacking in our diet. You can get vitamin A and D in fish oils as well as beta carotene. B-complex is essential for digestion and helps the liver to detoxify. It provides strength to the immune system. Vitamin C with bioflavonoids

helps the body produce interferon to protect against pneumonia. Vitamin E protects the cells from damage.

Minerals are important for lung health. Zinc protects the immune system and heals infections. A mineral supplement works with vitamins to heal infections.

Liquid chlorophyll helps the body produce its own interferon for efficient immune function. Blue-green algae is healing and will kill germs and viruses. Acidophilus provides the body with nutrients to protect the digestive system. It protects against yeast infestations. It helps eliminate toxins.

Germanium and CoQ10 protects the arteries, helps the body produce interferon, and increases lung capacity. Flaxseed oil and salmon oil protect the immune system and prevent infections.

POST POLIOMYELITIS SYNDROME

SYMPTOMS

Chronic Pain—Decreases Stamina—Fatigue—Fibrositis—Debilitation—Joint Pain—Muscle Twitching—Muscle Weakness—Respiratory Problems—Sciatica—Scoliosis—Swallowing Problems—The major complaints of post-polio victims are Pain (neck and back)—Weakness and Fatigue—

CAUSES

There are 500,000 American who survived the polio epidemic, and more than 125,000 are estimated to have post-polio syndrome. It is a condition that results in progressive muscle weakness. Swallowing problems are becoming a common sign of the syndrome. Many are often unaware of this condition, which could cause the risk of choking. It is called dysphagia.

Causes stem from polio ten, twenty, thirty or more years ago.

NUTRITIONAL THERAPY

A cleansing and building program is necessary. Foot reflexology strengthens the muscles. It takes a long time and is painful to get the muscles working again, but it is worth it.

Foods high in fiber such as whole grains, beans, fruit and vegetables are building.

Herbs help in building muscles such as: Oatstraw, Horsetail, Comfrey and Kelp.

HERBAL FORMULAS

Blood Cleansers—Circulatory System—Allergy — Colon Cleansers — Digestive System—Energy and Stamina—Immune Builders—Nervous System and Brain—Structural—Urinary System—Female or Male Formulas—

VITAMINS, MINERALS AND SUPPLEMENTS

Vitamins A, D, C, E, and minerals selenium and zinc are antioxidants to protect the immune system. B-complex is essential for the nervous system. It helps repair damaged nerves.

Calcium, magnesium, potassium and silicon are strengthening for the muscles and nerves. They are found in sea vegetables in richer amounts than other sources.

Chlorophyll and blue-green algae are rich in minerals and clean and nourish the blood. They build the immune system.

Acidophilus protects the colon and digestive system.

Bee pollen is rich in vitamins, minerals and amino acids for building the bones and muscles. Germanium and CoQ10 help protect the immune system. They provide oxygen and nutrients to the cells. Germanium helps the body produce it own interferon.

PREGNANCY
(Discomforts)

SYMPTOMS

Anemia—Constipation—Morning Sickness—Leg Cramps—Indigestion—Fatigue—Swollen Ankles — Backache — Varicose Veins — Toxemia—Insomnia—

CAUSES

Constipation and malnutrition are the most common causes of discomfort in pregnancy. It is vital to become aware of the importance of nutrition before becoming pregnant. Both men and women need to learn which foods build and nourish and help prevent birth defects in the new born, and how to eliminate the discomforts that can accompany pregnancy.

NUTRITIONAL THERAPY

Anemia is caused from a lack of iron. Natural iron formulas using yellow dock, and dandelion will build up the blood. Chlorophyll is rich in iron. Foods that contain iron are: kelp, dulse, rice bran, pumpkin and sesame seeds, whole grains, soybeans, beans, dried apricots, green leafy vegetables, and blackstrap molasses.

Constipation can be dangerous for the mother and baby. It can lead to toxemia (toxic blood), high blood pressure, and water retention. It also can lead to fatigue, leg cramps, backache and varicose veins. Morning sickness is a cleansing of the body to prepare a clean environment for the fetus.

A healthy diet would be fruit, two a day, seven vegetables, including salads, grains, which will prevent constipation and provide proteins, complex carbohydrates, vitamins and minerals. When grains are cooked in a thermos, it prevents the nutrients from being destroyed.

Indigestion can be helped with acidophilus, a food enzyme formula, Aloe Vera Juice, Peppermint Tea or

Ginger are recommended. Eating smaller meals and chewing well will help prevent indigestion.

HERBAL FORMULAS

Blood Cleansers—Circulatory System—Colon Cleansers—Digestive System—Immune Builders—Structural—Female Formulas—

VITAMINS, MINERALS AND SUPPLEMENTS

Vitamin A is important to protect the immune system. A deficiency has been linked with abnormalities of the eyes in babies and cleft lip and cleft palate.

Thiamine, B-1, is essential in preventing stillbirths and low-birth weight babies. A lack of B1 can also cause heart disorders in the baby.

Riboflavin B-2 is needed in larger amounts during pregnancy along with all the B vitamins. Deficiencies have been related to short limbs and cleft palate.

Niacin and Niacinamide B-3 deficiencies can cause nervousness, insomnia, irritability, depression, disorientation, fatigue and muscular weakness.

Pyridoxine, B-6, deficiencies have been linked with fetal abnormalities. It is related to a cleft lip and cleft palate.

Seizures in the new born are seen as a vitamin B-6 deficiency.

Folic Acid is needed to prevent anemia and is involved in DNA synthesis and is needed for rapidly growing cells. It helps prevent birth defects.

Vitamin C is needed to prevent infections and improve immune response. Low vitamin C levels are associated with smaller babies. It is needed every day.

Magnesium is needed to prevent miscarriage and birth abnormalities. It is seen as a common deficiency in pregnancy.

Calcium is important to prevent premature births. It is needed for healthy growth of bones and teeth. It is essential for the nervous system.

Phosphorus is important but a high intake can cause a disturbance in the calcium balance. Too much phosphorus can prevent the absorption of iron. Cow's milk is high in phosphorus. Soda pop is high in phosphorus. This imbalance can cause congenital abnormalities.

Manganese is important in the central nervous system and can cause brain abnormalities.

Iodine need is increased in pregnancy a lack of it can cause the fetus to fail to develop normally.

Zinc is essential to stabilize RNA. It is needed to prevent dwarfism and defects of the limbs.

Acidophilus is useful to prevent yeast infestations. It helps in the digestion of nutrients. Chlorophyll is rich in iron and other minerals. It helps nourish the blood and prevents toxemia.

Bee pollen is rich in amino acid, vitamins and minerals. Germanium and CoQ10 is needed to provide oxygen to the blood.

PREMENSTRUAL SYNDROME

SYMPTOMS

PMS is not a disease, nor a neurosis, although it has the symptoms of both. There are over 150 symptoms linked to PMS, the most common ones are —Depression—Irritability—Faintness—Restlessness—Sluggishness—Impatience—Lethargy—Delusions—Indecisiveness—Dizziness—Nervousness—Anxiety—Swelling Breasts—Swelling Feet—constipation—Hemorrhoids—skin Eruptions—Migraines—Backaches—

CAUSES

An irregular cycle often indicates the general state of a woman's health and is usually the result of nutritional deficiencies or autointoxication caused by constipation.

An imbalance in the system could stem from

genetic predisposition, an organic malfunction, a vitamin or mineral deficiency, stress, drugs, chemicals, or a combination of these.

Hormonal imbalance is seen in PMS. The liver is responsible for regulating hormone balance. It is involved with eliminating blood levels of estradiol, the 'unfavorable' type of estrogen. This estrogen can build up in the body. Constipation is the main cause of preventing the liver from filterin the unwanted estrogen. It enters the bloodstream and can reach the brain and cause depression and bizarre mental manifestations.

Lack of B vitamins is another cause. They are lacking in the typical American diet. They help the liver convert the excess estrogen to a harmless form. Magnesium is necessary to help the body eliminate unwanted estrogen. Fried foods interfere with magnesium absorption.

Eliminate chocolate, caffeine, sugar and excess sodium.

NUTRITIONAL THERAPY

With PMS, it would be helpful to avoid all foods that relate to the reproductive system of animals or contains artificial hormones. This includes milk, and all milk products such as sour cream, whipping cream, half-half, milk, cottage cheese, cheese, and all products of the cow's reproductive system. Eggs, a product of the chicken's reproductive system should also be avoided. All meat of animals that have been raised on hormones and antibiotics are potentially harmful.

A high fiber diet is beneficial. A lot of salads, using green leafy vegetables, almonds and millet which are rich in calcium and magnesium is beneficial. The diet should consist of more fruits, vegetables, sprouts, whole grains such as brown rice, millet, buckwheat, rye,wheat, barley, and herbs that are rich in vitamins, and minerals.

Colon cleansing is necessary in order for the liver to eliminate toxins. A good herbal liver formula is beneficial for restoring its function.

Exercise helps to alleviate stress and tension.

Herbs that help in PMS problems are Red Raspberry, Chamomile, Black Cohosh, Dong Quai, Licorice, and Parsley.

HERBAL FORMULAS

Blood Cleansers—Colon Cleansers—Digestive System—Glandular System—Immune Builders—Female Formulas—

VITAMINS, MINERALS AND SUPPLEMENTS

Vitamin A is needed to protect the lining of the reproductive organs. Endocrine glands associated with the reproductive organs need vitamin A to function properly. It also protects monthly skin disorders.

The B-complex vitamins play a major role in preventing women's problems. Tests have shown that the amount of estrogen metabolized by the liver can be controlled through sufficient intake of B vitamins. They help prevent depression, fatigue, sugar cravings, weight fluctuation and bloating.

Vitamin C helps alleviate stress by providing nutrients for the adrenal glands (stress glands). It is a natural diuretic. It is needed each day to help regulate menstrual flow and relieve pain associated with monthly cramps.

Vitamin E functions in easing breast tenderness and preventing fibrocystic breast disease. It also helps in equalizing blood circulation, reducing fluid retention and eliminating cramps.

Vitamin D helps the body absorb calcium properly. It assists in calming the nerves and aids in promoting restful sleep.

Calcium is essential during menstrual periods. Blood calcium drops ten days prior to menstruation. It happens when the ovaries are not producing much estrogen or progesterone and continues until after menstruation starts. A lack of calcium causes tension, headaches, nervousness, insomnia and depression. Magnesium and vitamin D aid in calcium absorption.

Magnesium along with calcium are needed to eliminate cramps. They increase B-complex absorption and help eliminate bad estrogen from the blood stream. They prevent spasms in the uterus wall, legs, and eliminate irritability and depression. They also help prevent indigestion and constipation.

Iron is vital for women because of the loss of blood each month. It helps prevent fatigue, weakness and depression stemming from low red blood cell count. Vitamin C helps the body assimilate iron.

Chromium helps stabilize blood sugar levels. It prevents the accumulation of fatty deposits in the veins and arteries.

Iodine help to keep estrogen levels from becoming too high. This helps the body regulate menstrual periods and prevent water retention.

Manganese is vital for normal reproduction and mammary glands. It is important to prevent osteoporosis.

Potassium helps regulate water balance in the tissues.

Selenium is an antioxidant and is excellent to help prevent menstrual cramps and breast tenderness.

Chlorophyll helps purify and enrich the blood. Blue-green algae is rich in nutrients to help prevent menstrual problems.

Acidophilus is needed to help in the digestion of nutrients. It provides the friendly bacteria to prevent candida which is common in some women who have eaten a high sugar diet or have been on antibiotics or birth control pills.

Germanium and CoQ10 are beneficial to provide oxygen to the cells and increase immune function.

Flaxseed oil and salmon oil help to regulate all body functions. They are needed for the reproductive system and are essential to regulate hormone function.

PROSTATE PROBLEMS
(Prostatis, Prostate Hypertrophy, Prostate Cancer)

SYMPTOMS

Pain—Discomfort—Prostate Enlargement—Frequent Urination—Painful Urination—Burning Sensation When Urinating—Blood or Pus in the Urine—Fever—

CAUSES

Prostatis is an inflammation of the prostate. It can cause urine retention which leads to infections. Bacteria builds up in the retained urine. The main cause is from bad diet, constipation and autointoxication. Not drinking enough water to keep the bladder clean can also be a problem. Too much alcohol, tobacco, sugar, coffee, cola drinks, sweet deserts, refined food and meat all contribute.

Constipation is the main reason toxins back up into the blood stream and create toxic blood. This will travel to all parts of the body.

Prostate hypertrophy is seen in men over the age of forty. Research on prostate problems with males who suffer form this disease show their diets are usually low in fatty acids (nuts, seeds, flaxseed oil and salmon oil), vitamin C and bioflavonoids, vitamin E and minerals such as zinc.

Prostate cancer is also linked to a deficient diet. Stress, anger, hate, and deep resentments can contribute to prostate problems. The body organs tighten up under stress and cause malfunctions and retention of toxic waste.

NUTRITIONAL THERAPY

Whole grains are rich in fiber which include: brown rice, whole wheat, millet, whole oats, barley, buckwheat, and quinoa and amaranth. Fruit, vegetables, beans, sea weeds and soups made with whole grains and vegetables using onions and garlic are very nourishing. Cooking grains in thermos will retain the enzymes for better assimilation.

Exercise is important to improve circulation, lower blood pressure and reduce toxins to prevent cancer. It also helps with depression and negative thinking.

Cleansing diet is essential to keep the prostate healthy. Eliminate coffee, alcohol, tobacco, caffeine drinks, and white sugar products. Cancer thrives on sugar. Drink lots of pure water.

Echinacea is an excellent herb for enlargement and weakness of the prostate glands. Cayenne is great for circulation. Kelp is rich in minerals and cleans the prostate. Saw Palmetto helps an enlarged prostate to reduce inflammation, pain and swelling. Parsley and herbal combinations designed for men are excellent. Burdock is excellent for enlarged prostate. The following herbs help the body produce its own natural hormones. Sarsaparilla, Ginseng, Licorice, Saw Palmetto, and Damiana.

HERBAL FORMULAS

Blood Cleansers—Circulatory System—Colon Cleansers—Digestive System—Glandular System—Immune Builders—Infection Fighters—Urinary System—Male Formulas—

VITAMINS, MINERALS AND SUPPLEMENTS

Vitamins A and D promote liver health, heal mucous membranes, and assist in producing natural steroids. They also protect against free radical damage.

B-complex vitamins are essential for healthy nerves, energy, digestion and depression. B 12 prevents nerve damage and helps maintain fertility. All B vitamins help nourish, protect and heal prostate problems.

Vitamin C with bioflavonoids helps prevent free radical damage, increases sperm count and mobility, and helps calcium and other minerals to absorb. It heals infections, promotes healthy blood vessels and capillaries, and protects against prostate problems.

Vitamin E is an antioxidant to protect against free radical damage to the prostate. E works with iodine for absorption. It increases hormone production and promotes the function of the sexual glands.

Calcium and magnesium are necessary for healthy nerves, bones and muscles. They increase resistance to infections.

Chlorine helps the body expel waste and purifies and disinfects against germs and viruses. Iodine is essential for regulating the thyroid gland and manufacturing the hormone thyroxin to control the metabolism of the body. Potassium prevents cancer and tumors from growing. It repairs the liver and aids in waste elimination. Selenium is believed necessary for sperm production. It works with vitamin E, an antioxidant, to protect against toxins. It helps to prevent chromosome breakage causing birth defects. Sulphur is essential in stimulating egg and sperm production. Zinc is essential for a healthy prostate gland. It helps to manufacturer male hormones and ensures the proper development of the genital organs.

Chlorophyll and blue-green algae contain cleansing properties to prevent prostate problems. They protect against infections as well as heal inflammation in the prostate.

Essential fatty acids found in flaxseed oil and salmon oil work with vitamin E to reduce the amount of urine retention in the bladder after urinating. EFA's are the building blocks from which prostaglandins are made. They are hormone-like substances that regulate every organ, tissue and cell in the human body. They help dissolve brown body fat, the kind that lies deep in the body and surrounds the heart, kidneys and adrenal glands.

Lecithin helps eliminate fatty deposits and protect the nerves. Germanium and CoQ10 provide oxygen to the cells and improve circulation. They help keep the capillaries and veins in the prostate healthy.

Acidophilus helps keep the bad bacteria under control. It improves digestion and assimilation of all nutrients.

RADIATION POISONING

SYMPTOMS

The human body accumulates low level radiation over a period of years. This causes the body to weaken and become very susceptible to many diseases. Cancer—Brain, nerve, endocrine and reproductive problems. Cataracts—Muscle Weakness—Bone Cancer—Miscarriage—Birth Defects—It can effect Mood and causes Autoimmune Diseases—

CAUSES

It is called electromagnetic impulses and is a new kind of radiation. It is found in tobacco smoke which contains polonium-210 due to a fertilizer used on the tobacco plant. Medical and dental X-rays, nuclear medicine (diathermy and radiation therapy), air travel, video display terminals, nuclear power (by-products), microwaves, satellites, high-voltage electric lines, electronic games, radar devises, satellite dishes, and televisions are all causes.

These waves are emitted in low doses and are absorbed deep into the body. Breathing these causes them to be absorbed faster than when ingesting them.

NUTRITIONAL THERAPY

Foods that limit our ability to protects against radiation are meats, poultry, dairy products, sugar, fats, refined foods and foods with chemical additives.

Foods that protect against radiation are whole grains, vegetables, beans, soy products (miso, tofu and tempeh), seeds, nuts and sea vegetables. Grains contain phytic acid and fiber that bind radioactive and toxic elements and eliminate them. Vegetables like broccoli, cabbage, and brussels sprouts contain amino acids which function as antioxidants and free radical deactivators and neutralize toxins. Root vegetables are rich in minerals.

In 1977, the Senate Select Committee on Nutrition and Human Needs published Dietary Goals for the United States. It strongly urged Americans to reduce their intake of fat, red meat, refined grains, sugar and salt and to increase their intake of whole grains, fresh vegetables, fish and fruit. This diet was recommended to reduce the leading causes of death in the U.S, which are cancer, heart disease, and diabetes. This diet is also very effective against radiation, air and chemical pollution.

Herbs are the best protection against radiation. Kelp contains algin, which eliminates strontium 90 from the body. Siberian Ginseng is as "adaptogen," which protects the body against toxins that lower our immunity and vitality. Aloe Vera helps in aiding the growth and repair of body tissues. It helps dissolve adhesions and heals radiation burns. Burdock purifies blood and prevents toxins from invading the cells. Garlic is a natural antibiotic. Echinacea cleans the blood and lymphatic system. Golden Seal is healing. Pau D'Arco protects the liver and cleans blood. Red clover is a blood cleanser.

HERBAL FORMULAS

Blood Cleansers—Circulatory System—Colon Cleansers—Digestive System—Energy And Stamina—Immune Builders—Nervous System and Brain—Urinary System—Female and Male Formulas—

VITAMINS, MINERALS AND SUPPLEMENTS

Vitamins A is essential for the immune system. It protects against radiation, air and chemical pollution. It helps the thymus to produce more T cells, which fight germs, viruses, and invading toxins.

B-complex vitamins have been found to prevent lead poisoning. They produce antibodies for the immune system. The B vitamins are essential for the liver to destroy toxins. Pantothenic acid , B6, B12, and folic acid have been found effective in stimulating the repair of red blood cells and protecting against radiation.

Vitamin C with bioflavonoids helps counteract radiation and chemical toxins. It is essential to protect against air pollutants, lead, mercury, DDT, cadmium, nitrates, nitrites, aluminum, chlorine, cigarette smoke, arsenic, carbon monoxide, pesticides, and the toxic side effects of drugs.

Vitamin D works with vitamin A and the B-complex vitamins to help remove radioactive isotopes such as strontium-90 from the bones. It works with calcium to protect against lead and cadmium which are found in the air. It also promotes the assimilation of calcium, phosphorus, magnesium, and other essential minerals. It helps in the regulation of the thyroid in maintaining calcium levels in the blood.

Vitamin E is an antioxidant which prevents free radical damage. It provides oxygen to the tissues, protects against cancer, circulatory diseases and strengthens the immune system. Vitamin E prevents the destruction of essential fatty acids, and vitamin A by radiation. It protects against toxins we breathe, drink and eat.

Calcium along with vitamin D help protect against strontium-90, radioisotopes and lead. It is especially beneficial for children, who have rapidly growing bones and are vulnerable to lead and strontium-90. Bone health is important for its skeletal support, formation of blood cells and immune response.

Iron is essential to protect the liver, bone marrow, ovaries, testes, and lungs. Excess phosphorus found in soft drinks and meat depletes iron.

Magnesium works with calcium and helps protect the body against aluminum poisoning. It protects against kidney disease, muscle cramps and seizures, confusion, nervous disorders, depression, PMS and circulatory problems.

Potassium protects against radioactive material. It works with sodium to protect the kidneys from damage, and keeps a proper acid-alkaline balance in the blood.

Selenium and zinc are antioxidants to protect the body from radiation damage. They protect against cancer of the colon, lungs, ovaries, pancreas, prostate, bladder and breast.

Acidophilus helps in the digestion and assimilation of necessary vitamins and minerals. It protects against yeast infections.

Chlorophyll and blue-green algae protect against radiation. They are similar in structure to human blood and are a beneficial tonic.

Bee pollen is rich in B-vitamins, amino acids, vitamins and minerals that protect against damage from radiation. Germanium and CoQ10 help the immune system and the production of the body's own interferon. They are classified as immuno-stimulating oxides which bind up or chelates and removes harmful toxic compounds.

RAYNAUD'S DISEASE

SYMPTOMS

Cold Hand or Feet—Numbness—Tingling—Fingers can turn pale and to red later—Brittle Nails caused form impaired Circulation—

CAUSES

The small arteries constrict or tighten in the extremities and this is brought on by exposure to cold or emotional upset. Lack of oxygen to the blood causes cold and blue fingers or toes. This could be caused by high blood pressure, emotional disturbances, drugs, connective tissue disease, inflammation of the arteries, or from vibrations of powerful equipment causing injury to the blood vessels.

NUTRITIONAL THERAPY

A high fiber diet is important including psyllium combinations to help rid the body of toxins in the arteries. Foods high in fiber are: grains, beans, lentils, vegetables, fruit, sprouts, seeds, nuts and herbs. Slow cooking of grains retains the enzymes for proper digestion. Grains such as brown rice, whole oats, millet, buckwheat, and barley, wheat, yellow cornmeal can be cooked in a wide mouth thermos or slow cooked in an oven of 200 degrees.

One doctor recommends swinging the arms like a windmilling propeller. Swing arms downward behind the body and upward in front of the body pulls gravity and forces the blood into the fingers.

Ginkgo is very effective in improving blood flow to the arteries. Suma and Butcher's Broom also improve circulation and strengthen the veins. Hawthorn, Ephedra, Ginger, Ginseng, Gotu Kola, and Horsetail are very beneficial.

HERBAL FORMULAS

Blood Cleansers—Circulatory System—Colon Cleansers Digestive System—Energy and Stamina—Glandular System—Immune Builders—Nervous System and Brain—Structural System—Female and Male Formulas—

VITAMINS, MINERALS AND SUPPLEMENTS

Vitamin A and E are important to improve circulation and prevent damage to the arteries. Vitamin B-complex helps the body eliminate fat from the arteries. Niacin improves circulation by dilating the small arteries. Vitamin C and bioflavonoids clean and strengthen the small arteries. It works with A and E to prevent free-radical damage in the arteries.

A multi-mineral supplement helps to prevent damage to the arteries. Calcium, vitamin D and magnesium help prevent lead, cadmium and other toxins from accumulating in the arteries, bones and brain. Selenium and Zinc are antioxidants which prevent damage to the arteries.

Germanium has improved poor circulation and has stopped the progress of advanced cases of Raynaud's disease. It may be seen as an effective treatment against stroke.

CoQ10 can prevent cell damage and protect the arteries and heart from damage. It can also prevent

tissue damage during surgery. Chlorophyll and blue-green algae protect the arteries from damage. They supply nutrients and strengthen the arteries.

Salmon oil and flaxseed oil reduce fatty deposits in the veins and prevent excess blood clotting. They also help in stress when emotions are the cause of restriction in the veins.

Bee pollen is rich in nutrients to feed and nourish the nerves and prevent toxins from accumulating in the veins. Canadian Elk antler increases stamina, heals the veins and improves circulation.

RHEUMATIC FEVER ———

SYMPTOMS

Pain—Inflammation—Stiffness—Joint Pain—Fever—Skin Rash—A child who is listless should be seen by a doctor. If left untreated, it can affect heart, brain or joints. It is a disease that is rarely seen, but never take chances with a small child who is listless and unresponsive. It most frequently occurs between the ages of three and eighteen. Residual heart disease is a possible complication.

CAUSES

Rheumatic fever is caused from a streptococcal bacteria which can also cause infection, strep throat, tonsillitis, scarlet fever and ear infections. When the body accumulates mucus and toxins, it becomes a breeding ground for germs and bacteria. When the body is clean, germs bacteria and viruses cannot accumulate because they have nothing to feed on.

Acute diseases are nature's way of cleansing the body of toxins. When they are not treated naturally and are suppressed by drugs such as aspirin, tylenol, cough suppressants and other drugs, they are pushed further into the organs of the body and stay there until the body provides another acute disease in the form of colds, coughs or fevers. This accumulates and provides an environment for germs, viruses and bacteria to breed on.

Rheumatic fever can be very serious and needs medical attention. Strep throat does not usually cause rheumatic fever. Treating acute diseases naturally will help prevent serious complication of disease.

Rheumatic fever introduces millions of bacteria to the walls, valves and muscle of the heart. The fever is actually a blessing and will drive the bacteria from the body. If there is not sufficient vitamin E in the body, it will cause damage to the heart covering and scarring. This is very harmful to the heart and surrounding tissues.

NUTRITIONAL THERAPY

To prevent a build-up of mucous and toxins in the body, eliminate mucous forming foods. They are: dairy products, meat, white flour products and sugar. Eat more fruits and vegetables, grains, nuts, seeds, sprouts, herbs, vitamins and minerals.

When treating acute diseases, avoid eating and drink only citrus juices, pure water and herbal teas. The body is attempting to eliminate toxins from the cells, which are squeezed into the stomach to be eliminated through the colon. When eating during an acute disease, the elimination process is stopped in order for the body to digest the food. It is better to fast for three days or more if needed and help nature cleanse the body.

Garlic, Red Clover, Echinacea, and Burdock are nature's antibiotics to kill bacteria. Comfrey and Fenugreek help eliminate mucus from the body. Catnip, Hops, and Chamomile help relax the body for proper healing.

HERBAL FORMULAS

Blood Cleansers—Colds, Flu, Fever and Allergies Cleansers—Colon Cleansers— Glandular System—Immune Builders— Infection Fighters—Nervous System and Brain—Urinary System—

VITAMINS, MINERALS AND SUPPLEMENTS

Vitamin A protects the mucous membranes against invading bacteria. It is essential for healthy mucous membranes. B-complex vitamins are needed every day. They are water soluble vitamins and cannot be stored in the body. They are essential for the nervous system and to protect the digestive tract and the immune system.

Vitamin C with bioflavonoids will help eliminate toxins from the liver. It should be taken at least four times a day because the kidneys eliminate it quickly.

Vitamin E is needed to prevent scar tissue from forming. It also provides oxygen to the cells to increase healing.

Calcium relaxes the muscles to speed healing. The body pulls calcium and magnesium from the body during acute diseases and fever. Potassium will protect the heart from damage. Prolonged fevers, vomiting and diarrhea cause a loss of potassium.

Selenium and zinc are healing for the body. Zinc speeds healing and prevents scarring. Silicon is healing for acute diseases.

Chlorophyll and blue-green algae heal and purify the blood. Acidophilus aids digestion and protects against bacteria.

SEASONAL AFFECTIVE SYNDROME

SYMPTOMS

Depression—Withdrawal—Social Isolation— Cravings—Weight Gain—Loss of Energy— Oversleep—Decreases Sexual Drive—

CAUSES

The lack of light through the pineal, pituitary and hypothalamus glands can cause this syndrome. It is common in areas that have less sunlight in the winter months. Excessive stress and nutritional deficiency reduce the function of the pineal gland. The winter months bring dark and dreary days and increases this syndrome. Mood changes occur with the seasons. It is also called "Winter Blues" and is recognized by the American Psychiatric Association as a psychiatric syndrome.

NUTRITIONAL THERAPY

Humans have seasonal rhythms, like bears and migratory birds, and need sunlight during their waking hours. Strong artificial light can have a positive effect on mental health as well as natural sunlight.

Wholesome, natural food and supplements can help the negative aspects of depression. In most cases, it is caused by an undernourished nervous system. It is caused by nutrient deficiency, toxemia, negative attitude and can be hereditary. Heredity is a problem because we inherit nutritional deficiencies.

Foods rich in B-complex vitamins will help in SAS syndrome. Almonds, rice bran, wheat germ, sunflower seeds, potatoes, millet, buckwheat, brown rice, barley, green vegetables, beans, molasses, and soybeans are beneficial. Complex carbohydrates found in whole grains contain tryptophan which has a calming effect. They stimulate the production of serotonin, a neurotransmitter that promotes feelings of well-being and counteracts depression. Fresh and steamed vegetable are rich in minerals which are needed for the nervous system and brain.

Gotu Kola, Ginkgo and Suma are brain foods. Capsicum helps clean and nourish the blood. Dong Quai relaxes the nerves. Chamomile, Hops, Scullcap, and Passion Flower help feed and nourish the nerves and brain. St. Johns Wort has been found effective for mood swings.

HERBAL FORMULAS

Blood Cleansers—Circulatory System—Colon Cleansers—Digestive System—Energy and Stamina—Glandular System—Immune Builders—Nervous System and Brain— Urinary System—Female or Male Formulas—

VITAMINS, MINERALS AND SUPPLEMENTS

Vitamins A and D are necessary for the proper assimilation of minerals. Vitamin A helps counteract the harmful effect of the toxic environment on the mucous membranes.

Vitamin C with bioflavonoids protects vitamins A, E and the B-complex vitamins from oxidation. It is essential for the formation of the adrenal and thyroid hormones. It helps the body deal with depression.

The B-complex vitamins are essential to prevent depression. They feed the nerves and brain. They help the liver eliminate toxins. They help in the digestion and assimilation of food to prevent malnutrition. Prolonged malnutrition can cause depression.

Minerals are important for the nervous system, especially calcium and magnesium. Silicon found in oatstraw and horsetail will help the body assimilate calcium and other essential minerals. Selenium and zinc help prevent free radical damage, along with vitamins A, C and E.

Lecithin is important for the health of the myelin sheath that protects the nerves. Chlorophyll and blue-green algae provide energy and help in depression. Essential fatty acids found in flaxseed oil and salmon oil work with vitamin E to help protect the body against depression.

SENILITY

SYMPTOMS

Also called Dementia—Secondary dementias are treatable. Memory Loss—Inability to think Straight and Reason to where it will interfere with family, social life and job. Depression—Loss of interest in Sex—

CAUSES

Malnutrition and drug use are the main causes of senility. Toxemia causes malnutrition, clogs the blood vessels and capillaries in the brain, and prevents nutrition from reaching the brain.

The brain is very sensitive and reacts to poor nutrition, drugs, air pollution, chlorine and toxins in water. Autopsies on individuals with senility disclosed very low brain levels of biochemical raw material essential for synthesizing neurotransmitters, which help make brain function possible.

NUTRITIONAL THERAPY

Malnutrition is usually caused by toxemia and lack of proper digestion. Food intake should consist of raw or slowly cooked foods to retain all the nutrients and enzymes. Lack of enzymes puts a burden on the digestive system. Raw nuts and seeds help brain function.

Millet and buckwheat are high in protein, calcium and magnesium and are easy to digest. A high fiber diet will help in toxemia and prevent toxic build-up. Foods that help nourish the brain are salmon, sardines, soybeans, wheat germ and lentils.

Fresh fruit and vegetables provide the body with enzymes to aid in digestion. Fruit are cleansers of the body, while vegetables are builders.

Gotu Kola, Ginkgo, Ginseng, Suma, Kelp, Pau D'Arco, and Hawthorn are foods for the brain. Ginkgo shows promise in preventing further deterioration of mental capacities.

HERBAL FORMULAS

Blood Cleansers—Circulatory System—Colon Cleansers—Digestive System—Energy and Stamina—Immune Builders—Nervous System and Brain—Structural Builders—Urinary System—Female and Male Formulas—

VITAMINS, MINERALS AND SUPPLEMENTS

Supplements are very critical for senility. The brain becomes starved when nutrients fail to reach the brain because of clogged veins. Free radical damage prevention is helped with vitamins A, C, E, and the minerals selenium and zinc. A lack of B-complex vitamins is often seen in the elderly. They prevent deterioration of the brain, especially B-12, which is involved in the production of myelin that covers the nerves and brain. Prolonged lack of B vitamins can cause neurological changes in the brain. Vitamin C with bioflavonoids helps keep the capillaries healthy and clean. It can help prevent them from clogging.

Lecithin is considered brain food. Choline, found in lecithin, is involved in the synthesis of acetylcholine in the body, which is involved with nerve impulses. It plays a major role in emotional behavior and health. Deficiencies increase with age, and supplements are necessary. Bee pollen increases energy and brain function. Chlorophyll and blue-green algae clean and nourish the blood vessels. Germanium and CoQ10 increase oxygen to the brain and improve memory.

SEXUALLY TRANSMITTED DISEASES

SYMPTOMS

Anal pain—Blisters around Vagina—Burning when urinating — Itching — Pelvic Inflammation—Penile discharge—Sore Throat—Flu-like Symptoms—The disease Chlamydia does not always have warning signs and couples can trade the infection back and forth. Other sexually transmitted diseases are Chancroid, Venereum, Granuloma, Inguinal, Genital Herpes, Trichomoniasis and AIDS.

CAUSES

Venereal diseases are transmitted as a result of intimate contact through sexual intercourse. They can cause sterility in women along with urinary tract problems, and in men, they can cause prostatic inflammation. These diseases are reaching epidemic proportions and the sad part is they can be prevented.

Each year, one in four sexually active teenage girls gets a sexually transmitted disease. Chlamydia is seen without symptoms in most cases. It can cause serious complications. It can cause urinary tract infections and adhesions results in infertility.

NUTRITIONAL THERAPY

The best protection to prevent STD's is abstinence. Condoms can give some protection but they are not fool proof. Three to four million Americans each year contact chlamydia. These women are very likely to have reproductive problems.

Education is the only way these diseases are going to be stop. STD's can kill newborn babies.

Syphilis can cause miscarriage, stillbirth and birth defects. Neurological damage is very common in some newborn babies.

Wholesome food can help to overcome the symptoms of these diseases. These viruses are in the body for life and can be transmitted to others. A high fiber diet will help prevent auto-intoxication. Fresh fruit and vegetables, whole grains, sprouts, fresh seeds and nuts will help keep the body clean.

Blood cleansers are Burdock, Chaparral, Pau D'Arco, Garlic and Echinacea which act like an antibiotic. A vegetarian diet has been beneficial to AIDS patients.

Sugar is very harmful to the body because it robs essential nutrients. Calcium and other minerals are depleted along with the B-complex vitamins.

HERBAL FORMULAS

Blood Cleansers—Colon Cleansers—Immune Builders—Infection Fighters—Nervous System and Brain—Urinary System—Female and Male Formulas—

VITAMINS, MINERALS AND SUPPLEMENTS

Vitamins A and C, in large doses, can help infections. Vitamins E and K provide oxygen to the cells and help purify the blood. The B-complex vitamins help to detoxify the liver.

Minerals are essential for the immune system. Selenium and zinc help protect the immune system. Calcium, magnesium, manganese and potassium are needed to balance the pH factor in the body.

Supplements to protect the immune system are: acidophilus, chlorophyll, blue-green algae, lecithin, bee pollen, germanium and CoQ10.

SHINGLES

(Herpes Zoster)

SYMPTOMS

Intense Pain—Rash—Fever—Itching—Blister—Shingles is the same virus that causes Chicken pox and can be serious. It can affect the ophthalmic nerves and cause temporary blindness or permanent scarring of the cornea. Paralysis can result if the facial nerves are affected.

Fever and pain occur for days before the rash appears. Small red areas appear and puff up with fluid the size of a quarter. The skin tightens over the blisters until they erupt.

The disease is increasing by a million cases each year.

CAUSES

The virus in shingles lies dormant in the nerve cells near the spinal cord and can be activated by a weak immune system, stress or trauma. It is considered a relapse of the childhood disease chicken pox and is usually seen after the age of 50.

A weak immune system is the main cause. Lack of proper digestion and assimilation can cause malnutrition and weaken the immune system. Autointoxication is common in the elderly because of bad diet and poor elimination.

NUTRITIONAL THERAPY

When the eruptions appear, wear cotton clothing so the skin can breathe. The skin is the largest elimination organ and is trying to eliminate toxins from the cells. It should be treated as an acute disease; stop eating and use orange, grapefruit, lemon and lime juices. Herbs will help the cleansing process and ease the pain and discomfort. Use a lower bowel cleanser to speed the elimination process.

Applying vitamin E to the skin will help heal and relieve the pain. It will also help prevent scarring. Aloe vera juice will also help.

Use the nervine herbs in extract or capsules to relax and heal the nerve endings. St John's Wort, Hops, Scullcap, Passion Flower, Valerian Root, Black Cohosh, Black Walnut, Comfrey, Fenugreek and Golden Seal will all help shingles.

HERBAL FORMULAS

Blood Cleansers—Circulatory System—Colds, Flu, Fevers and Allergy Formulas—Colon Cleansers—Digestion—Immune Builders—Infection Fighters—Nervous System and Brain—Urinary System—Female and Male Formulas—

VITAMINS, MINERALS AND SUPPLEMENTS

Antioxidants, will help keep shingles under control. They are vitamins A, C, D, E, and minerals selenium and zinc. They help prevent free radical damage to the cells. Vitamin C, taken every hour for the first few days will ease the pain and help healing. 1,000 milligrams should be taken every hour at the beginning. Vitamin A in fish oils and beta-carotene will also help the healing. 50,000 I.U. units a day has been recommended.

Calcium and magnesium are relaxing and soothing for the nerves. Silicon is essential for the assimilation of calcium and other minerals. Potassium promotes healing and builds resistance to infection. Sodium helps dissolve poisons in the body. Zinc is healing. Kelp is an herb that contains a high content of vitamins and minerals.

Lecithin is healing and protects the nerves. Acidophilus protects the immune system. Germanium and CoQ10 help in healing and provide oxygen to the cells. Chlorophyll and blue-green algae clean the blood and provide nutrients.

SILVER FILLINGS
(Mercury Amalgam)

SYMPTOMS

Some symptoms are allergies—Anxiety—Confusion—Depression—Fatigue—Facial and Back Pain—Headaches—Irritability—Indigestion—Lack of Self Control—Loss of self confidence—Metallic Taste—Nervousness—Personality Change—Tremors—uncontrollable Crying— Uncontrollable Eye Movement—Vertigo—

Mercury kills cells and interferes with their ability to exchange oxygen, nutrients and waste products through the cell membrane. Mercury lodged in the cells causes the immune system to destroy its own tissue. Autoimmune diseases are increasing.

Diabetes, multiple sclerosis, chronic fatigue syndrome, and lupus are examples of autoimmune diseases.

CAUSES

There are nearly 100 chemicals that are placed daily into dental patients' mouths. Some of them are mercury, copper, nickel, beryllium, zinc, phenol, formaldehyde, disocyanate and acetone.

Mercury has been scientifically proven to cause damage to the developing fetus, cell walls, immune system, nervous system, heart, lungs, muscles, liver, kidneys, mouth, thyroid, adrenals, pituitary, pancreas and the spleen.

Mercury vapor exposure is very high during periods when people chew gum, grind or clench their teeth. Mercury vapor from amalgam fillings has an adverse affect on the T-lymphocytes involved in immunity. It can build up over a number of years and lead to progressive degeneration of the brain, liver, kidneys, and intestines. It is readily absorbed in the lungs and then distributed to other parts of the body.

Some of the most common sources of mercury poisoning are silver amalgam fillings, pesticides, pharmaceutical drugs, cosmetics, and large ocean fish such as swordfish and tuna. We ingest and inhale mercury through our food, air, water and soil. It can even be absorbed through the skin. Our bodies convert it into a toxic form called methyl mercury.

NUTRITIONAL THERAPY

Vegetables are important, especially cabbage, broccoli, carrots, asparagus and brussels sprouts. They are rich in minerals. Mercury can accumulate when minerals are lacking. Eat lots of vegetables, both raw and lightly steamed. Brown rice contains B-complex vitamins and will protect the nerves. Millet is rich in protein, calcium and magnesium which nourishes the brain and nerves.

Fruit are cleansers, especially citrus, lemons, limes, oranges and grapefruit. Apples contain pectin and protect against heavy metal poisoning.

Whole grains are rich in fiber and will prevent the accumulation of toxic metals. Whole wheat, whole oats, barley, buckwheat, millet, quinoa, and amaranth are all high in fiber.

Herbs that will help counteract metal poisoning are the sulphur herbs: Alfalfa, Burdock, Cayenne, Catnip, Chaparral, Comfrey, Dandelion, Echinacea, Eyebright, Fennel, Garlic, Juniper, Kelp, Lobelia and Watercress.

HERBAL FORMULAS

Blood Cleansers—Circulatory System—Colon Cleansers—Digestive System—Immune Builders—Nervous System and Brain—Structural—Urinary System—Female and Male Formulas—

VITAMINS, MINERALS AND SUPPLEMENTS

Vitamin A is necessary for the cells to throw off the poisons from chemicals in the air, food and water. A deficiency of vitamin A can cause lesions from radiation, antibiotics and metal poisoning. B-complex vitamins protect the nervous and immune systems. They are needed daily. Deficiencies of B6 suppress the immune system. A weak immune system has a difficult time eliminating mercury. B-complex vitamins are necessary for the liver to detoxify.

Vitamin C with bioflavonoids stimulates natural interferon production in the body. When a virus or foreign material invades the cells, interferon keeps the virus or toxic material from multiplying. Vitamin C needs to be replaced daily.

Vitamin E, an antioxidant, prevents free radical damage. It prevents B-complex from oxidizing when present in the digestive tract. It provides oxygen from the cells and protects from mercury poisoning.

Calcium and magnesium are natural chelating minerals. They protect against mercury poisoning as an alkaline forming mineral.

Selenium works with vitamin E to enhance it's metabolic reactions. Zinc is an effective free radical inhibitor. It helps in the proper utilization of vitamin A.

Chlorophyll and blue-green algae are effective in eliminating toxins and heavy metals from the body. Lecithin is necessary to protect the nerves from damage. Acidophilus protects against the accumulation of bad bacteria. It helps in the absorption of nutrients. Germanium and CoQ10 help prevent the accumulation of toxins in the body. They nourish and supply oxygen to the cells. Bee pollen is rich in nutrients to protect against cell damage from toxic metals.

SINUSITIS

(Sinus Infection)

SYMPTOMS

Facial Pain — Earache — Headache — Toothache—Tenderness on the Cheekbones, Face and Forehead—Dry cough—Bad Breath—Fever—Hazy Feeling in the Head—It can cause burning and tearing eyes.

When the sinuses drain down the throat, if there is infection, it can affect the lungs and cause asthma, bronchitis, laryngitis or even pneumonia.

CAUSES

Acute sinusitis is usually caused by colds or bacterial and viral infections of the upper respiratory tract nose or throat. It occurs in the nasal sinuses, which are located in the bones surrounding the eyes and nose. Injury to the nasal bone, irritants such as fumes, air pollution, smoking and growths in the nose can cause chronic sinusitis.

An over-acid condition in the stomach will cause sinus infections. Infections are suspected when the mucus drainage is greenish or yellowish. Poor digestion of starch, sugar and dairy products will cause a runny nose. Metal poisoning such as mercury and lead can cause irritation to the stomach and sinus and cause infections.

Sinusitis is usually caused by suppressing a cold, flu, sore throat, infected tonsils, or other acute diseases. The mucus and toxins are trying to eliminate, and when they are suppressed, it hardens in the throat, sinuses, head or wherever there is an acute disease. There are eight sinus cavities located in the vicinity of the eyes and nose. Anyone of them can accumulate mucus and become inflamed.

Decayed teeth, enlarged and infected adenoids, cigarette smoke, and dusty air can irritate the delicate sinuses.

NUTRITIONAL THERAPY

Sinusitis ia an acute disease and needs to be treated naturally. A short fast using citrus juices, herbal teas and extracts to help the body eliminate the toxins can be beneficial.

Nose drops and antihistamines only increase the problem. They may stop the drainage, but they drive the infection further into the cavities, the mucus becomes hardened.

A cleansing fast, using herbal teas, extracts, citrus juices and herbs that loosen and clean the sinuses will assist nature in cleaning naturally. Allergies are implicated with sinus infections. The irritants can continually irritate the delicate sinus membranes and cause infections. An elimination diet will help find the food or irritants that cause the problems. Perfume, household cleansers, and other air pollutant can cause irritations.

A humidifier will benefit especially during the winter months. The air inside is dry and causes the sinuses to become dry and brittle, which creates an environment for germs and viruses.

Eliminate congesting foods such as meat, dairy products, white flour products and sugar.

Carrots, and carrot and celery juice, chard, spinach, string beans, broccoli, squash, apricots, and sweet potatoes are high in vitamin A. Grains such as buckwheat, wheat, whole oats, rye, and brown rice, cooked in a thermos, will retain enzymes and B-complex vitamins. Slow cooking of grains, and steamed vegetables retain their vitamin and mineral content.

Herbs that help sinuses congestion are Comfrey, Fenugreek, Yerba Santa, Marshmallow, Mullein, Slippery Elm, Lobelia, Aloe Vera, Ephedra, Burdock, Red Clover and White Oak Bark.

HERBAL FORMULAS

Blood Cleansers—Circulatory System—Colds, Flu, Fever and Allergic Formulas—Immune Builder—Infection Fighters—Nervous System and Brain—

VITAMINS, MINERALS AND SUPPLEMENTS

A deficiency of vitamin A can cause mucus to harden and destroy the cilia which protects against invading toxins. It strengthens the immune system. B-complex are important for the nervous system and are needed for healthy mucous membranes. They are important for overall health. Vitamin C with bioflavonoids helps stimulate interferon production to fight infections. Vitamin E is an antioxidant to protect the cells against carcinogens and toxins which include mercury, lead, carbon tetrachloride, nitrites and nitrates found in cigarette smoke, air pollution, and cured meats.

Minerals regulate the flow of bodily fluids. They work with vitamins to prevent infections. Calcium and magnesium are involved in nerve transmissions. They help to build cells. Selenium and zinc are antioxidants and work with vitamin E to protect the immune system. They help speed the healing of infections.

Acidophilus is a natural antibiotic. It is needed to restore natural, internal, good bacteria. Chlorophyll and blue-green algae help the body produce natural interferon. Germanium and CoQ10 increase immune response and protect the body from bacteria and viruses.

SKIN PROBLEMS

(Acne, Eczema, Dermatitis, Psoriasis)

SYMPTOMS

*Acne—Blackheads—Pimples—Whiteheads—
Itching—Flaking—Redness—Dryness—
Bumps—*

CAUSES

The skin's health depends on the health of the inner organs. If the glands in the walls of the stomach do not secrete sufficient hydrochloric acid, the skin can lose its surface acidity which increases the chance of infection. Digestion, assimilation and elimination are vital to a healthy skin. If the skin is abused with frequent washing with harsh soaps that are highly alkaline, it removes all the protective oil as well as the acidity.

Skin diseases are a sign of toxic irritations. The colon, liver and kidneys are responsible for eliminating toxins from the body, but when they are overloaded with mucus and poisons, the skin and lungs take over. The skin is not supposed to eliminate these toxins and when it does, it causes irritations.

Dead cells accumulate along with perspiration, gases, wastes, rancid oils, bacteria and viruses and irritations can occur. When not properly cleaned, blackheads, pimples, whiteheads in the clogged pores can result. Dirt and pollution accumulate daily on the surface of the skin.

A combination of fat and protein are the most common causes of pimples, acne and boils. Foods responsible for clogging the skin pores are sugar, milk, cheese, ice cream, fatty meats, peanut butter, fried foods and processed salty nuts.

Excess fat, protein and malfunctioning of protein metabolism can also discharge in the form of callouses, moles, tumors and warts. It is also felt that too much sugar in the diet surfaces to the outer skin in the form of brown spots and freckles brough out by the heat of the sun.

Constipation is associated with skin problems. A diet high in fried foods, salt, sugar and refined carbohydrates is irritating to the skin. Chocolate is high in molecular carbons, sugar and xanthines which causes diminished fluidity of the surface skin. Xanthines are found in coffee, tea, chocolate and cola drinks.

NUTRITIONAL THERAPY

Use natural cleansers that are pH balanced and won't dry the skin. Use natural ingredients in skin cleansers such as lanolin, cocoa butter or glycerine. Avoid colorings, perfumes, harmful dyes and chemicals in skin cleansers. Avoid cleansing creams containing mineral oil, which destroys vitamin A and clogs the pores.

A change of diet using whole grains, beans, fresh fruit and vegetables, sprouts, seeds and nuts will help. Fresh carrot juice with parsley and celery is rich in vitamin A and zinc and are necessary for healthy skin and healing.

Skin brushing helps rid the skin of dead cells. It also cleans the lymphatic system. It helps with poor circulation. Dry skin brushing using a brush made with natural bristles is best.

Aloe Vera is used effectively for treating dry skin, burns, skin irritations,and acne. Black Walnut, Golden Seal, Echinacea, Red Clover, and Yellow Dock help in maintaining healthy skin.

HERBAL FORMULAS

Blood Cleansers—Circulatory System—Colon Cleansers—Digestive System—Immune Builders—Infection Fighters—Urinary System—

VITAMINS, MINERALS AND SUPPLEMENTS

Vitamin A is essential in maintaining the health of the skin. It has a healing effect on acne and psoriasis. The antioxidants, including vitamin C maintain and restore the health of the tissues.

The B-complex vitamins are necessary for healthy skin. Vitamin E prevents fats stored in body from causing harmful effects.

A multi-mineral supplement works with vitamins for healthy skin. Zinc is healing for acne and other skin problems. Chlorophyll and blue-green algae keep the blood and skin clean. Acidophilus helps in proper digestion and acts as an antibiotic. Germanium and CoQ10 help in protecting the immune system. Flaxseed oil and salmon oil help in keeping the skin soft and prevent dry skin.

SMOKING ⸻

SYMPTOMS

Lung irritation—Inflammation and Excess Mucus—Chronic Cough—Chronic Bronchitis—Emphysema—Lung Cancer—High Blood Pressure—Heart Disease—Stroke—

CAUSES

Nicotine is a very toxic drug. It is very addictive. It is powerful and harmful, therefore; the body quickly develops tolerance to it to protect itself. Tobacco is the most addictive drug in the form of cigarette smoking and is harder to quit the habit than to stop drinking alcohol or heroine. Dr. Andrew Weil, M. D, & Winifred Rosen, in their book, *Chocolate To Morphine,* says, "Smoke from cigarettes inhaled deeply delivers concentrated nicotine to vital brain centers within a few seconds-faster than heroine reaches the brain when it is injected into a vein in the arm. This fact probably explains why tobacco in the form of cigarettes is so addictive."

Tobacco smoke contains lead, cadmium, and carbon monoxide which causes deposits in the artery walls. It contains hydrogen cyanide which irritates the lining of the lungs and bronchi and can cause pneumonia or bronchitis.

It works like heroin, cocaine and alcohol. It isn't relaxing; it makes the heart pump faster and work harder and causes palpitations.

Withdrawal symptoms are depression, cough, anxiety, headaches, stomach cramps, irritability, hunger, and cravings for tobacco that lasts for about two weeks.

It is very harmful during pregnancy. It can cause abortion, stillbirth, premature births and smaller birth weight. Women also are at risk of cancer and osteoporosis.

NUTRITIONAL THERAPY

Smoking is considered a very serious health problem which is preventable. It causes premature death and disability from heart disease, lung cancer, and respiratory illnesses.

A cleansing diet will help rid the cells of nicotine. Drink lots of liquids. Citrus juices and herbal teas will help the cleansing process.

Eat nutritional foods such as grains, beans, vegetables and fruit. Strengthen the nervous system by eating calcium rich, and B-complex rich foods. Calcium foods are abundant and some are kelp, almonds, parsley, dandelion greens, beans, fresh vegetables, sesame and sunflower seeds. B vitamins are found in whole grains, seeds, nuts, beans, wheat, almonds, wheat germ, millet, brown rice, molasses, honey, egg yolk, sprouts, yogurt, fish, lecithin, and oatmeal.

Carrot, celery and parsley juice will protect the lungs from damage.

Herbs to help quit smoking are Ephedra, Lobelia, Ginseng, Ginkgo, and Suma.

HERBAL FORMULAS

Blood Cleansers—Circulatory System—Colon Cleansers—Energy and Stamina—Glandular System—Immune Builders—Nervous system and Brain—Structural—Urinary System—Female and Male Formulas—

VITAMINS, MINERALS AND SUPPLEMENTS

Antioxidant vitamins and minerals are essential because of the free-radical damage smoking causes. These include vitamins A, D, C, E, and the minerals selenium and zinc. Vitamin B-complex protects the nervous system and damage to the cells. Vitamin C is depleted rapidly when smoking and is needed in large amounts. Vitamin E protects the veins.

Minerals are essential to protect the immune system.

Acidophilus will help protect against digestive problems which can accompany cigarette smoking and protect the colon. Chlorophyll and blue-green algae clean the blood and help the body produce interferon to prevent germs and viruses from invading. It also protects against cancer. Germanium and CoQ10 are necessary to improve oxygen to the cells and are free radical scavengers.

STRESS ————

SYMPTOMS

Anxiety — Depression — Chronic Fatigue — Irritability—Low Stress Tolerance—Unable to Cope—Nervous Exhaustion—Insomnia— Panic Attacks—Unable to Relax—Illness, because the immune system is weakened.

Physical symptoms of stress are stomach muscles tightens and causes nausea or digestive problems.

Blood pressure increases, sweaty palms, trembling without being cold, tense muscles in the neck and shoulders. A shaky feeling, when almost in an accident. Dry mouth, this happens to speaker, who are nervous.

Emotional symptoms of stress are inability to retain information, poor concentration, negative thoughts, stubborn attitude to prevent being taken advantage of, loss of sense of humor, demanding attitude, situations

become magnified, withdrawn or leaving family and a critical attitude.

CAUSES

Lack of essential nutrients causes a weakened immune system and put a strain on the adrenal and thymus glands. A low immune response causes the nervous system to fail which prevents the body from handling stress. A strong nervous system is essential to protect against stress.

Negative emotions have a harmful effect on immune response. So positive thoughts and images can help restore immune function. Laughter has a positive benefit on hormones, lung and heart function. An imbalance in the hormonal and nervous system can cause kidney damage, cardiovascular diseases and even death. A balance in work, relationships, self-worth, religious beliefs and recreation are seen in people who can handle stress.

Everyone has to deal with stress. It is how we choose to handle stress that determines its effect on our bodies.

NUTRITIONAL THERAPY

A diet change is needed to restore a healthy immune and nervous system. Whole grains are high in fiber and B-vitamins needed for a healthy immune system and enhanced digestion and intestinal function. Fruit are cleansers of the body and will boost the immune system. Fresh vegetable salads improve enzyme function. Vegetables boost the immune system such as: broccoli, carrots, squash, onions, garlic, leeks, chives, watercress, cauliflower, Brussels' sprouts, cabbage and kale. Sea vegetables are rich in minerals, kelp and dulse. Shiitake mushrooms have anti-tumor and enhance the immune system. If you can purchase organic food, it will help protect the immune function from pesticides and herbicides.

Pinto beans, lentils and dried peas are nourishing. Raw seeds and nuts contain anti-stress nutrients. Sprouts are considered live food to help the body handle stress.

Emotional helps for stress can change your outlook on life. Seek for peace and serenity through meditation and prayer which will help to establish self-control. Stress your good points and learn to be less critical. This will increase self confidence. If a situation is overwhelming, take time to evaluate and respond. Don't worry about pleasing everyone, which is impossible, but try to see the other person's point of view. Relationships with others will improve.

Herbs that help the body deal with stress are Ginseng, Dong Quai, Echinacea, Ginkgo, Gotu Kola and Suma. The nervine herbs will strengthen the nervous system such as Hops, Scullcap, Passion Flower, Lobelia, Valerian Root, Wood Betony and Lady's Slipper.

HERBAL FORMULAS

Blood Cleansers—Circulatory System—Colds, Flu, Fever and Allergy Formulas—Colon Cleansers—Digestive System—Energy and Stamina—Glandular System—Immune Builders—Nervous System and Brain— Urinary System—Female and Male Formulas—

VITAMINS, MINERALS AND SUPPLEMENTS

The antioxidants protect the cells from free radical damage. They are vitamin A, D, C, and E and the minerals selenium and zinc. The B-complex vitamins are vital for a healthy immune system. High amounts of vitamin C are needed when under stress. It protects the body when it is weak and under stress. Vitamin E protects the cells from damage.

Minerals are important when under stress. Immunity is increased with selenium, zinc, manganese, calcium, magnesium and copper. Zinc deficiency can cause the thymus gland to shrink and reduce immunity.

Acidophilus is important as an antibiotic and to improve digestive problems. Chlorophyll and blue-green algae can rebuild the thymus, and detoxify and enhance the immune system. Lecithin breaks down fatty deposits and strengthens the nervous system. Flaxseed and salmon oil increase the white blood cells which attack foreign cells. Amino acids such as tyrosine protect against stress. Glutamine protects the brain by eliminating the waste ammonia, a by-product of protein breakdown, which is toxic to the brain.

STROKE

SYMPTOMS

Early Warnings: Fainting—Stumbling— Numbness or Paralysis of the finger of one hand—Blurring of Vision—Loss of Speech— Loss of Memory—A mild Attack can cause temporary confusion—Light Headedness— Speech Difficulty—Loss of Consciousness— Amnesia—Coma for short or long periods.

CAUSES

A Thrombus is a clot inside an artery that blocks the flow of blood to the brain are Embolism is a wandering clot carried in the bloodstream until it wedges in one of the arteries leading to the brain. Aneurysms are blood-filled pouches that balloon out from weak spots in the artery wall and burst. A hemorrhage is a defective artery in the brain that bursts flooding the surrounding tissue with blood.

The main cause of a stroke is a toxic blood stream from autointoxication and constipation. The blood containing poisons circulates through the arterial system which consists of nearly a thousand miles of arteries, veins and capillaries. The walls of the arteries collect toxins, thicken and harden. When they become brittle, pieces break off and clog the arteries. The artery wall can also burst under pressure.

The Chinese see strokes as being caused by "blood stasis" and "stagnation of liver-qi." Chinese medical practitioners prevent strokes and also treat them by treating constipation. American health doctors and naturopaths have known that constipation causes many illnesses including strokes.

Smoking, birth control pills and high stress lifestyle are some factors that lead to stroke. Also a lack of exercise, high-fat, high-sodium diet, and certain drugs and medication contribute to strokes.

NUTRITIONAL THERAPY

Treating constipation is very important in preventing a stroke. Grains are high in fiber such as wheat, rye buckwheat, millet, whole oats and brown rice. Fresh fruit and vegetables, nuts, seeds, sprouts, beans and fresh vegetable juices help to clean the blood stream and also provide nutrients for healthy blood and veins.

A natural oral chelation cleans the entire system and helps the blood flow more freely and improves circulation so nutrition and oxidation can function normally. A good chelation formula contains vitamins, minerals, glandular extracts, amino acids and herbs that supply nutrition vital for maximum circulation. These chelating elements work in a bonding reaction and surround the plaque, much like a magnet attracts metals. The chelation elements remove the deposits on the arterial wall. Cholesterol and other fatty substances in the arteries that make up the plaque are softened and exposed to the blood, which is then able to metabolize these deposits, breaking them into smaller molecules. The toxins are bound to the chelating elements and pass through the bloodstream and are excreted in the urine by the kidneys. This chelating combination is effective in removing high levels of toxic metals.

Many people using this formula have found that it improves memory, increases energy, smooths skin, lowers high blood pressure, and in some cases has reduced diabetics need for insulin.

Cayenne is one of nature's best herbs for nourishing the heart and keeping the veins and arteries in good condition. Bugleweed, Burdock, Butcher's Broom, Garlic, Ephedra, Ginkgo, Hawthorn, Suma, and Gotu Kola are all nourishing for the veins.

HERBAL FORMULAS

Blood Cleansers—Circulatory System—Colon Cleansers—Digestive System—Energy and Stamina—Immune Builders—Nervous System and Brain—Urinary System—Female and Male Formulas—

VITAMINS, MINERALS AND SUPPLEMENTS

Vitamin E is essential for the heart. It supplies oxygen to the heart muscles and protects the veins and dissolves toxins. Vitamin A is an antioxidant along with vitamins D and C and the minerals selenium and zinc. They protect the immune system and cells from free-radical damage.

Minerals work with vitamins for pure blood. They are essential in keeping the body's chemistry in balance. Iron is essential to supply oxygen to the cells. Silicon helps the body utilize calcium and prevent deposits from adhering to the veins. Potassium is necessary for a healthy heart. Calcium and magnesium are needed for the function of the nerves and brain.

Lecithin is necessary to prevent fatty deposits. Chlorophyll and blue-green algae protect the immune system by stimulating the body to produce interferon. Flaxseed oil and salmon oil are essential for healthy arteries. They help eliminate toxins from the blood. Germanium and CoQ10 improve oxygen to the tissues and organs. They help rebuild heart damage and prevent strokes. L-carnitine helps to dissolve fatty deposits in the veins around the heart.

SUDDEN INFANT DEATH SYNDROME

SYMPTOMS

There are no visible symptoms to predict this syndrome. With this, the babies don't seem to cry out as they do when they are hurting, or hungry.

CAUSES

It is one of the leading causes of infant death in the United States. The winter is when most deaths occur. Underweight babies from poor families are prone. The mothers are usually under 20. The babies who die from SIDS death seem to be healthy.

There is evidence linking infant formulas to high blood lead levels and SIDS. (Robert S. Mendelsohn, M.D., *How to Raise A Healthy Child, In Spite of Your Doctor.*) Dr. M. Erickson reported in (*Pediatric Research,* October 1983). He says that there are high levels of lead in infants who die of SIDS.

There are 10,000 SIDS deaths that occur in the United States each year. The central nervous system is effected and suppresses the involuntary act of breathing. Dr. Mendelshon suggested that breast fed babies are less susceptible to SIDS. They have less allergies, respiratory diseases, gastroenteritis, hypoglycemia, obesity, hypoglycemia and SIDS.

There is evidence that SIDS is caused by the pertussis vaccine administered to new born babies at two, four and six months of age. (Harris L. Coulter and Barbara Loe Fisher, *A Shot In The Dark*, Avery Publishing Group, Inc., pp 50-57).

NUTRITIONAL THERAPY

Mothers should nurse their babies if possible. If they cannot, they need to be aware of the high content of protein baby formulas. It is possible to make your own formulas from raw almonds, cashews, or sesame seeds. See *Health Handbook,* page 131 to 145 for more information on feeding infants.

Mothers should be aware of the importance of a nutritional diet when they are pregnant. Using foods rich in minerals, steamed and fresh vegetables, fruit, whole grains such as millet, brown rice, whole wheat, whole oats, and buckwheat strengthen the veins and supply vitamins. Pinto beans help eliminate toxic metals and supply fiber and protein. Raw almonds are high in calcium, magnesium and protein.

Avoid chemicals when pregnant, for they overwork the liver. Avoid drugs during pregnancy, even aspirin, it interferes with the clotting of blood, so bleeding could develop, It could also cause damage to the fetus. Caffeine, alcohol and smoking interfere with the development and growth of the baby. Avoiding these harmful substances will help build a stronger baby and prevent SIDS.

Herbs are rich in minerals and help strengthen the uterus and provide nutrients for the growing fetus. Red raspberry is rich in calcium and iron. Alfalfa contains protein, vitamins and minerals. It is also a blood cleanser. It is high in vitamin K which is necessary to clot the blood and prevent hemorrhage. Kelp is rich in minerals and Dandelion cleans and protects the liver. Herbal calcium formulas containing Oatstraw and Horsetail will nourish the bones and teeth. Slippery Elm is nourishing.

HERBAL FORMULAS

These are formulas mothers can take to nourish, clean and build her health and the health of her baby. Blood Cleansers (in small amounts)—Colon Cleansers (in small amounts)—Immune Builders—Structural—Female Formulas—

VITAMINS, MINERALS AND SUPPLEMENTS

Vitamin A is needed, especially after the first three months, if the mother is nursing. Vitamin C is needed every day. A baby can get this through the nursing mother if she takes supplements. Bottle fed babies are most likely to be deficient in vitamins A and C, calcium and iron.

Babies need essential fatty acids. A flaxseed oil supplement or cooked flaxseeds using the liquid can help.

Mothers can take supplements to help a baby with a cold. I have seen nursing mothers use immune formulas, and vitamins A and C to heal the baby of an eye infection.

TICKS, LICE, BED BUGS, FLEAS _____

(Lyme Disease, Rocky Mountain Spotted Fever)

SYMPTOMS

Head lice are most often found on the scalp and hair, behind the ears and the back of the neck—The tiny nits (eggs) are laid at the base of a hairshaft, the attached egg moves away from the scalp as the hair grows. Itching is one symptom—The lice and eggs may look like dandruff.

Symptoms of Lyme disease are rash—Flu-like symptoms—Headaches—Fever—Chill—Stiff Neck—Aching Muscles—Joint Aches—Fatigue—Lyme disease can be treated in the early stages—Symptoms can appear months after the tick has bitten. The tick can inject a disease-causing bacteria.

CAUSES

The disease is most active during June and July. Not everyone who is bitten with a tick gets the disease. Internal and external conditions of the body can supply food to support their life. When the blood is pure and the body clean, the ticks, bed bugs, and lice will not invade.

A high sugar and fat diet will attract insects. The skin is the largest elimination organ and will eliminate toxins and attract bugs when the diet is unnatural.

NUTRITIONAL THERAPY

Prevention is the only sure way to avoid tick bites. Wear long sleeved shirts, boots or put socks over pants. Wear a hat to prevent them from getting in the hair. Check thoroughly after being in the woods.

To release a tick, pour rubbing alcohol or oil, use tweezers and gently twist out. This is a method I used when my children were young. Disinfect the area with soap and water and then disinfect with alcohol.

A diet high in fiber and natural food will help keep the body clean and protect against infections. Sugar attracts insects.

Herbs are important to prevent infections. Golden Seal, Echinacea, Burdock, and Garlic will help in infections. Rubbing with Lobelia will disinfect and prevent infections. Lemon or lime juice rubbed on the area will help prevent infections. Aloe Vera rubbed on the area will help the healing.

HERBAL FORMULAS

Blood Cleansers—Colon Cleansers—Immune Builders—Infection Fighters—

VITAMINS, MINERALS AND SUPPLEMENTS

Vitamins A and C protect against infections. Vitamin E prevents scarring from bites. Use both inside and out. B-complex vitamins help keep the blood clean.

Minerals are important to keep the body clean inside and out. Sulphur works with the B-vitamins as an oxidizing agent. Foods rich in sulphur are cabbage, cauliflower, horse radish, brussels sprouts, watercress, parsley, celery and kale.

Chlorophyll and blue-green algae act as an antibiotic to clean the blood.

TMJ

(Temporomandibular Joint Syndrome)

SYMPTOMS

Pain in the muscles and joints of the jaws—It can radiate to the face—and neck—Frequent clenching of jaws—Clicking sounds when eating—Headaches—Ringing in the Ears—Locked Jaws—Pain when chewing or yawning—

CAUSES

A misaligned bite causes tension and stress which puts pressure on the jaw area and the muscles and nerves around it. Bone loss in the jaws can cause damage in that area.

Tension and stress are implicated with TMJ. When some people are under stress, they clench or grind their teeth. An injury, osteoarthritis, or poor dental work can cause this problem.

NUTRITIONAL THERAPY

A dentist can determine if a series of dental adjustments can help relieve tension on the teeth and joints. Many people have found improvement by wearing a splint while sleeping. This takes the strain off the joints.

A diet rich in B-vitamins, calcium and magnesium feeds and nourishes the nervous system. Buckwheat, millet, wheat, whole oats, rye, barley, and other grains provide B vitamins and other nutrients. Eliminating sugar helps to restore bone and nerve health. Sugar depletes calcium, other minerals and B vitamins from the body. Smoking and high meat diet causes bone loss.

Stress and relaxation therapy are beneficial to relax the jaw muscles.

Herbs that help in building strong bones and nerves are: Horsetail, Oatstraw, Comfrey, Hops, Scullcap, Passion Flower, Lady's Slipper, Wood Betony and Valerian Root.

HERBAL FORMULAS

Blood Cleansers—Colon Cleansers—Energy and Stamina—Immune Builders—Nervous System and Brain—Structural—Female or Male Formulas—

VITAMINS, MINERALS AND SUPPLEMENTS

Antioxidants will strengthen the immune system Vitamin A, C, D, and E along with minerals are important, especially selenium and zinc. Magnesium, calcium and silicon are important for healthy bones.

Lecithin will nourish the nerves. Acidophilus will help in the assimilation of calcium. Chlorophyll and blue-green algae are nourishing

Flaxseed oil and salmon oil help in every function of the body. Germanium and CoQ10 help in providing oxygen to the cells. They protect the immune system.

TINNITUS

SYMPTOMS

Sounds of Ringing in Ears—Whistling—Roaring—Buzzing—Cricket sounds when no physical outside sounds are present. First they come and go and later in advanced stages the sound is constant. The noise is only heard by the sufferer.

CAUSES

One cause of tinnitus is an irritation of the nerve endings in the inner ear by loud noises. Chemicals and drugs can injure the internal ear which is very sensitive. Prescription drugs can effect hearing loss and tinnitus which can be temporary or permanent. An overdose of Quinine can cause hearing loss. Aspirin used in large amounts has been known to cause tinnitus and hearing loss in many people. Nicotine is a vasoconstrictor and inhibits the flow of blood by causing the blood vessels to narrow. Mercury poisoning is another cause of tinnitus.

It can also be caused by ear accumulations, glandular problems, and high blood pressure.

NUTRITIONAL THERAPY

Exercise, a change of diet and learning stress reduction has helped with tinnitus. Stress reduction will help. Stress causes the adrenal glands to secrete the hormone adrenalin. Its main function is in the constriction of blood vessels, and toxic waste is not eliminated when blood vessels are constricted.

A clean colon will assure that nutrients will be absorbed and assimilated. A blood and colon cleanse will help dissolve catarrh and eliminate toxins from the body.

Foods that will help are grains, beans, sprouts, fresh and steamed vegetables. Vegetable juices supply minerals in concentration for easily assimilation. Fruit are cleansers and help in cleaning the toxins especially the citrus fruits.

Herbs for ear health are Bugleweed, which equalizes circulation in head area, Butcher's Broom to improve circulatory health, Garlic dissolves toxins, Ginkgo, Ginseng, Gotu Kola and Suma improve circulation and help to combat fatigue. Capsicum and Prickly Ash increase circulation in the head area.

HERBAL FORMULAS

Blood Cleansers—Circulatory System—Colon Cleansers—Digestive System—Energy and Stamina—Immune Builders—Structural—Urinary System—Female and Male Formulas—

VITAMINS, MINERALS AND SUPPLEMENTS

Lack of B-vitamins is associated with hearing problems. They fight stress and strengthen the nerves. Pantothenic acid prevents over-stimulation of the adrenal glands. Vitamin C with bioflavonoids strengthens the capillaries and cleans toxins. It also acts as an antihistamine. Vitamin E and choline help in circulatory problems. They provide oxygen and strengthen the tiny ear arteries. Lecithin, choline and vitamin E work together to dissolve fatty deposits in the capillary walls.

Minerals speed healing of damaged veins and capillaries. Minerals increase the absorption of nutrients and eliminate metals from the body. Zinc speed healing. Calcium and magnesium improve nerve health. A magnesium deficiency is seen in tinnitus sufferers. Chromium helps regulate glucose metabolism.

Flaxseed oil and salmon oil help to improve blood flow in the inner ear. Chlorophyll and blue-green algae help in cleansing the blood and improving circulation. Germanium and CoQ10 improve circulation and blood flow to the head and ear areas.

TONSILLITIS AND STREP THROAT

SYMPTOMS

Sore Throat—Fever—Hard to Swallow—Swollen Tonsils—Headache—Vomiting—

CAUSES

Sore throat is an acute disease; nature's way of cleansing toxins from the body. The tonsils protect the body against airborne bacteria entering the system through the mouth and nose. The tonsils protect the body, and when they become inflamed, it is a signal to clean and nourish the body.

Food allergies are common; usually cow's milk, chocolate or too much white flour or sugar products are to blame. The lymphatic system, which is part of the tonsils, becomes congested from producing lymphocytes which surround the toxins produced by junk food.

Antibiotics weaken the body further. Developing rheumatic fever is one excuse the doctors give for using penicillin. Dr. Robert S. Mendelsohn, a former pediatrician, said that after treating 150,000 patients during a 15 year period, only 1 case of rheumatic fever appeared. He said, "Obviously, risking damage to all the other children who had sore throats by treating them with penicillin, in order to prevent one case of rheumatic fever, would have been a poor trade-off."(*How to Raise A Healthy Child...In Spite of Your Doctor*, page. 134)

Dr. Mendelsohn also said that strep infection responds within 24-48 hours to treatment with penicillin, and without treatment, strep will surrender to antibiotics produced in the bloodstream and will usually disappear in less than a week. Penicillin merely speeds the process a bit.

NUTRITIONAL THERAPY

Cleansing and healing the body naturally will speed the strep or tonsillitis infections. Using citrus juices, with vitamin C and herbal teas and extracts will clean. A garlic formula will act as an antibiotic and speed healing.

Changing to a natural food diet will help the tonsils to shrink and heal. Make soups with carrots, celery, onions and garlic, blend and warm up, and use just the broth.

Lemon or lime juice in warm water with honey and ginger will help the cleansing process. Peppermint tea will help settle the stomach.

Golden Seal, Echinacea and Garlic act as antibiotics. Tea Tree Oil will help heal throat infections. It will not cause irritation to the skin. Fenugreek and Comfrey loosen mucus and eliminate it from the body. Lobelia is excellent to clean the tonsils, stomach and relax at the same time. Herbs to relax the body are Chamomile, Catnip, Passion Flower and Hops. An extract containing these nervine herbs will help relax a child which speeds healing.

A natural herbal laxative tea will speed the removal of toxins from the body. Cleansing the colon is important when infections are in the system.

HERBAL FORMULAS

Blood Cleansers—Colds, Flu, Fever and Allergies Formulas-Glandular System—Immune Builders—Infection Fighters—Nervous System and Brain—

VITAMINS, MINERALS AND SUPPLEMENTS

Vitamin A is needed in high amounts at first. Vitamin C with bioflavonoids will help the body produce interferon, to fight infections. B-complex vitamins rebuild the health of the tonsils.

Calcium, magnesium, potassium, selenium and zinc are healing and nourishing and will strengthen the nervous system.

Liquid chlorophyll and blue-green algae both stimulate the body to produce interferon for infections. Acidophilus helps protect from bad bacteria and aids in digestion. Flaxseed oil will help protect the body from infections. It essential for all body functions.

TUBERCULOSIS (T.B.) ___

SYMPTOMS

Malaise—Fever—Cough with Bloody Sputum—Chest Pain—Fatigue—Anorexia—Night Sweats—General Weakness of the Whole Body—Shortness of Breath—

CAUSES

The bacillus can lie dormant within the tubercle for years and reactivate when the immune system is low. It is often found in underdeveloped countries where poor sanitation is common. Brazil is having an outbreak and the doctors are using Thalidomide to treat it as well as leprosy. They claim that thalidomide is inexpensive and easy to dispense.

T.B. is prevalent in poverty-stricken countries where there is hunger and starvation. Cases are increasing in the United States because of poor nutrition and not because of the lack of nourishing food.

It is seen in impaired immune function from chronic illnesses such as AIDS. Chronic constipation and autointoxication are a constant irritation to the respiratory system and can contribute to the development of diseases like leprosy or T.B.

NUTRITIONAL THERAPY

Rest, proper nutrition and time are very beneficial for healing tuberculosis. Fresh juices, such as fresh pineapple juice, orange, grapefruit, lemon and lime, carrot and celery provide cleansing and healing properties.

Soups containing fresh vegetables using onions and garlic are strengthening to a weak body. Short fasts are beneficial. Using cleansing and building therapies are beneficial for chronic diseases like T.B.

Eliminate all mucus forming foods such as meat, dairy products, white flour and white sugar products. They overload the body and cause weakness and toxins to form and irritate the lungs.

Colon cleansing is vital. When the colon isn't eliminating properly, the lungs take over. It irritates the lungs and toxins build up causing chronic asthma, bronchitis or T.B.

Eat as much raw food as possible especially fruit and vegetables. Use brown rice, millet, buckwheat, yellow corn meal, amaranth, quinoa and tofu.

The healing herbs are: Garlic, Echinacea, Burdock, Red Clover, Horsetail, Eucalyptus (used in vaporizer and inhaled), Gotu Kola, (acts as a sedative and is healing). Hops has antibacterial and sedative properties. Horehound is a tonic and laxative. Myrrh and Gentian are healing.

HERBAL FORMULAS

Blood Cleansers—Circulatory System—Colds, Flu, Fevers and Allergy Formulas—Colon Cleansers—Digestive System—Infection Fighters—Nervous System and Brain—Structural—Urinary System—Female and Male Formulas—

VITAMINS, MINERALS AND SUPPLEMENTS

Vitamin A is essential for the lungs. Take 100,000 IU a day to start. Vitamin C with bioflavonoids is healing and promotes interferon production in the body. B-complex with extra B12, B6 and B5 is building and helps the liver detoxify, repair tissue, and improve digestion. Vitamin E is a free-radical scavenger. It provides oxygen to the cells and heals scars in the lungs that are common with T.B.

All minerals are needed for healing. Calcium and magnesium are needed for building the nerves. Silicon helps in the absorption of calcium and other minerals. Selenium and zinc speed healing and protect the immune system.

Chlorophyll and blue-green algae speed healing by helping the body produce interferon. It is nourishing and healing for the lungs. Germanium and CoQ10 heal by providing oxygen to the cells. Acidophilus restores friendly bacteria for quicker healing. It helps in the digestion of nutrients. Lecithin helps in repairing the nerves.

ULCERS

SYMPTOMS

Heartburn—Nausea—Burning Sensation or Discomfort in the upper abdomen relieved when eating food but can reoccur two to three hours after a meal—Bleeding or Vomiting can occur—

CAUSES

Liver stagnation, constipation and auto-intoxication are the main causes of ulcers. Stress is also implicated in ulcers which increases stomach acid. Peptic ulcers small open sores on the inner wall of the stomach or section of the intestine.

When the lower colon is congested and delays the passage of food from the system, fermentation and acid conditions irritate the stomach and can result in ulcers.

Frequent meals have been suggested, but that only stimulates more frequent gastric-acid secretion. Ulcers can be caused by white flour and sugar products, fats, coffee, aspirin, steroids, tobacco, alcohol, and tea, all of which increase stomach acid.

NUTRITIONAL THERAPY

Fresh cabbage juice is rich in vitamin U, which is very healing and rich in pepsin, an enzyme essential for digestion. Also cabbage, celery, carrot and parsley juice are beneficial. Add fresh ginger, which is also healing. Clarified butter can be used for cooking to prevent acid upset. It is high in butyric acid, a fatty acid that has antiviral and anti-cancer properties. It also stimulates interferon which is an antiviral chemical.

Buckwheat, millet and brown rice are healing and easy to digest. Soups made with grains and vegetables are rich in minerals and B-complex vitamins. Bananas, avocados, tofu, yogurt, and almond milk are all nourishing for ulcers. Lightly steamed vegetables are nourishing

Proper chewing is essential so that food can be digested properly. Proper food combining is vital to give the stomach time for healing and restoring vitality.

A high fiber diet is recommended. A little raw honey in water is healing. Red Raspberry and Chamomile tea are healing and relaxing. Milk Thistle and Pau D'Arco are healing for liver stagnation. Slippery Elm, Comfrey, Garlic, Burdock and Cayenne are healing for ulcers. Aloe Vera is healing and prevents scarring. Licorice is healing and contains anti-inflammatory properties. Saffron and Dandelion are also healing. Saffron helps in the digestion of fats and Dandelion is cleansing for the liver. Nervine herbs strengthen the nervous system and prevent stress.

Barley water helps to rebuild the lining of the stomach. Rejuvelac is a healthy enzyme drink and acts as a protection against harmful organisms in the intestinal tract. Thermos cooking is nourishing and contains enzymes for proper digestion.

HERBAL FORMULAS

Blood Cleansers—Colon Cleansers—Digestive System (ulcer formulas)—Glandular System—Immune Builders—Infection Fighters—Nervous System and Brain—Urinary System—

VITAMINS, MINERALS AND SUPPLEMENTS

Vitamins A and E are very healing for ulcers. They also prevent scarring and adhesions. B-complex vitamins are seen deficient in ulcer patients. They are needed for cleansing the liver and aiding in digestion. Vitamin C may also be deficient. It is healing and cleansing for ulcers.

Selenium and zinc are healing. Calcium and magnesium heal the nerves. Potassium helps balance excess stomach acid. Silicon helps in the assimilation of calcium and other minerals. Kelp is rich in minerals and is cleansing and healing for ulcers.

Acidophilus is healing and helps in the digestion of food. Chlorophyll and blue-green algae are healing. They contain vitamin U for healing and K for controlling bleeding.

VACCINATIONS ⸺

SYMPTOMS

Fever—Cold and Flu like symptoms—The body is trying to throw off the shots because it consider it foreign to the health of the body. Dr. Robert S. Mendelsohn, M.D., felt that the wide use of vaccinations along with antibiotics are the main cause of the auto-immune diseases today. He also said that the DPT shots can cause brain damage. Vaccinations are also implicated in SIDS deaths.

CAUSES

Side effect of vaccinations are caused because the shots go directly into the bloodstream by-passing the liver which is the body's filter system. The shots put a shock on the system, and if a child is weak with a low immune system, this could cause serious problems. The following are linked with vaccinations: cancer, leukemia (common in small children), paralysis, multiple sclerosis, arthritis, and brain damage.

Childhood diseases are nature's way of eliminating inherited or acquired toxins. When the childhood diseases are treated properly, the body is healthier and cleaner than before they had the disease. Natural cleansing with herbs, citrus juices, and vegetables juices will help the body heal faster and without side effects.

Sugar products have been implicated in the severity of childhood diseases. Sugar invites germs and viruses and creates a deficiency in vitamins and minerals.

If you decide to be immunized, take massive doses of vitamins A and C at least two weeks before and after the shots.

Disease can be controlled if you live in accordance with Natural Laws. Feed yourself and your children as much natural food as possible. Use white sugar and flour products sparingly. Proper rest, positive attitude, laughter, and relaxation are important.

Read the chapter on Childhood Diseases for herbs and other nutrients to help with healing and preventing complications from diseases.

The following books will give you documented information on the side effects of vaccinations. *Immunization, The Reality Behind The Myth*, by Walene James and *A Shot In The Dark*, by Harris L. Coulter and Barbara Loe Fisher.

VARICOSE VEINS

SYMPTOMS

Blue, Bulging Veins on the legs—Pain—Swelling—Leg Cramps—Sores—Heavy feeling in the legs—Tired Legs—Dull Aches and Pains—Swollen Ankle Leg Tenderness—Varicose veins is considered the leading circulatory disorder in this country. If varicose veins are left untreated can lead to phlebitis, leg ulcers, permanently swollen legs, pulmonary emboli (or clots in the lungs), and even surface leg hemorrhaging.

CAUSES

Varicose veins are caused by residue deposits of clotting blood within the vein interiors. Constipation and a lack of fiber are the main causes of the residue accumulation. Liver congestion from constipation which produces only half the amount of bile, can cause chronic indigestion and a vicious cycle of constipation. Lack of exercise and weight gain can contribute to varicose veins. Poor circulation in the legs and thighs can cut off circulation in the legs. The blood stream can become thick, sluggish and plugged with toxins and causes autointoxication and stagnation in the blood.

Anything that interferes with or stops the normal blood flow through the major veins of the leg can cause varicose veins. Pregnancy often causes varicose veins. The weight gain and less exercise contribute. At this time, vitamins and minerals are needed in larger amounts.

People whose jobs require sitting or standing for long periods are more prone to varicose veins.

Sugar leaches the calcium in the body. Alcohol, tobacco and white flour products also contribute. One of the first places calcium and minerals are leached from the body are the veins and this can cause varicose veins and may develop into phlebitis.

NUTRITIONAL THERAPY

Add grains, vegetables and fruit to the diet. Millet is rich in calcium and magnesium and protein. It is easy to digest. Brown rice is rich in B-complex. Buckwheat contains rutin which is healing for varicose veins. Use fresh vegetable juices to clean the blood and provide minerals for healing.

Eliminate sugar, it turns to fat in the liver, and causes the little capillaries to become plugged. Fried and rancid fats and food are harmful to the veins. Sodium chloride (table salt) is harmful to the veins. Substitute herbs or natural salt for seasoning food. Use beans, sprouts, and a lot of fresh vegetable salads. Use flaxseed oil along with lemon juice for a salad dressing. It will nourish the veins. Capsicum aids the body in strengthening the veins and arteries by increasing circulation. It is rich in calcium.

Eat figs, raisins and prunes soaked in pure water. Citrus fruit, using the inner skin, will strengthen and heal the veins. Okra, is rich in silicon and selenium and helps to open clogged veins and strengthen capillaries.

Herbs that help varicose veins are: Butcher's Broom, Capsicum, Kelp, Golden Seal, White Oak Bark, Comfrey, Horsetail and Oatstraw. A White Oak Bark salve will help heal the veins when used externally. It can also help ease the pain.

HERBAL FORMULAS

Blood Cleansers—Circulatory System—Colon Cleansers—Digestive System—Immune Builders—Infection Fighters—Structural—Urinary—

VITAMINS, MINERALS AND SUPPLEMENTS

Vitamin A strengthens the veins and prevents infections. Vitamin E helps prevent blood clots and embolisms that block circulation. Clots are common in pregnancy when there is a deficiency of vitamin E. Vitamin E can be used externally as well as internally. B-complex vitamins with extra B-12 and B6 are beneficial. Vitamin C with bioflavonoids feeds and strengthens the veins.

Minerals are very important for vein health. Silicon is nourishing for the veins. Calcium and magnesium are essential for healthy veins. Zinc is healing.

Lecithin is nourishing and helps prevent clogged veins. Chlorophyll and blue-green algae help in cleaning the blood and prevent bleeding. They provide nutrients for a healthy immune system. Germanium and CoQ10 help provide oxygen to the blood and veins.

BIBLIOGRAPHY

Balch, James F., M.D. and Phyllis A. Balch, CNC. *Prescription For Nutritional Healing*, Garden City Park, N.Y.: Avery Publishing Group, Inc., 1990.

Bradstreet, Karen. *Overcoming Infertility Naturally*, Pleasant Grove, UT: Woodland Books, 1993.

Braly, James, M.D., "A Scientific Herb For The Symptoms of Agins," *Doctor's Best*, Laguna Hills, Ca.

Breggin, Peter R., M.D., *Toxic Psychiatry*, New York, NY: St. Martin's Press, 1991.

Calbom, Cherie and Maureen Keane. *Juicing For Life*, Garden City Park, NY: Avery Publishing Group, Inc., 1992.

Cameron, Myra. *Lifetime Encyclopedia of Natural Remedies*, West Nyack, NY: Parker Publishing Co., 1993.

Carr, Ann et. al. *Rodale's Illustrated Encyclopedia of Herbs*, Emmaus, Pennsylvania: Rodale Press, Inc., 1987.

Castleman, Michael. *The Healing Herbs*, Emmaus, Pennsylvania: Rodale Press, Inc., 1991.

Cayetoano, J.H.M., *Building Vital Health*, Eastern Publishing Association, Manila: 1988.

Challem, Jack Joseph and Renale Lewin - Challem, *What Herbs Are All About*, New Canaan, Connecticut: Keats Publishing, 1980.

Chishti, Hakim G.M., N.D. *The Traditional Healer's Handbook*. Rochester, Vermont: Healing Arts Press, 1988.

Christopher, John R., "Red Raspberry." *Herbalist Magazine*, Vol. 1, No. 4, 1976.

Colbin, Annemarie. *Food and Healing*, New York, NY: Balantine Books, 1986.

Coulter, Harris L. and Barbara Loe Fisher, *A Shot In The Dark*, Garden City, NY: Avery Publishing Group, Inc., 1991.

Culbreth, David M.R., Ph.G., M.D., *A Manual of Materia Medica and Pharmacology*, Philadelphia, PA: Lea & Febiger, 1927.

Davis, Dr. Stephen and Dr. Alan Stewart, *Nutritional Medicine*, New York, NY: Avon Books, 1987.

Duke, James A., *Handbook of Medicinal Herbs*, Boca Raton, Florida: CRC Press, Inc., 1985.

Foster, Steven. "Milk Thistle." *Nutrition News*, Vol. XII, No. 10, 1985.

Galland, Leo, M.D., with Dian Dincin Buchman, Ph.D. *Superimmunity for Kids*, New York, NY: Dell Publishing, 1988.

Gittleman, Ann Louise. *Guess What Came To Dinner*, Garden City Park, NY: Avery Publishing Group, Inc., 1993.

Graedon, Joe and Teresa. *Graedon's Best Medicine*, New York, NY: Bantam Books, 1991.

Grieve, Mrs. M., F.R.H.S. *A Modern Herbal*, London, England: Cresset Press, 1992.

Griggs, Barbara. *Green Pharmacy*, Rochester, Vermont: Healing Arts Press, 1981.

Health World Magazine, "The Best of Health World." 1993.

Hobbs, Christopher. *"Let's Live,"* april, 1994.

Hobbs, Christopher. "St. John's Wort," *Herbalgram*, Fall/Winter, 1988.

Hobbs, Christopher. *Foundations of Health, The Liver and Digestive Herbal*. Capitola, CA: Botanica Press, 1992.

Holmes, Peter. *The Energetics of Western Herbs*, Boulder: Artemis Press, 1989.

Huggins, Dr. Hal A. *It's All In Your Head*, Garden City Park, NY: Avery Publishing Group, Inc., 1993.

Hutchens, Alma R. *Indian Herbology of North America*, Ontario, Canada: Merco, 1969.

Inlander, Charles, Lowell S. Levin, Ed Weiner. *Medicine On Trial*, New York, NY: Prentice Hall Press, 1988.

Israel, Richard. *The Natural Pharmacy Produced Guide*, Garden City Park, NY: Aver Publishing Group, Inc., 1991.

James, Walene. *Immunization, The Reality Behind The Myth*, South Hadley, Mass.: Bergin & Gravey Publishing, Inc., 1988.

Journal of Ethmopharmacology. 1986.

Kamen, Betty. "Gymnema Extract." *"Let's Live,"* September, 1989.

Kellogg, John Harvey, M.D. *Colon Hygiene*, Battle Creek Michigan: Good Health Publishing, Co., 1916.

Kloss, Jethro. *Back to Eden*, Loma Linda, CA: Back to Eden Books, 1971.

Lawrence Review of Natural Products The, St. Louise: *Facts and Comparisons*, March 1988, April 1994, November 1991, May 1987, June 1989, Dec. 1991, September 1989, July 1990, April 1993, December 1987, January 1990, October 1992, March 1991.

Lieberman, Shari, M.A., R.D., and Nancy Bruning. *Design Your Own Vitamin & Mineral Program*, Garden City Park, NY: Avery Publishing Group, Inc., 1990.

Lieberman, Shari, M.A., R.D., and Nancy Bruning. *The Real Vitamin and Mineral Book*. Garden City Park, NY: Avery Publishing Group, Inc., 1990.

Lindlahr, H., M.D. *Nature's Cure*, Chicago, IL: The Nature Cure Publishing Co., 1917.

Lines, Anni Airola, R.D. *Vitamin and Minerals: The Health Connection*, Phoenix, AZ: Health Plus Publishers, 1985.

Long, James W., M.D. *The Essential Guide to Prescription Drugs*, New York, NY: Harper Perennial, 1992.

McCaleb, Rob. "Bilberry, Health From Head to Toe." *Better Nutrition For Today's Living*, June, 1991.

Meyer, Joseph E. *The Herbalist,* Glenwood, Illinois: Meyer Books, 1918.

Michaud, Ellen, Lila L. Anastas and The Editors of Prevention Magazine. *Listen to Your Body*, Emmaus, Pennsylvania: Rodale Press, 1988.

Miller, Benjamin F., M.D. with Lawrence Galton. *The Complete Medical Guide*, New York, NY: Simon and Schuster, 1978.

Mills, Simon Y. *Out of the Earth*, London, England: Penguin Group, 1991.

Montagna, Joseph F. *The People's Desk Reference,* Lake Oswego, OR: Quest for Truth Publishing, Inc., 1979.

Monte, Tome and The Editors of East West Natural Health. *World Medicine*, New York, NY: The Putnam Publishing Group, 1993.

Mowry, Daniel B., Ph.D. *The Scientific Validation of Herbal Medicine*, New Canaan, Connecticut: Keats Publishing, 1986.

Murray, Michael, N.D. and Joseph Pizzorno, N.D. *Encyclopedia of Natural Healing,* Rocklin, CA: Prima Publishing, 1991.

Murray, Michael, N.D. and Joseph Pizzorno, N.D. *The Healing Power of Foods,* Rocklin, CA: Prima Publishing, 1993.

Murray, Michael, N.D. *The Healing Power of Herbs,* Rocklin, CA: Prima Publishing, 1992.

Ody, Penelope. *The Complete Medicinal Herbal,* London: Dorling Kindersley, 1993.

Olsen, Cynthia B. *Australian Tea Tree Oil*, Pagosa Springs, CO: Kali Press, 1991.

Pitchard, Paul. *Healing with Whole Foods*, Berkeley, CA: North Atlantic Books, 1993.

Professional Guide to Diseases, Bethleham, PA: Intermed Communications, Inc. 1982.

Reader's Digest: Family Guide to Natural Medicine, Pleasantville, NY: The Reader's Digest Association, Inc., 1993.

Ritchason, Jack. *The Little Herb Encyclopedia,* Pleasant Grove, UT: Woodland Books, 1994.

Ritchason, Jack. *The Vitamin and Health Encyclopedia*, Pleasant Grove, UT: Woodland Books, 1994.

Schechter, Steven R., N.D. "Schizandra." *Let's Live*, September 1994.

Schechter, Steven R., N.D. *Fighting Radiation and Chemical Pollutants with Foods, Herbs and Vitamins*, Encinitas, CA: Vitality, INK, 1988.

Schmidt, Michael A., Lendon H. Smith, Keith W. Schnert. *Beyond Antibiotics,* Berkeley, CA: North Atlantic Books, 1993.

Sharon, Michael, Dr. *complete Nutrition*, United Kingdom: Prion, 1989.

Shook, Dr. Edward E. *Advanced Treatise in Herbology,* Lakemont, Georgia: CSA Press, 1978.

Shook, Dr. Edward E. *Elementary Treaties in Herbology*, Lakemont, Georgia: CSA Press, 1978.

Spencer, Mike. "Yucca, New Hope for Arthritics." *Let's Live*, February 1975.

Stevens, Dr. John. *Medical Reform*, London, England: Whittaker and Co., 1847.

Tenney, Louise, M.H. *Health Handbook*, Pleasant Grove, UT: Woodland Books, 1994.

Tenney, Louise, M.H. *Modern Day Plagues, Revised*, Pleasant Grove, UT: Woodland Books, 1994.

Tenney, Louise, M.H. *Nutritional Guide with Food Combining*, Pleasant Grove, UT: Woodland Books, 1994.

Tenney Louise, M.H. *Today's Healthy Eating*, Pleasant Grove, UT: Woodland Books, 1986.

Tenney, Louise, M.H. *Today's Herbal Health, 3rd Edition*, Pleasant Grove, UT: Woodland Books, 1992.

The PDR Family Guide to Prescription Drugs, Based on Physicians' Desk Reference. Montvale, NJ: Medical Economics Data Inc., 1993.

Tierra, Michael C.A., N.D. *Planetary Herbology*, Santa Fe, New Mexico: Lotus Press, 1988.

Vogel, Dr. H.C. *The Nature Doctor*, New Canaan, Connecticut: Keats Publishing, Inc., 1952, 1991.

Weil, Andrew, M.D., and Winifred Rosen. *Chocolate to Morphine*, Boston, Mass.: Houghton Mifflin Co., 1983.

Weiner, Michael, A., Ph.D. and Janet A. Weiner. *Herbs That Heal*, Mill Valley, CA: Quantum Books, 1994.

Weiss, Rudolf Fritz, M.D. *Herbal Medicine*, Beaconsfield, England: Beaconsfield Publishers Ltd, 1988.

Wentzler, Rich. *The Vitamin Book*, New York, NY: Gramercy Publishing Co., 1978.

INDEX